Lysosomal Storage Diseases

Early Diagnosis and New Treatments

Fondazione Pierfranco e Luisa Mariani
Viale Bianca Maria 28
20129 Milan, Italy

Telephone: +39 02 795458
Fax: +39 02 76009582
Publications coordinator: Valeria Basilico
e-mail: publications@fondazione-mariani.org
www.fondazione-mariani.org

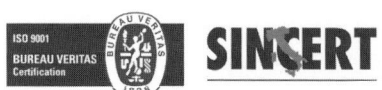

Lysosomal Storage Diseases
Early Diagnosis and New Treatments

Edited by

Rossella Parini and Generoso Andria

Mariani Foundation Paediatric Neurology Series: 23
Series Editor: Maria Majno

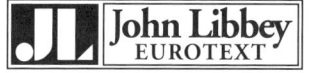

ISBN: 978-2-7420-0779-0

Cover illustration: by Christian Montenegro from the book *The Creation*. Courtesy of Christian Montenegro and publisher Gestalten.

Technical and language editor: Justine Cullinan.

Published by

Éditions John Libbey Eurotext
127, avenue de la République, 92120 Montrouge, France
Tél. : +33 (0)1 46 73 06 60
Fax : +33 (0)1 40 84 09 99
e-mail : contact@jle.com
www.jle.com

© 2010 John Libbey Eurotext. All rights reserved.

Unauthorized duplication contravenes applicable laws.

It is prohibited to reproduce this work or any part of it without authorization of the publisher or of the Centre Français d'Exploitation du Droit de Copie (CFC), 20, rue des Grands Augustins, 75006 Paris, France.

Contents

General aspects

Chapter 1   Lysosomal storage disorders: commonalities and differences
Luca Astarita, Michelina Sibilio and Generoso Andria   3

Chapter 2   Lysosomal storage disorders—epidemiology, biochemistry, and genetics: how to read and interpret biochemical and molecular tests
Mirella Filocamo and Amelia Morrone   13

Chapter 3   Organizational and ethical aspects of newborn screening for lysosomal storage diseases
Carlo Corbetta and Luisella Alberti   27

Chapter 4   Pathophysiologic aspects of lysosomal storage disorders
Cinzia Maria Bellettato, Rosella Tomanin and Maurizio Scarpa   31

**Clinical presentations in detail:
Mucopolysaccharidoses
and Anderson-Fabry disease**

Chapter 5   Early signs and symptoms for the timely diagnosis of mucopolysaccharidosis
Maria Luisa Melzi, Francesca Furlan and Rossella Parini   45

Chapter 6   Anderson-Fabry disease in children
Rossella Parini and Francesca Santus   59

**Mucopolysaccharidoses
from the specialists' point of view**

Chapter 7   Epilepsy in mucopolysaccharidosis: clinical features and outcome
Daniele Grioni, Margherita Contri, Francesca Furlan, Miriam Rigoldi, Attilio Rovelli and Rossella Parini   73

Chapter 8	Psychological assessment and support for patients with mucopolysaccharidosis *Milena Marini and Alessio Gamba*	81
Chapter 9	Mucopolysaccharidosis: radiologic findings *Marco Grimaldi, Daniela Di Marco and Paolo Remida*	89
Chapter 10	Anaesthesia for children with mucopolysaccharidosis *Pablo Mauricio Ingelmo and Emre Sahillioğlu*	99
Chapter 11	Neurosurgical complications and their management in mucopolysaccharidosis *Carlo Giussani, Sara Miori and Erik P. Sganzerla*	107

Specific treatments for lysosomal storage diseases

Chapter 12	Enzyme replacement therapy in lysosomal storage disorders: clinical effects and limitations *Michael Beck*	123
Chapter 13	Gaucher disease: clinical follow-up and management with individualized treatment *Elena Cassinerio, Irene Motta and Maria Domenica Cappellini*	133
Chapter 14	Enzyme replacement therapy in glycogenosis type II *Giovanni Ciana and Bruno Bembi*	147
Chapter 15	Haematopoietic stem cell transplantation for lysosomal storage diseases *Giovanna Lucchini, Paola Corti and Attilio Rovelli*	155
Chapter 16	Allogeneic stem cell transplantation for Hurler syndrome: graft outcome and long-term clinical outcomes *Jaap Jan Boelens and Mieke Aldenhoven*	163
Chapter 17	Haematopoietic stem cell gene therapy for metachromatic leukodystrophy *Alessandra Biffi and Luigi Naldini*	171

General aspects

Chapter 1

Lysosomal storage disorders: commonalities and differences

Luca Astarita, Michelina Sibilio and Generoso Andria

Department of Paediatrics, Università 'Federico II', via Sergio Pansini 5, 80131 Naples, Italy
andria@unina.it

Summary

Lysosomal storage disorders, like many other groups of metabolic diseases, show a wide range of clinical phenotypes. Physical signs can be a clue to suspect and to potentially diagnose a lysosomal storage disorder, but in the early stages, signs can be mild and nonspecific and are often not easily recognized. As the disease progresses, some clinical manifestations, such as coarse facies, skeletal dysplasia, and developmental delay, can alert the physician to the possible diagnosis of a lysosomal storage disorder. Different lysosomal storage disorders share common signs and symptoms. We will consider the five main groups of these: involvement of the central nervous system (CNS), visceromegaly, a Hurler-like phenotype, haematologic findings, and the presence of a macular cherry-red spot. Various combinations of these signs can give a rather precise indication of the further diagnostic procedures that are needed to identify specific groups of lysosomal storage disorders. A high index of suspicion should be maintained so that diagnosis can be made quickly, followed by appropriate treatment. This is of great importance since innovative therapeutic approaches have been developed for some of these conditions, and these modalities are more effective if started at the earliest stages of the disease.

General features of lysosomal storage disorders

This chapter is aimed at helping physicians, particularly paediatricians, to raise their awareness of lysosomal storage disorders (LSDs) and start, as early as possible, the appropriate actions needed to take care of the patient and his or her family in the framework of a multidisciplinary team approach.

Genetics

LSDs are rare genetic diseases with a combined incidence of 1 in 7, 000 to 10, 000 live births. About 50 different LSDs are known. Almost all LSDs are transmitted in an autosomal recessive fashion, whereas only a few are inherited with an X-linked mechanism, either recessive (in Hunter disease or in Fabry disease) or dominant (in Danon disease). A positive family history can help to raise the physican's awareness of a possible genetic disorder. Autosomal recessive disorders can be suspected when two or more siblings are affected or parents are consanguineous or when the family comes from a small isolated community, whereas in X-linked conditions only males are affected (*e.g.*, brothers or male proband and maternal uncle) and the disease is transmitted through female carriers.

Phenotypic variability

LSDs, like many other groups of metabolic diseases, show a wide range of clinical phenotypes, even within a single disease type or subtype. Because of the progressive nature of LSDs, in the early stage, symptoms are mild, nonspecific, and not readily recognizable.

The age of onset and the clinical course of LSDs can be variable, even amongst patients with the same enzymatic defect. Many LSDs have different forms, defined as infantile (early and late), juvenile, and adult. We also know that affected sibs who share the same genetic mutation(s) can present at different ages and have symptoms that progress at different rates (Fig. 1) (Andria *et al.*, 1979). Many LSDs, as well as other monogenic diseases, behave as multifactorial conditions, where unknown modifying genes or environmental factors influence the individual clinical presentation in spite of the identical molecular basis of the disease.

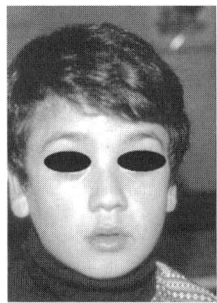 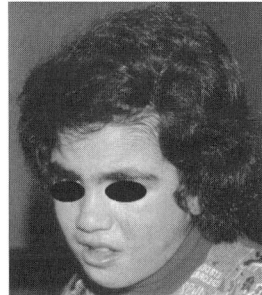

Fig. 1. Phenotypic variability in two sibs with MPS IIIB. The 13-year-old girl shown at the right displays mild coarse facies with hirsutism, prominent supraorbital ridges and thick lips, associated with severe mental retardation and visceromegaly. The 9-year-old boy at the left did not show apparent dysmorphic features of the face after many years; his mental retardation was very mild and visceromegaly absent. Even mucopolysacchariduria in this boy was intermittent and in most instances undetectable.

From suspicion to the specific diagnosis

If there is no positive family history for LSDs, physical signs are the only way for the physician to suspect these diseases at an early stage. When an LSD is suspected, biochemical confirmation must be ascertained by testing blood, urine, or cultured fibroblasts in order to determine the specific enzyme/protein deficiency. Molecular diagnosis is now available for most LSDs to more precisely define the case.

Prenatal diagnosis (when indicated) is available for the majority of LSDs through enzymatic or molecular testing or ultrastructural examination of amniocytes and chorionic villus cells.

From diagnosis to treatment

For the majority of LSDs there are currently no specific therapeutic approaches, and the objective thus far has been to delay or treat the clinical manifestations or complications of the disease.

However, early diagnosis of LSDs is becoming more and more important nowadays, because several innovative therapeutic approaches have become available that could be much more effective if started early.

Specific treatments for some of these diseases include:
(1) bone marrow transplantation;
(2) enzyme replacement therapy, with the infusion of recombinant enzyme molecules;
(3) substrate reduction therapy, with small molecules inhibiting the synthesis of the substrate stored as a consequence of the genetic defect;
(4) enzyme enhancement therapy, with pharmacologic chaperones.

Gene therapy is also under investigation in several LSD animal models for future transfer to human patients (Beck, 2007).

Prognosis

Prognosis for LSDs is often unfavorable, with a progressive worsening of the clinical status, but depends on many factors, such as type of disease, age of onset, and age at start of therapy. Genotype–phenotype correlations usually are not strong, but sometimes specific mutations or types of mutations are related to disease outcome, as in the case of the N370S mutation of the β-glucocerebrosidase gene, which confers a mild non-neuronopathic course on patients with Gaucher disease.

Common signs and symptoms of lysosomal storage disorders

Phenotypes of LSDs are highly heterogeneous, but it is possible to find some commonalities in the clinical expressions and presentations of some groups of LSDs.

Age of onset

A first helpful indication comes from the age of clinical presentation. Because of the progressive nature of LSDs, a neonatal diagnosis, suspected only on clinical grounds, is uncommon. A coarse facies, generally considered a hallmark of LSDs, is only rarely present at birth (exceptions are, for example, newborns or infants with mucolipidosis II, GM1 gangliosidosis, or infantile sialic acid storage disease) (Wraith, 2002). Only after several months do dysmorphic facial features become easily recognizable (Fig. 2). A rather pathognomonic presentation at birth in infants with various LSDs is a nonimmune hydrops foetalis, although various groups of inborn errors of metabolism other than LSDs may affect the foetus similarly, but less commonly (Table 1) (Brunetti-Pierri *et al.*, 2009).

Disorders with an early age of onset (first year of life) include Krabbe disease, Tay-Sachs disease, and Sandhoff disease (with predominant neurologic involvement), I-cell disease, sialidosis and galactosialidosis type 2, and GM1 gangliosidosis, severe infantile type (with neu-

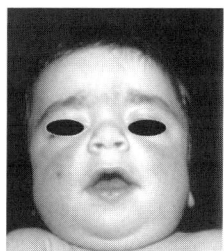 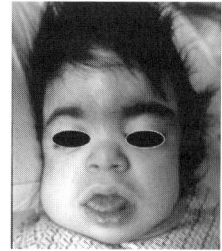

Fig. 2. Progression of facial dysmorphism in a child with MPS IH at (left) 1 year and (right) at 6 years of age.

rologic involvement, hepatosplenomegaly, coarse facies, and joint limitations), Pompe disease (with cardiomyopathy and hypotonia), and the severe forms of Niemann-Pick disease (type A) and Gaucher disease (type 2 and 3).

Disorders with age of onset after the first year of life are mucopolysaccharidoses, mucolipidoses, Fabry disease, Gaucher disease type 1, fucosidosis, Farber disease, and the late infantile and juvenile forms of galactosialidosis, GM2 gangliosidosis, and metachromatic leukodystrophy.

Table 1. Lysosomal disorders associated with nonimmune foetal hydrops

Disease	Defective enzyme/protein
Oligosaccharidoses	
GM1 gangliosidosis	β-galactosidase
Sialidosis	Neuraminidase
Galactosialidosis	Protective protein/cathepsin A deficiency
Gaucher disease type 2	Acid β-glucosidase
Niemann-Pick disease, type A	Sphingomyelinase deficiency
Niemann-Pick disease, type C	NPC1
Farber lipogranulomatosis	Acid ceramidase
Wolman disease	Lysosomal acid lipase
I-cell disease	Multiple defects affecting mannose-6-phosphate receptor
Infantile sialic storage disease	Sialin
Multiple sulphatase deficiency	Sulphatase-modifying factor-1
Mucopolysaccharidoses	
Hurler disease (MPS I)	α-L-iduronidase
Sly disease (MPS VII)	β-glucuronidase
Morquio A disease (MPS IVA)	Galactosamine-6-sulphate sulphatase

Signs and symptoms suggestive of lysosomal storage disorders

There are no signs or symptoms that are really pathognomonic of a single disease, but a physician must suspect an LSD and plan further diagnostic investigations when some 'cardinal' signs and symptoms are observed in a child. Table 2 lists selected signs and symptoms that should alert the physician and suggest an LSD (Wilcox, 2004). Only for the less frequent clinical abnormalities is the specific disease reported in parentheses. Table 3 summarizes in more detail the phenotypic variability with reference to the involvement of the main organs in selected LSDs.

Figures 2 to 4 illustrate some of the classical findings seen in LSDs that are the bases for the clinical algorithm proposed in the next section.

Generally, early presentations with life-threatening symptoms are promptly diagnosed (or suspected), but attenuated phenotypes with later onset cannot be diagnosed for many years. In these cases, anything that suggests a progressive disease, such as loss of acquired developmental skills, progressive dementia, worsening behavioural abnormalities, or signs of muscular or neurologic degeneration should be promptly recognized, because they might be the first manifestations, among other causes, of an LSD.

Table 2. Selected signs and symptoms suggestive of a lysosomal storage disorder[a]

FACIES	SKIN
• Coarse facial features • 'Doll-like face' (*GM2-gangliosidosis*) • Macroglossia	• Hirsutism • Angiokeratoma (*Fabry disease, fucosidosis*) • Ichthyosis, collodion baby (*Gaucher disease type 2*) • Subcutaneous nodules (*Farber disease*) • Extensive mongolian spots
SKELETAL	BLOOD
• Skeletal dysplasia, dysostosis multiplex with or without short stature • Joint stiffness • Bone crisis (*Gaucher disease type 1*)	• Vacuolated lymphocytes • Foamy histiocytes • Anemia, thrombocytopenia
HEART	EYE
• Cardiomyopathy (*Pompe disease, Danon disease*) • Valvular heart disease	• Macular cherry-red spot • Corneal opacities • Vertical supranuclear ophthalmoplegy
ABDOMEN	CNS
• Hepatomegaly • Splenomegaly • Cholestasis (*Niemann-Pick disease type C, neonatal*) • Umbilical, inguinal hernias	• Progressive mental retardation/dementia • Peripheral neuropathy • Leukodystrophy (TC scan) (*Krabbe disease, metachromatic leukodystrophy*) • Seizures • Startling reaction (*GM2 gangliosidosis*) • Myoclonus • Ataxia • Hypotonia (*Pompe disease, Danon disease*) • Acroparesthesias (*Fabry disease*) • Cataplexy (*Niemann-Pick disease type C*)
KIDNEY	
• Proteinuria, isosthenuria (*sialidosis, late infantile*) • Nonimmune hydrops foetalis, neonatal ascites (see Table 1) • Renal failure (*Fabry disease*)	

Cataplexy: episodes of loss of muscle tone during strong emotions such as laughing or anger; angiokeratoma: raised reddish-purple vascular skin lesions.

[a] Examples of diseases in which signs/symptoms are less frequently found are given in italics in parentheses.

A proposal for a clinical algorithm

Phenotypes of different LSDs usually overlap each other and it is difficult to suspect a specific disease based only on physical examination. A proposal has been made to divide signs and symptoms into five main groups according to their various associations in order to aid in clinical suspicion, even for specific groups of LSDs (Andria & Parenti, 2004).

These groups are:

- involvement of CNS and/or mental retardation;
- visceromegaly;
- 'Hurler-like' phenotype (coarse facial features and/or skeletal dysplasia);
- haematologic signs (*e.g.*, vacuolated lymphocytes, foamy histiocytes in the bone marrow) (Fecarotta & Andria, 2006);
- ocular signs (in particular macular cherry-red spot).

The observed associations of the aforementioned groups of signs and symptoms are the following:

(1) Isolated involvement of CNS in infancy represents the main clinical presentation of:

(*a*) GM2 gangliosidoses (Tay-Sachs and Sandhoff disease) associated in all cases with macular cherry-red spot;

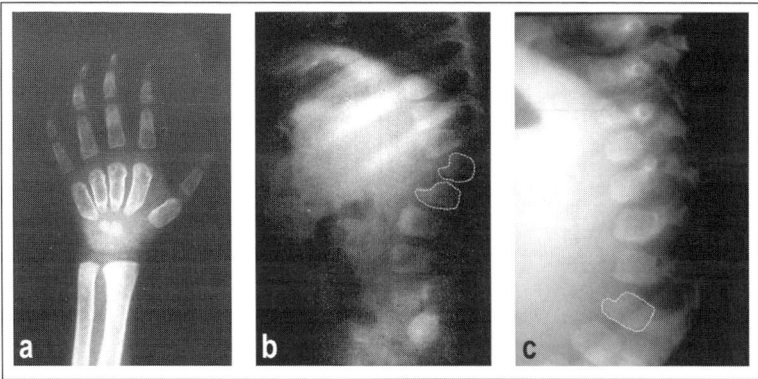

Fig. 3. Typical features of dysostosis multiplex in different examples of LSDs. X-ray of left hand and wrist (a) in a boy with the intermediate form of MPSI (formerly classified as Hurler-Scheie phenotytpe). Note the metacarpals with wide diaphysis and pointed distal extremities and 'bullet-shaped' phalanges. Lateral view of the spine of a child with galactosialidosis (b) and GM1 gangliosidosis (c), showing the typical deformity of lumbar vertebral bodies (hypoplasia of the anterior-superior portion) that leads in most cases to a dorsal-lumbar gibbus.

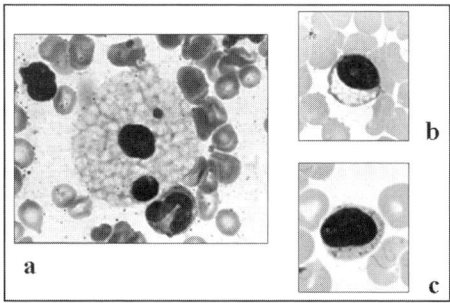

Fig. 4. Typical haematologic findings in some LSDs: (a) foamy histiocyte in the bone marrow smear of a boy with galactosialidosis; (b) lymphocyte with vacuolated cytoplasm in Niemann-Pick disease type A; and (c) metachromatic granules in the cytoplasm of a lymphocyte in the blood smear of a boy with MPS I.

(b) Schindler disease type I, Krabbe disease, and metachromatic leukodystrophy, without macular cherry-red spot.

(2) In a patient in whom mental retardation, visceromegaly and haematologic signs are associated (Fig. 5), it is crucial to evaluate the presence of a macular cherry-red spot. If it is present, a diagnosis of Niemann-Pick type A disease can be suspected; if it is absent, Gaucher disease (type 2 or 3) or Niemann-Pick disease type C (classic type) must be considered.

(3) Visceromegaly and haematologic signs, without mental retardation and skeletal dysplasia (Fig. 6), could suggest a diagnosis of Niemann-Pick type B disease (with macular cherry red spot a rare finding) or Gaucher disease type 1 (without macular cherry-red spot).

(4) The association of all groups of signs and symptoms (Fig. 8), including the macular cherry-red spot, is suggestive of the early infantile forms of sialidosis, galactosialidosis, or GM1 gangliosidosis. Without the macular cherry-red spot, these signs are suggestive of α-mannosidosis, fucosidosis, aspartyl-glucosaminuria (with only hepatomegaly), GM1 gangliosidosis, late infantile (without visceromegaly) mucolipidosis II and III, infantile sialic acid storage disease, mucolipidoses II and III, mucopolysaccharidoses IH, II, III, and VII, or multiple sulphatase deficiency.

Table 3. Phenotypic variability relative to main organs in selected LSDs with early onset

Disease	Facies	CNS			Eye		Liver	Spleen	Heart	Skeleton		Laboratory findings
	Hurler-like phenotype	Mental retardation	Seizures	Myoclonus	Corneal opacities	Cherry-red spot	Hepatomegaly	Splenomegaly	Cardiomyopathy Valvular heart disease	Short stature	Dysostosis multiplex	Haematologic signs
Mucopolysaccharidoses (specific disease)												
MPS I (Hurler, Scheie)	+→++	-→++	+		+		++	++	++	++	++	+
MPS II (Hunter)	+→++	-→++	+		-		++	++	++	++	++	+
MPS III (Sanfilippo)	-→+	++	+		±		+	+		±	+	+
MPS IV (Morquio)	+	-			+		+			++	+	+
MPS VI (Maroteaux-Lamy)	+→++	-			+		++	++	++	++	++	±
MPS VII (Sly)	+	-→+	±		+		++	++	+	+	+	+
Multiple sulphatase deficiency	+	++	+		±		+	+		+	+	+
Sphingolipidoses												
Fabry disease					+				+			
Gaucher disease, neuronopathic		++	+→++	+			++	++	++			++
Globoid cell leukodystrophy		+	+	+		±	±	±		+		±
Niemann–Pick A disease		++				+	++	++				++
Niemann–Pick B disease		±				±	++	++				++

Disease	Facies	CNS			Eye		Liver	Spleen	Heart	Skeleton		Laboratory findings
	Hurler-like phenotype	Mental retardation	Seizures	Myoclonus	Corneal opacities	Cherry-red spot	Hepatomegaly	Splenomegaly	Cardio-myopathy Valvular heart disease	Short stature	Dysos-tosis multiplex	Haematologic signs
Niemann–Pick C disease		++	+	+			+	+				++
GM1 gangliosidosis (severe infant)	+	++	+			+	+	+		+	+	+
GM2 gangliosidosis (Tay–Sachs)		++	++			+						
GM2 gangliosidosis (Sandhoff)		++	++			+	±	±				±
Oligosaccharidoses												
Fucosidosis	+	+	+		±		±	±		+	+	+
α-Mannosidosis	++	+	+		+		+	+		±	++	+
β-Mannosidosis	+	+	+							±		
Sialidosis	++	++	+	+	+	±	++	++		+	++	++
Schindler disease		++	+	+								
Galactosialidosis	++	±→+	±	–→+	±	±	+	+	+	+	+	++
Aspartylglucosaminuria	+	+	+		±		±	±		±	±	+
Other												
Pompe disease							+		++			+
Mucolipidosis II	++	+			+		++	±	++	++	+	+
Mucolipidosis III	+	±	±		±		±	±	±	+	+	+

Symbols (from – to ++) indicate the degree of severity. The arrow between two symbols indicates the range of severity observed in individual patients or in different types of the same genetic disorder. A blank box means that the sign/symptom has not been reported.

(5) The absence of mental retardation, but the presence of visceromegaly, haematologic signs, Hurler-like phenotype, and macular cherry-red spot (Fig. 8) could suggest galactosialidosis (late infantile). Mucopolysaccharidoses IS or VI must be considered in the presence of associated visceromegaly, haematologic signs, and Hurler-like phenotype, without either CNS involvement or macular cherry-red spot.

Finally, there are genetic syndromes and diseases presenting with a coarseness of the face that might resemble that seen in the dysmorphic LSDs. However, these syndromes do not generally show the typical associations with dysostosis multiplex, visceromegaly, haematologic findings, or ocular features, as indicated in Figures 5-8 for LSDs. Table 4 lists such genetic syndromes and diseases with Hurler-like features of the face and the respective OMIM number for further documentation.

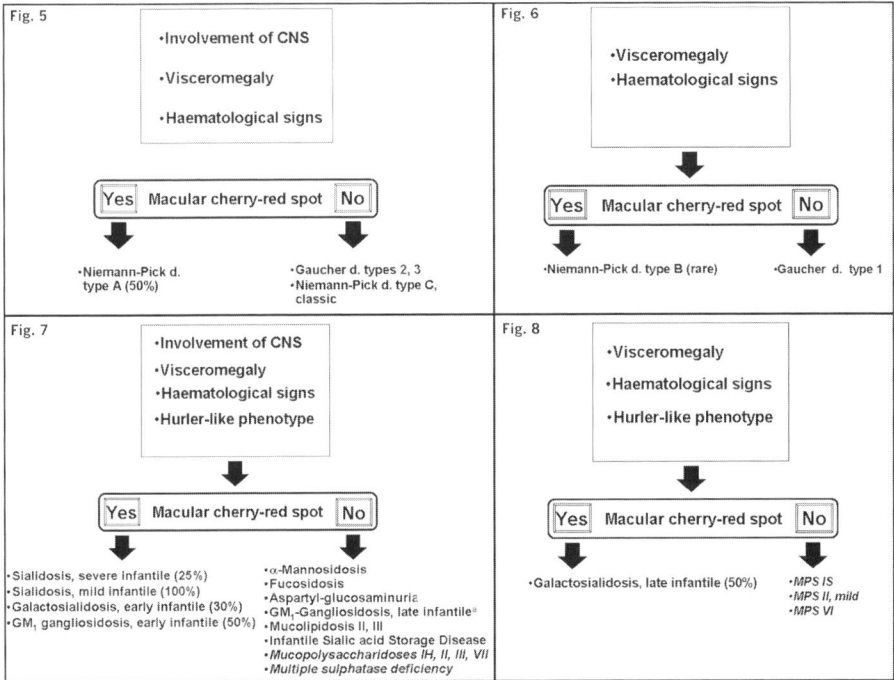

Figs. 5-8. Clinical approach to the diagnosis of oligosaccharidoses, mucopolysaccharidoses, sphingolipidoses, and related disorders with early (infantile) onset. The variable association of four cardinal signs or symptoms is first considered, namely: CNS involvement of various types, visceromegaly, Hurler-like phenotype, including facial dysmorphism and/or skeletal (vertebral) involvement suggestive of dysostosis multiplex, and haematologic findings in peripheral blood or bone marrow smears. The presence or absence of macular cherry-red spot is considered next, although the percentage of patients showing this spot, when described in a given disorder, is variable (as indicated in parentheses). Roman typeface shows conditions associated with abnormal oligosacchariduria whereas italics indicates conditions associated with abnormal mucopolysacchariduria.
[a] *Absence of visceromegaly (Fig. 7).*

Conclusion

LSDs are a heterogeneous group of about 50 diseases that share a common pathogenesis. Phenotypes of LSDs show a wide spectrum of variability from the neonatal, usually severe and rapidly progressive course to a more attenuated one. Early diagnosis is crucial because new therapies are available for many LSDs that are more effective if started in the earliest stages

Table 4. Genetic syndromes and diseases presenting with coarse Hurler-like face, not associated with dysostosis multiplex, visceromegaly, haematologic findings, or ocular features typical of LSDs

Syndrome/disease	OMIM number[a]
Coffin-Lowry syndrome	303300
Coffin-Siris syndrome	135900
Frontometaphyseal dysplasia	305620
Sotos syndrome	117550
Williams syndrome	194050
Multiple neuroma syndrome	171400
Pachydermoperiostosis	167100
Patterson-David syndrome	169170
Fountain syndrome	229120
Costello syndrome	218040
Acromegaloid facial appearance syndrome	102150
Schinzel-Giedeon syndrome	269150
Simpson-Golabi-Behmel syndrome	312870
Pallister-Killian syndrome	601803
Beckwith-Wiedemann syndrome	130650
Perlman syndrome	267000
Congenital hypothyroidism	

[a] The OMIM number refers to the online Catalogue of Mendelian Inheritance in Man (http://www.ncbi.nlm.nih.gov/sites/entrez?db=OMIM&itool=toolbar)

of the disease, before progressive and irreversible damage has occurred. There are no signs or symptoms pathognomonic of a single disease but, with scrupulous physical examination, 'atypical signs' (*e.g.*, coarse facial features, visceromegaly, loss of developmental skills) can be noticed. They should suggest a possible diagnosis of LSDs, especially if they occur in association, and must be further investigated with disease-specific laboratory procedures.

References

Andria, G. & Parenti, G. (2004): Oligosaccharidoses and related disorders. In: *Physician's guide to the laboratory diagnosis of metabolic diseases* (2nd ed.), eds. N. Blau, M. Duran, M.E. Blaskovics & K.M. Gibson, pp. 399–410. Heidelberg: Springer Verlag.

Andria, G., Di Natale, P., Del Giudice, E., Strisciuglio, P. & Murino, P. (1979): Sanfilippo B syndrome (MPS III B): mild and severe forms within the same sibship. *Clin. Genet.* **15,** 500–504.

Beck, M. (2007): New therapeutic options for lysosomal storage disorders: enzyme replacement, small molecules and gene therapy. *Hum. Genet.* **121,** 1–22.

Brunetti-Pierri, N., Parenti, G. & Andria, G. (2010): Inborn errors of metabolism. In: *Neonatology, a practical approach to neonatal diseases*, eds. G. Buonocore, R. Bracci & M. Weindling. Heidelberg: Springer Verlag. In press.

Fecarotta, S. & Andria, G. (2006): Hematological manifestations in inborn errors of metabolism. *Ital. J. Pediatr.* **32,** 241–250.

Wilcox, W.R. (2004): Lysosomal storage disorders: the need for better pediatric recognition and comprehensive care. *J. Pediatr.* **144** (Suppl.), S3–14.

Wraith, J.E. (2002): Lysosomal disorders. *Semin. Neonatol.* **7,** 75–83.

Chapter 2

Lysosomal storage disorders—epidemiology, biochemistry, and genetics: how to read and interpret biochemical and molecular tests

Mirella Filocamo and Amelia Morrone*

'Diagnosi Pre e Post-natale Malattie Metaboliche' Laboratory, Department of Neurosciences, IRCCS G. Gaslini, largo G. Gaslini 5, 16147 Genova, Italy
* Metabolic and Muscular Unit, Department of Sciences for Woman and Child's Health, University of Florence, Clinic of Paediatric Neurology, Azienda Ospedaliero-Universitaria Meyer, viale Pieraccini 24, 50139 Florence, Italy
mirellafilocamo@ospedale-gaslini.ge.it; a.morrone@meyer.it

Summary

About 60 lysosomal storage disorders (LSDs) have been identified up to now. All of them are clinically heterogeneous, and often include neurologic involvement. The diagnosis of most LSDs, after accurate clinical/paraclinical evaluation including analysis of some urinary metabolites, is based mainly on the detection of a specific enzymatic deficiency. In these cases, molecular genetic testing (MGT) can refine the enzymatic defect. Once the genotype of an individual LSD patient has been ascertained, genetic counseling should include prediction of the possible phenotype and the identification of the carriers in the family at risk. MGT is essential for the identification of genetic disorders resulting from nonenzymatic lysosomal protein defects and is complementary to biochemical genetic testing (BGT) in complex situations such as enzymatic pseudodeficiency. Prenatal diagnosis is performed on the most appropriate samples, which include fresh or cultured chorionic villus sampling (CVS) or cultured amniotic fluid (AF). The choice of the test, enzymatic and/or molecular, is based on the characteristics of the defect to be investigated. Prenatal MGT requires the genotype of the family index case to be known. The availability of both tests, enzymatic and molecular, enormously increases the reliability of the entire prenatal diagnostic iter. Thus, biochemical and molecular genetic testing are mostly complementary for postnatal and prenatal diagnoses of LSDs. Whenever genotype/phenotype correlations are available, they can be helpful for prognosis and decision-making on therapeutic approaches, including use of pharmacologic chaperone/active-site-specific chaperones (ASSCs).

Introduction

Lysosomal storage disorders (LSDs) are a group of about 60 different inherited metabolic diseases resulting from defective function, in the great majority, of a specific lysosomal protein or, in few cases, of non-lysosomal proteins involved in lysosomal biogenesis. The common biochemical hallmark of these diseases is the accumulation of undegraded molecules in the lysosome. This can arise through several mechanisms as a result of defects in any aspect of lysosomal biology that hampers the catabolism of molecules in the lysosome or the egress of molecules from the lysosome. Lysosomal accumulation results in complex clinical pictures characterized by multisystemic involvement (Futerman & van Meer, 2004; Vellodi, 2004; Wraith, 2002). In general, the extremely variable phenotypic expression depends on the specific macromolecule accumulated, the site of production and degradation of the specific metabolites, the residual enzymatic activity, and the general genetic background of the patient. Many of the lysosomal disorders have phenotypes that have been recognized as infantile, juvenile, and adult (Wraith, 2002).

Review of the topic

The endolysosomal system

The original concept that the lysosome is only one component of a series of unconnected intracellular organelles of the endolysosomal system (De Duve & Wattiaux, 1966) has been widely modified by more recent studies requiring the lysosomal function to be considered in the larger context of the endosomal/lysosomal system (Maxfield & McGraw, 2004). In this highly dynamic system, which mediates the internalization, recycling, transport, and breakdown of cellular/extracellular components and facilitates dissociation of receptors from their ligands, the lysosome represents the greater degradative compartment of endocytic, phagocytic, and autophagic pathways. Although hydrolytic enzymes are present in endosomes and lysosomes, they function optimally in the lysosome as it is the most acidic compartment.

Lysosomal enzymes: synthesis and trafficking

The lysosomal enzymes, synthesized in the rough endoplasmic reticulum (ER), move across the ER membrane to the lumen of the ER with an N-terminal signal sequence–dependent translocation. Once in the ER lumen they are N-glycosylated and their signal sequence is cleaved. They then proceed to the Golgi compartment and, at this stage, the lysosomal enzymes, which require the mannose 6-phosphate (M6P) marker to enter the lysosome, acquire the M6P ligand (Hickman & Neufeld, 1972) by the sequential action of a phosphotransferase and a diesterase (Reitman & Kornfeld, 1981; Waheed et al., 1981). The receptor–protein complex then moves to the late endosome, where dissociation occurs; the hydrolase translocates into the lysosome and the receptor is recycled either to the Golgi or to the plasma membrane. The final steps in the maturation of the lysosomal enzyme include proteolysis, folding, and aggregation.

However, not all lysosomal enzymes depend on the M6-P pathway. Recently, it has been shown that the lysosomal integral membrane protein type 2 (LIMP-2), a ubiquitously expressed transmembrane protein mainly found in the lysosomes and late endosomes, is a receptor for lysosomal M6-P-independent targeting of the glucocerebrosidase (Reczek et al., 2007).

Epidemiology

To date, worldwide epidemiologic data are not available or are limited to distinct populations. Apart from selected populations presenting a high prevalence for specific diseases, such as the Ashkenazi Jewish population at high risk for Gaucher disease (Beutler & Grabowski, 2001), Tay-Sachs disease, and Niemann-Pick disease (Vallance & Ford, 2003), the Finnish population at a high incidence of aspartylglucosaminuria (Arvio et al., 1993) and infantile/juvenile neuronal ceroid lipofuscinosis (Santavuori, 1988), as far as we know, prevalence data on the LSDs, as a group, have only been reported in Greece (Michelakakis et al., 1995), the Netherlands

Chapter 2 Lysosomal storage disorders—epidemiology, biochemistry, and genetics

(Poorthuis *et al.*, 1999), Australia (Meikle *et al.*, 1999), Italy (Dionisi-Vici *et al.*, 2002), and Portugal (Pinto *et al.*, 2004). As a group, overall incidence of LSDs is estimated at around 1:5,000–1:8,000.

The main problems associated with gathering accurate epidemiologic data for these individually rare disorders are, on the one hand, the clinical heterogeneity of LSDs, leading to missed diagnoses and diagnostic confusion, and, on the other hand, the dispersion of the diagnoses in countries where there is more than one diagnostic centre, such as Italy. This said, LSDs have been diagnosed at the laboratory of the Gaslini Institute (Genova) since the 1970s and from 1976 biological samples from most of Italian patients with LSDs have been preserved in a biobank (<http://dppm.gaslini.org/biobank/>) and the related data registered in a database. Fig. 1 reports data extrapolated from this database and compared with data from the Australian population (Meikle *et al.*, 1999), confirming that Gaucher disease is the most frequent LSD in the Italian population as it is in the Australian population.

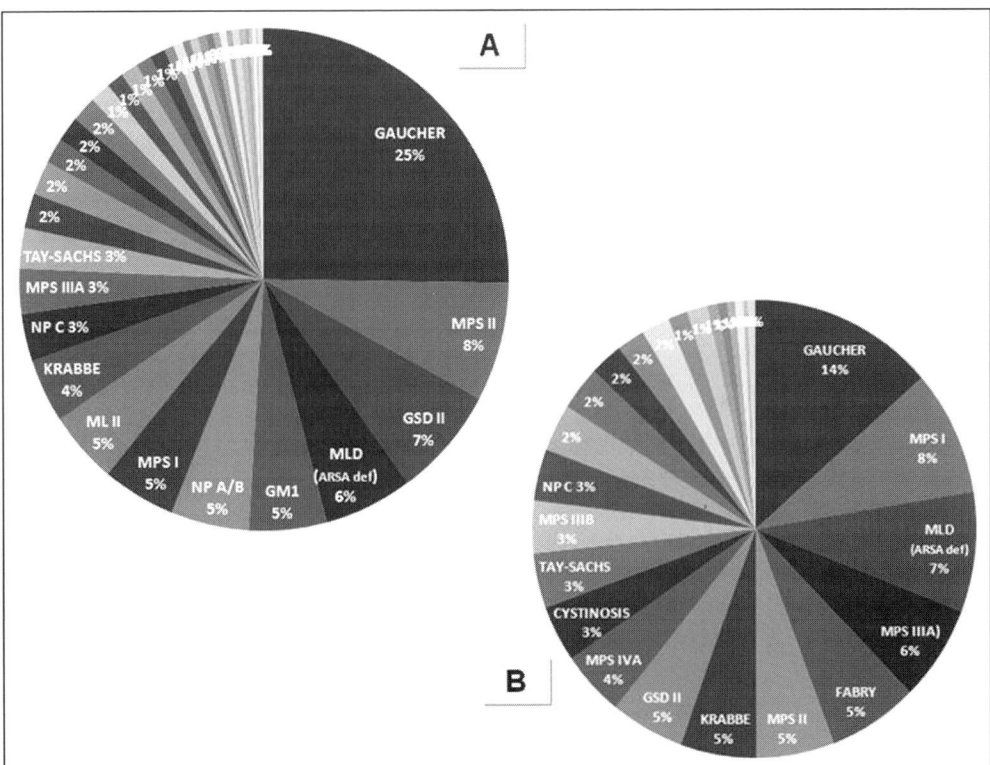

Fig. 1. Comparison of data extrapolated from the Gaslini Biobank database (A) and from the Australian population (B) (Meikle et al., *1999).*

Classification: biochemical and molecular defects

LSDs can be grouped according to various classifications. While in the past they were classified on the basis of the nature of the accumulated substrate(s), more recently they tend to be classified by the molecular defect (Table 1). A classic example of LSDs grouped by storage is the mucopolysaccharidoses group, in which the impaired function of 1 of 11 lysosomal enzymes results in the accumulation of glycosaminoglycans (or mucopolysaccharides). In the group of

15

sphingolipidoses, undegraded sphingolipids accumulate because of an enzyme deficiency or an activator protein defect (this latter is classified in the table as a subgroup according to the molecular defect). In the oligosaccharidoses (also known as glycoproteinoses), single lysosomal hydrolase deficiency causes storage of oligosaccharides. In some cases, a deficiency in a single enzyme can result in the accumulation of different substrates. Such example includes GM1 gangliosidosis and Morquio B disease, which are both caused by an acid β-galactosidase activity defect resulting in GM1 ganglioside and keratan sulphate accumulation, respectively.

Table 1. Classification of lysosomal storage disorders

Disease	Defect
Mucopolysaccharidoses	
MPS I (Hurler, Scheie)	α-iduronidase
MPS II (Hunter)	Iduronate sulphatase
MPS III A (Sanfilippo A)	Heparan sulphamidase
MPS III B (Sanfilippo B)	Acetyl α-glucosaminidase
MPS III C Sanfilippo C)	Acetyl CoA: α-glucosaminide N-acetyltransferase
MPS III D (Sanfilippo D)	N-acetyl glucosamine-6-sulphatase
MPS IV A (Morquio A)	Acetyl galactosamine-6-sulphatase
MPS IV B (Morquio B)	β-galactosidase
MPS VI (Maroteaux-Lamy)	Acetyl galactosamine-4-sulphatase (arylsulphatase B)
MPS VII (Sly)	β-glucuronidase
MPS IX (Natowicz)	Hyaluronidase
Sphingolipidoses	
Fabry	α-galactosidase A
Farber	Acid ceramidase
Gangliosidosis GM 1	β-galactosidase
Gangliosidosis GM2, Tay-Sachs	β-hexosaminidase A
Gangliosidosis GM 2, Sandhoff	β-hexosaminidase A+B
Gaucher	Glucosylceramidase
Krabbe	β-galactosyl ceramidase
Metachromatic leukodystrophy	Arylsulphatase A
Niemann-Pick A and B	Sphingomyelinase
Oligosaccharidoses (glycoproteinoses)	
Aspartylglycosaminuria	Glycosylasparaginase
Fucosidosis	α-fucosidase
α-Mannosidosis	α-mannosidase
β-Mannosidosis	β-mannosidase
Schindler	N-acetylgalactosaminidase
Sialidosis	α-neuraminidase

Glycogenoses	
Glycogenosis II/ Pompe	α1,4-glucosidase
Lipidoses	
Wolman / CESD	Acid lipase
Non-enzymatic lysosomal protein defect	
Gangliosidosis GM 2, activator defect	GM2 activator protein
Metachromatic leukodystrophy	Saposin B
Gaucher	Saposin C
Transmembrane protein defect	
Transporters	
ISSD/ Salla	Sialin
Cystinosis	Cystinosin
Niemann-Pick C1	NPC1 and NPC2
Structural proteins	
Danon	Lysosome-associated membrane protein 2 (LAMP2)
Mucolipidosis IV	Mucolipin
Lysosomal enzyme protection defect	
Galactosialidosis	Protective protein cathepsin A (PPCA/CTSA) (β-galactosidase and neuraminidase defects)
Post-translational processing defect	
Multiple sulphatase deficiency	Multiple sulphatase
Trafficking defect in lysosomal enzymes	
Mucolipidosis II/IIIαβ	UDP-*N*-acetylglucosamine-1-phosphotransferase (various lysosomal enzyme defects)
Mucolipidosis IIIγ	UDP-*N*-acetylglucosamine-1-phosphotransferase (various lysosomal enzyme defects)
Polypeptide degradation defect	
Pycnodysostosis	Cathepsin k
Others	
Neuronal ceroid lipofuscinoses	
NCL 1	Palmitoyl protein thioesterase (PPT1)
NCL 2	Tripeptidyl peptidase 1 (TPP1)
NCL 3	CLN3, lysosomal transmembrane protein
NCL 5	CLN5, soluble lysosomal protein
NCL 6	CLN6, transmembrane protein of ER
NCL 7	MFS8, lysosomal transmembrane protein of MFS family
NCL 8	CLN8, transmembrane protein of ER
NCL 10	Cathepsin D

Table 1 also reports the emerging subclassification of the diseases based on the recent understanding of LSD molecular bases. This subclassification includes groups of disorders due to: (1) non-enzymatic lysosomal protein defects; (2) transmembrane protein defects (transporters and structural proteins); (3) lysosomal enzyme protection defects; (4) post-translational processing defects of lysosomal proteins; (5) trafficking defects in lysosomal enzymes; and (6) polypeptide degradation defects. Finally, a subgroup includes the neuronal ceroid lipofuscinoses (NCLs), which are considered as lysosomal disorders even though distinct characteristics exist. In the classic LSDs, the deficiency or dysfunction of an enzyme or transporter leads to lysosomal accumulation of specific undegraded substrates or metabolites, whereas accumulating material in NCLs is not a disease-specific substrate, but the subunit c of mitochondrial ATP synthase or sphingolipid activator proteins A and D (Jalanko & Braulke, 2008).

With respect to the molecular subclassification, multiple sulphatase deficiency (MSD) is worth noting. It has been shown that MSD results from a post-translational processing defect due to the failure of the Cα-formylglycine-generating enzyme to convert a specific cysteine residue, at the catalytic centre of all sulphatases, to a Cα-formylglycine residue (Cosma *et al.*, 2003; Dierks *et al.*, 2003). Another rare LSD, galactosialidosis, is associated with the defective activity of two enzymes, β-galactosidase and α-neuraminidase. In these diseases, subclassified as a 'lysosomal enzyme protection defect', a multi-enzyme complex between the two lysosomal enzymes and the protective protein, cathepsin A (PPCA/CTSA), forms improperly (D'Azzo, *et al.*, 2001).

The breakdown of certain glycosphingolipids by their respective hydrolases requires the presence of activator proteins, known as sphingolipid activator proteins or saposins, encoded by two different genes. The defective function of the GM2 activator protein results in the AB variant of GM2 gangliosidosis (Conzelmann *et al.*, 1978). The prosaposin is processed to four homologous saposins (Sap A, Sap B, Sap C and Sap D) (O'Brien *et al*, 1988). Deficiency of Sap A, Sap B, and Sap C results in variant forms of (1) Krabbe disease, with an abnormal storage of galactosylceramide (Spiegel *et al.*, 2005); (2) metachromatic leukodystrophy with sulphatide storage (Wenger *et al.*, 1989); and (3) Gaucher disease with glucosylceramide storage (Christomanou *et al.*, 1989), respectively. Rarely a total deficiency of prosaposin has been reported that results in a very severe phenotype (Bradova *et al.*, 1993).

Mucolipidoses result from defects in the enzyme UDP-*N*-acetylglucosamine-1-phosphotransferase, which plays a key role in lysosomal enzyme trafficking (Kornfeld & Sly, 2001). This enzyme is responsible for the initial step in the synthesis of mannose 6-phosphate (M6P) recognition markers, essential for receptor-mediated transport of newly synthesized lysosomal enzymes to the endosomal/prelysosomal compartment. Failure to attach this recognition signal leads to the mistargeting of all lysosomal enzymes that require the M6P marker to enter the lysosome.

Laboratory diagnosis

Diagnosis of LSDs relies on close collaboration between laboratory specialists and clinicians. Samples and diagnostic tests are different for each group of disorders and often are specific for a given disease. Laboratory diagnosis requires the clinician to select the appropriate test to be performed on the basis of a comprehensive evaluation that includes a physical assessment of the patient as well as paraclinical test results (peripheral blood smears, radiologic/neurophysiologic findings, *etc.*).

Before specific analyses (enzymatic and/or molecular) are considered, preliminary screening tests should be performed. Increased urinary excretion of glycosaminoglycans is mainly found in the mucopolysaccharidoses group; abnormal urinary oligosaccharide excretion patterns mostly characterize the oligosaccharidoses (glycoproteinoses). There are also more specific preliminary tests, such as the qualitative assessment of urinary sulphatide storage, which can indicate metachromatic leukodystrophy (due to arylsulphatase A enzyme deficiency or saposin B activator defect). Increased urinary excretion of free sialic acid is suggestive of the sialic acid storage disorders, the severe infantile form (ISSD) or the slowly progressive adult form (Salla). However, urinary tests have a risk of false-positive/-negative results, which then requires specific diagnostic analyses to be performed on suitable samples, leukocytes, and or cell lines (fibroblasts and lymphoblasts).

Each sample sent to the laboratory should be accompanied by a detailed clinical anamnesis and family history. This history is fundamental if the sample is referred for molecular genetic testing (MGT).

About the 75 per cent of LSDs are due to a deficiency of lysosomal hydrolase activity, hence the demonstration of a reduced/absent lysosomal hydrolase activity by a specific enzyme assay is an effective and reliable method of diagnosis. In these cases, molecular analysis can refine the enzymatic diagnosis. The remaining LSDs, resulting from nonenzymatic protein defects, require molecular analysis to be performed on the specific gene for a conclusive diagnosis to be made.

Pseudodeficiency

Generally an inherited deficiency of a lysosomal enzyme is associated with a disease. There are, however, individuals who show greatly reduced enzyme activity, but remain clinically healthy. This condition, termed a 'pseudodeficiency', is known in some lysosomal hydrolases. At the same time, there are circumstances in which affected individuals with a clinical/paraclinical picture resembling some glycosphingolipidoses show normal activity of the relevant lysosomal enzyme. These patients should be investigated for a possible defect of some activator protein involved in glycosphingolipid breakdown.

To date pseudodeficiencies, due to polymorphic genetic variants, have been reported to occur in at least nine lysosomal enzymes including: arylsulphatase A (*ARSA* gene) (Gieselmann *et al.*, 1989; Gieselmann, 1991), β-hexosaminidase (*HEXA* gene) (Cao *et al.*, 1997), α-iduronidase (*IDUA* gene) (Aronovich *et al.*, 1996), α-glucosidase (Nishimoto *et al.*, 1988), α-galactosidase (Froissart *et al.*, 2003; Hoffmann, 2005), β-galactosidase (*GLB1* gene) (Gort *et al.*, 2007), α-fucosidase (*FUCA1* gene) (Wauters *et al.*, 1992), and β-glucuronidase (*GUSB* gene) (Chabas *et al.*, 1991; Vervoort *et al.*, 1995).

While some of these genetic conditions are rare, arylsulphatase A pseudodeficiency (Pd) has been estimated to have a frequency of 7.3–15 per cent (Gieselmann *et al.*, 1991; Regis *et al.*, 1996). Since the Pd allele is more frequent than the alleles causing metachromatic leukodystrophy (MLD) (estimated to be 0.5 per cent), individuals presenting with neurologic symptoms and homozygous for the pseudodeficiency of arylsulphatase A are likely to be misdiagnosed as having MLD (Shen *et al.*, 1993). Additionally, it must be noted that Pd polymorphisms can occur on the same gene as MLD-causing mutations. It is therefore necessary to perform a combination of enzymatic and molecular analyses to determine the actual genetic make-up of MLD patients and their family members in order to distinguish individuals carrying Pd alleles from those carrying MLD alleles.

Activator proteins

Another complication, potentially leading to missed diagnoses, is represented by defects of those cofactors (mentioned above) required for the function of certain lysosomal enzymes involved in glycosphingolipid breakdown. Variant forms of GM2 gangliosidosis, Krabbe disease, metachromatic leukodystrophy, and Gaucher disease can result not only from the deficiency of an enzymatic activity, but also from defects of sphingolipid activator proteins or saposins. In these cases conclusive diagnosis requires a comprehensive evaluation based on a range of diagnostic procedures including neuroradiologic, neurophysiologic, and biochemical/ enzymatic and molecular tests.

Genetic counseling

All LSDs are inherited as autosomal recessive traits, except for Fabry disease, Hunter syndrome (MPSII), and Danon disease, which are X-linked disorders. Once the laboratory diagnosis (enzymatic and/or molecular) of an LSD patient is ascertained, genetic counseling for at-risk couples includes prenatal testing on chorionic villi (at 11–12 weeks) or amniocytes (at 16 weeks). Genotyping individual LSD patients also allows carriers in the family to be identified and can sometimes predict phenotypes in the patients.

From biochemical to molecular genetic testing and *vice versa*

Biochemical genetic testing (BGT) includes the analysis of human proteins and certain metabolites and is predominantly used to detect inborn errors of metabolism. BGT, feasible for most LSDs, is essential for the diagnosis of primary lysosomal enzyme deficiency.

Lysosomal enzymes are present in almost all tissues and biological samples. The choice of the sample type to be analyzed is based on (1) the level of an enzyme activity in a specific tissue; (2) the sample stability during its transfer to the referring lab; and (3) the time of diagnosis.

Theoretically, some biological fluids, such as plasma, serum, and urine, might be assayed for enzyme activity. However, since several enzymatic pseudodeficiencies have been reported in serum or plasma, their use can lead to pitfalls in diagnosis (Thomas, 1994; Hoffmann *et al.*, 2005). Leukocytes are often appropriate biological samples, although possible interferences between isoenzymes should be taken carefully into consideration. Fibroblast samples represent the gold standard in the diagnosis since they express the optimum enzyme activity, even though they require an invasive skin biopsy and culturing. Epstein-Barr virus–transformed B-lymphoblast culture obtained from noninvasive blood sampling can be useful if we keep in mind that lymphoblasts do not express some enzymatic activities, such as that of arylsulphatase A. Enzymatic assays are usually performed by synthetic (fluorimetric or colorimetric) substrates which show undetectable or very low enzyme activity in affected individuals. Screening tests of several LSDs by BGT on dried blood spot (DBS) using fluorescent methods (Chamoles *et al.*, 2001a, 2001b, 2002) or tandem mass spectrometry (Li *et al.*, 2004; Gelb *et al.*, 2006) have been reported and a DBS control quality for these tests has recently been developed (De Jesus *et al.*, 2009).

The availability of multiplex technology has facilitated the technical aspects of testing, making it easier to identify LSDs and to introduce screening programs for neonates for treatable LSDs (Fletcher, 2006; Zhang *et al.*, 2008). In this respect, attempts to widen screening programs covering other LSDs are essential in those cases in which an early and presymptomatic diagnosis can provide better outcomes for patients by reducing clinically significant disabilities (Dajnoki *et al.*, 2008).

It is important to remark, however, that a reduced residual enzyme activity detected in a presymptomatic patient at neonatal screening needs to be confirmed by standard laboratory diagnostic procedures.

Molecular genetic testing (MGT) is performed on human DNA or RNA to detect heritable genotypes and mutations for clinical purposes. Such analyses, always carried out with the informed consent of patients and/or their parents, comprise different molecular approaches aimed at investigating an entire gene coding region and its exon/intron boundaries.

While MGT is supportive in confirming an enzymatic diagnosis, it is essential for identifying defects of lysosomal non-enzymatic proteins such as membrane protein LAMP2, LIMP, protective protein/cathepsin A, saposin proteins, activator protein, *etc*. MGT is an important tool in postmortem diagnoses when only specimens suitable for DNA extraction are available. It is also an elucidative tool in the event of highly biochemical residual enzyme activity or in presence of some enzymatic pseudodeficiency.

The correct interpretation of molecular data, however, relies on a comprehensive evaluation that includes clinical and biochemical data. There are also circumstances in which a proved enzymatic deficiency and a significant clinical picture are not apparently accompanied by the detection of the underlying genetic lesion in the coding region and in the exon/intron boundaries. This circumstance calls for careful evaluation by additional molecular studies. Expression gene profiling or RNA and protein analyses can help to reveal both deletion/insertion in autosomal recessive diseases or in X-linked heterozygous female as well as possible transcriptional defects.

How to interpret molecular genetic testing

After excluding possible misincorporations with different PCR amplifications, a nucleotide change requires a careful interpretation. Available specific databases and/or updated literature should be checked to determine whether the change has already been described as disease-causative or as a polymorphic variant (SNP). If the detected nucleotide change is known, the patient's biochemical and clinical data should be compared with the literature. Even in the presence of known and well-characterized mutations, it should be remembered that additional nucleotide changes could be present 'in *cis*' on the same allele as part of a complex allele, which could therefore influence the phenotype. This makes genotype/phenotype correlation difficult and underlines the importance of an exhaustive evaluation of clinical and biochemical data in interpreting MGT (Caciotti *et al.*, 2003).

The identification of novel nucleotide changes or 'private mutations' is complicated and can be time-consuming. First, parallel methodologic approaches are necessary to demonstrate that these changes have a frequency of less than 1 per cent in a population with the same genetic background. Once the change is confirmed as deleterious, additional studies at the RNA and protein levels could be necessary for a conclusive diagnosis.

Routine techniques used during MGT can miss insertion/deletions, complex rearrangements, and uniparental disomy (UPD), resulting in incorrect genotyping of the patients. In particular, partial or total gene deletions have been reported as pitfalls leading to apparent homozygosity of the patients (Filocamo *et al.*, 2001). Therefore additional techniques, in conjunction with the conventional screening methods, are strongly recommended to discover accidental misgenotyping. Also, when a genetic lesion is identified in a patient at a homozygous level, the minimum ascertainment is confirmation in both parents.

It should be emphasized that sometimes the MGT results may require attention even in presence of a change previously reported as a deleterious mutation. In this context, it should be mentioned that for years the c.1151G>A (p.S384N) was considered a disease-causing mutation in patients with Maroteaux-Lamy syndrome. Recently a segregation study in a family at risk for the syndrome conclusively revealed c.1151G>A (p.S384N) to be a polymorphism (Zanetti *et al.*, 2009).

How to interpret biochemical genetic testing

The complete absence of lysosomal enzyme activity in the patient generally confirms the diagnosis. The detection of residual lysosomal enzyme activity should be carefully evaluated together with clinical, instrumental and molecular data, in order to reveal possible polymorphisms leading to a pseudodeficiency. However, the presence of a normal lysosomal enzyme activity cannot exclude that specific diagnosis if this normal result is accompanied by suggestive clinical symptoms and/or abnormal presence of metabolites in the urine. Such findings must be duly investigated. For example, a patient who presents with a clinical profile resembling that of Gaucher disease, with high levels of chitotriosidase activity and increased concentrations of glucosylceramide in plasma and normal beta-glucosidase activity in skin fibroblasts, should be referred for a molecular genetic study of the *PSAP* gene, which codes for the cofactor Sap C required for the function of beta-glucosidase (Tylki-Szymańska *et al.*, 2007).

Biobanking

Sample and clinical/instrumental data banking is crucial in genetic rare diseases, such as LSDs, which often lead to death at an early age. Since it is likely that our understanding of the diseases and testing methodology will improve in the future, consideration should be given to banking appropriate biological material from patients affected or suspected to be affected by LSDs.

Biological material such as urine, whole blood, plasma, serum, leukocytes, DNAs, and cell lines (fibroblasts from skin biopsy and/or lymphoblasts from blood) from a patient with an LSD should be stored in a biobank, especially when the diagnosis is uncertain or when a severely affected patient is to be investigated. In this respect, an effective interaction between clinicians and biobank staff is essential since the possibility of achieving results in the future results depends on the availability of the most appropriate biological samples as well as the associated clinical/paraclinical data. Not only does biobanking aid in postmortem diagnoses and retrospective studies, but it also allows basic, translational, and epidemiologic biomedical research to be carried out in lysosomal diseases.

Hydrops foetalis, which is an extreme presentation of many LSDs, represents the best example of a complex case in which the diagnosis can be achieved only if appropriate samples are stored. Foetal hydrops can be associated with a wide spectrum of phenotypes, including mucopolysaccharidosis VII and IVA (Cheng *et al.*, 2003; Venkat-Raman *et al.*, 2006), Gaucher disease (Church *et al.*, 2004), sialidosis (Loren *et al.*, 2005), GM1 gangliosidosis (Sinelli *et al.*, 2005), galactosialidosis (Malvagia *et al.*, 2004), infantile free sialic acid storage disease (ISSD) (Froissart *et al.*, 2005), Niemann-Pick disease type C (and A), mucolipidosis II (I-cell disease), Wolman disease, and disseminated lipogranulomatosis (Farber disease) (Stone & Sidransky, 1999; Staretz-Chachman *et al.*, 2009; Burin *et al.*, 2004; Kooper *et al.*, 2006). Frequently, these LSDs are only recognized after the recurrence of hydops fetalis in several pregnancies (Malvagia *et al.*, 2004; Venkat-Raman *et al.*, 2006). Hence, such a complex picture, potentially requiring a range of distinct methodologic approaches for a conclusive diagnosis, can only rely on a close interaction between skilled experts including, among others, clinicians, genetic biochemists, and molecular biologists to optimize the storage of the most appropriate biological material.

Conclusions

Biochemical and molecular genetic testing must be considered as complementary studies for the diagnosis of most LSDs, for genotype/phenotype correlation, and for prenatal diagnosis. Molecular genetic testing is essential for carrier detection, and it can sometimes predict the prognosis and support therapeutic choices including the application of new therapeutic approaches.

References

Aronovich, E.L., Pan, D. & Whitley, C.B. (1996): Molecular genetic defect underlying alpha-L-iduronidase pseudodeficiency. *Am. J. Hum. Genet.* **58**, 75–85.

Arvio, M., Autio, S. & Louhiala, P. (1993): Early clinical symptoms and incidence of aspartylglucosaminuria in Finland. *Acta Paediatr.* **82**, 587–589.

Beutler, E. & Grabowski, G. (2001): Gaucher disease. In: *The metabolic and molecular bases of inherited disease*, 8th ed., eds. C.R. Scriver, A.L. Beaudet, W.S. Sly & D. Valle, pp. 3635–3668. New York: McGraw-Hill.

Bradova, V., Smid, F., Ulrich-Bott, B., Roggendorf, W., Paton, B.C. & Harzer, K. (1993): Prosaposin deficiency: further characterization of the sphingolipid activator protein-deficient sibs. Multiple glycolipid elevations (including lactosylceramidosis), partial enzyme deficiencies and ultrastructure of the skin in this generalized sphingolipid storage disease. *Hum. Genet.* **92**, 143–152.

Burin, M.G., Scholz, A.P., Gus, R., Sanseverino, M.T., Fritsh, A., Magalhães, J.A., Timm, F., Barrios, P., Chesky, M., Coelho, J.C. & Giugliani, R. (2004): Investigation of lysosomal storage diseases in nonimmune hydrops fetalis. *Prenat. Diagn.* **24**, 653–657.

Caciotti, A., Bardelli, T., Cunningham, J., D'Azzo, A., Zammarchi, E. & Morrone, A. (2003): Modulating action of the new polymorphism L436F detected in the GLB1 gene of a type-II GM1 gangliosidosis patient. *Hum. Genet.* **113**, 44–50.

Cao, Z., Petroulakis, E., Salo, T. & Triggs-Raine, B. (1997): Benign *HEXA* mutations, C739T(R247W) and C745T(R249W), cause beta-hexosaminidase A pseudodeficiency by reducing the alpha-subunit protein levels. *J. Biol. Chem.* **272**, 14975–14982.

Chabas, A., Giros, M.L. & Guardiola, A. (1991): Low β-glucuronidase activity in a healthy member of a family with mucopolysaccharidosis VII. *J. Inherit. Metab. Dis.* **14**, 908–914.

Chamoles, N.A., Blanco, M. & Gaggioli, D. (2001): Fabry disease: enzymatic diagnosis in dried blood spots on filter paper. *Clin. Chim. Acta.* **308**, 195–196.

Chamoles, N.A., Blanco, M.B., Gaggioli, D. & Casentini, C. (2001): Hurler-like phenotype: enzymatic diagnosis in dried blood spots on filter paper. *Clin. Chem.* **47**, 2098–2102.

Chamoles, N.A., Blanco, M., Gaggioli, D. & Casentini, C. (2002): Gaucher and Niemann-Pick diseases: enzymatic diagnosis in dried blood spots on filter paper. Retrospective diagnoses in newborn-screening cards. *Clin. Chim. Acta* **317**, 191–197.

Cheng, Y., Verp, M.S., Knutel, T. & Hibbard, J.U. (2003): Mucopolysaccharidosis type VII as a cause of recurrent non-immune hydrops fetalis. *J. Perinat. Med.* **31**, 535–537.

Christomanou, H., Chabas, A., Pampols, T. & Guardiola, A. (1989): Activator protein deficient Gaucher's disease: a second patient with the newly identified lipid storage disorder. *Wien. Klin. Wochenschr.* **67**, 999–1003.

Church, H.J., Cooper, A., Stewart, F., Thornton, C.M. & Wraith, J.E. (2004): Homozygous loss of a cysteine residue in the glucocerebrosidase gene results in Gaucher's disease with a hydropic phenotype. *Eur. J. Hum. Genet.* **12**, 975–978.

Conzelmann, E., Sandhoff, K., Nehrkorn, H., Geiger, B. & Arnon, R. (1978): Purification, biochemical and immunological characterisation of hexosaminidase A from variant AB of infantile GM2 gangliosidosis. *Eur. J. Biochem.* **84**, 27–33.

Cosma, M. P., Pepe, S., Annunziata, I., Newbold, R.F., Grompe, M., Parenti, G. & Ballabio, A. (2003): The multiple sulphatase deficiency gene encodes an essential and limiting factor for the activity of sulphatases. *Cell* **113**, 445–456.

D'Azzo, A., Andria, G., Strisciuglio, P. & Galjaard, H. (2001): Galactosialidosis. In: *The metabolic and molecular bases of inherited disease*, eds. C.R. Scriver, A.L. Beaudet, W.S. Sly & D. Valle, pp. 3811–3826. New York: McGraw-Hill.

Dajnoki, A., Mühl, A., Fekete, G., Keutzer, J., Orsini, J., DeJesus, V., Zhang, X.K. & Bodamer, O.A. (2008): Newborn screening for Pompe disease by measuring acid alpha-glucosidase activity using tandem mass spectrometry. *Clin. Chem.* **54**, 1624–1629.

De Duve, C. & Wattiaux, R. (1966): Functions of lysosomes. *Annu. Rev. Physiol.* **28**, 435–492.

DeJesus, V.R., Zhang, X.K., Keutzer, J., Bodamer, O.A., Mühl, A., Orsini, J.J., Caggana, M., Vogt, R.F. & Hannon, W.H. (2009): Development and evaluation of quality control dried blood spot materials in newborn screening for lysosomal storage disorders. *Clin. Chem.* **55**, 158–164.

Dierks, T., Schmidt, B., Borissenko, L.V., Peng, J., Preusser, A., Mariappan, M. & von Figura, K. (2003): Multiple sulphatase deficiency is caused by mutations in the gene encoding the human Cα-formylglycine generating enzyme. *Cell* **113**, 435–444.

Dionisi-Vici, C., Rizzo, C., Burlina, A.B., Caruso, U., Sabetta, G., Uziel, G. & Abeni, D. (2002): Inborn errors of metabolism in the Italian pediatric population: a national retrospective survey. *J. Pediatr.* **140**, 321–327.

Filocamo, M., Regis, S., Mazzotti, R., Parenti, G., Stroppiano, M. & Gatti, R. (2001): A simple non-isotopic method to show pitfalls during mutation analysis of the glucocerebrosidase gene. *J. Med. Genet.* **38**, E34.

Fletcher, J.M. (2006): Screening for lysosomal storage disorders: a clinical perspective. *J. Inherit. Metab. Dis.* **29**, 405-408.

Froissart, R., Guffon, N., Vanier, M.T., Desnick, R.J. & Maire, I. (2003): Fabry disease: D313Y is an alpha-galactosidase A sequence variant that causes pseudodeficient activity in plasma. *Mol. Genet. Metab.* **80**, 307–314.

Froissart, R., Cheillan, D., Bouvier, R., Tourret, S., Bonnet, V., Piraud, M. & Maire, I. (2005): Clinical, morphological, and molecular aspects of sialic acid storage disease manifesting in utero. *J. Med. Genet.* **42**, 829–836.

Futerman, A.H. & van Meer, G. (2004): The cell biology of lysosomal storage disorders. *Nat. Rev. Mol. Cell Biol.* **5**, 554–565.

Gelb, M.H., Turecek, F., Scott, C.R. & Chamoles, N.A. (2006): Direct multiplex assay of enzymes in dried blood spots by tandem mass spectrometry for the newborn screening of lysosomal storage disorders. *J. Inherit. Metab. Dis.* **29**, 397–404.

Gieselmann, V. (1991): An assay for the rapid detection of the arylsulphatase A pseudodeficiency allele facilitates diagnosis and genetic counseling for metachromatic leukodystrophy. *Hum. Genet.* **86**, 251–255.

Gieselmann, V., Polten, A., Kreysing, J. & von Figura, K. (1989): Arylsulphatase A pseudodeficiency: loss of a polyadenylation signal and N-glycosylation site. *Proc. Natl. Acad. Sci. USA* **86**, 9436–9440.

Gieselmann, V., Fluharty, A.L., Tønnesen, T. & Von Figura, K. (1991): Mutations in the arylsulphatase A pseudodeficiency allele causing metachromatic leukodystrophy. *Am. J. Hum. Genet.* **49**, 407–413.

Gort, L., Santamaria, R., Grinberg, D., Vilageliu, L. & Chabás, A. (2007): Identification of a novel pseudodeficiency allele in the *GLB1* gene in a carrier of GM1 gangliosidosis. *Clin. Genet.* **72**, 109–111.

Hickman, S. & Neufeld, E.F. (1972): A hypothesis for I-cell disease: defective hydrolases that do not enter lysosomes. *Biochem. Biophys. Res. Commun.* **49**, 992–999.

Hoffmann, B., Georg Koch, H., Schweitzer-Krantz, S., Wendel, U. & Mayatepek, E., (2005): Deficient alpha-galactosidase A activity in plasma but no Fabry disease: a pitfall in diagnosis. *Clin. Chem. Lab. Med.* **43**, 1276–1277.

Jalanko, A. & Braulke, T. (2009): Neuronal ceroid lipofuscinoses. *Biochim. Biophys. Acta* **1793**, 697–709.

Kooper, A.J., Janssens, P.M., de Groot, A.N, Liebrand-van Sambeek, M.L., van den Berg, C.J., Tan-Sindhunata, G.B., van den Berg, P.P., Bijlsma, E.K., Smits, A.P. & Wevers, R.A. (2006): Lysosomal storage diseases in non-immune hydrops fetalis pregnancies. *Clin. Chim. Acta* **371**, 176–82.

Kornfeld, S. & Sly, W.S. (2001): I-cell disease and pseudo-Hurler polydystrophy: disorders of lysosomal enzyme phosphorylation and localization. In: *The metabolic and molecular bases of inherited disease*, eds. C.R. Scriver, A.L. Beaudet, W.S. Sly & D. Valle, pp. 3469–3505. New York: McGraw-Hill.

Li, Y., Scott, C.R., Chamoles, N.A, Ghavami, A., Pinto, B.M., Turecek, F. & Gelb, M.H. (2004): Direct multiplex assay of lysosomal enzymes in dried blood spots for newborn screening. *Clin. Chem.* **50**, 1785–1796.

Loren, D.J., Campos, Y., D'Azzo, A, Wyble, L., Grange, D.K., Gilbert-Barness, E., White, F.V. & Hamvas, A. (2005): Sialidosis presenting as severe nonimmune fetal hydrops is associated with two novel mutations in lysosomal alpha-neuraminidase. *J. Perinatol.* **25**, 491–494.

Malvagia, S., Morrone, A., Caciotti, A., Bardelli, T., D'Azzo, A., Ancora, G., Zammarchi, E. & Donati, M.A. (2004): New mutations in the *PPBG* gene lead to loss of PPCA protein which affects the level of the beta-galactosidase/neuraminidase complex and the EBP-receptor. *Mol. Genet. Metab.* **82**, 48–55.

Maxfield, F.R. & McGraw, T.E. (2004): Endocytic recycling. *Nat. Rev. Mol. Cell Biol.* **5**, 121–132.

Meikle, P.J., Hopwood, J.J., Clague, A.E. & Carey, W.F. (1999): Prevalence of lysosomal storage disorders. *JAMA* **281**, 249–254.

Michelakakis, H., Dimitriou, E., Tsagaraki, S., Giouroukos, S., Schulpis, K. & Bartsocas, C.S. (1995): Lysosomal storage diseases in Greece. *Genet. Couns.* **6**, 43–47.

Nishimoto, J., Inui, K., Okada, S., Ishigami, W., Hirota, S., Yamano, T. & Yabuuchi, H. (1988): A family with pseudodeficiency of acid a-glucosidase. *Clin. Genet.* **33**, 254–261.

O'Brien, J.S., Kretz, K.A., Dewji, N., Wenger, D.A., Esch, F. & Fluharty, A.L. (1988): Coding of two sphingolipid activator proteins (SAP-1 and SAP-2) by the same genetic locus. *Science* **41**, 1098–1101.

Pinto, R., Caseiro, C., Lemos, M., Lopes, L., Fontes, A., Ribeiro, H., Pinto, E., Silva, E., Rocha, S., Marcão, A., Ribeiro, I., Lacerda, L., Ribeiro, G., Amaral, O. & Sá Miranda, M.C. (2004): Prevalence of lysosomal storage diseases in Portugal. *Eur. J. Hum. Genet.* **12**, 87–92.

Poorthuis, B.J., Wevers, R.A., Kleijer, W.J., Groener, J.E., de Jong, J.G., van Weely, S., Niezen-Koning, K.E. & van Diggelen, O.P. (1999): The frequency of lysosomal storage diseases in the Netherlands. *Hum. Genet.* **105**, 151–156.

Reczek, D., Schwake, M., Schröder, J., Hughes, H., Blanz, J., Jin, X., Brondyk, W., Van Patten, S., Edmunds, T. & Saftig, P. (2007): LIMP-2 is a receptor for lysosomal mannose-6-phosphate-independent targeting of beta-glucocerebrosidase. *Cell* **131**, 770–783.

Regis, S., Filocamo, M., Stroppiano, M., Corsolini, F. & Gatti, R. (1996): Molecular analysis of the arylsulphatase A gene in late infantile metachromatic leukodystrophy patients and healthy subjects from Italy. *J. Med. Genet.* **33**, 251–252.

Reitman, M.L. & Kornfeld, S. (1981): UDP-N-acetylglucosamine:glycoprotein N-acetylglucosamine-1-phosphotransferase: proposed enzyme for the phosphorylation of the high mannose oligosaccharide units of lysosomal enzymes. *J. Biol. Chem.* **256**, 4275–4281.

Santavuori, P. (1988): Neuronal ceroid-lipofuscinoses in childhood. *Brain Dev.* **10**, 80–83.

Shen, N., Li, Z.G., Waye, J.S., Francis, G. & Chang, P.L. (1993): Complications in the genotypic molecular diagnosis of pseudoarylsulphatase A deficiency. *Am. J. Med. Genet.* **45**, 631–637.

Sinelli, M.T., Motta, M., Cattarelli, D., Cardone, M.L. & Chirico, G. (2005): Fetal hydrops in GM(1) gangliosidosis: a case report. *Acta Paediatr.* **94**, 1847–1849.

Spiegel, R., Bach, G., Sury, V., Mengistu, G., Meidan, B., Shalev, S., Shneor, Y., Mandel, H. & Zeigler M. (2005): A mutation in the saposin A coding region of the prosaposin gene in an infant presenting as Krabbe disease: first report of saposin A deficiency in humans. *Mol. Genet. Metab.* **84**, 160–166.

Staretz-Chacham, O., Lang, T.C., LaMarca, M.E., Krasnewich, D. & Sidransky, E. (2009): Lysosomal storage disorders in the newborn. *Pediatrics* **123**, 1191–1207.

Stone, D.L. & Sidransky, E. (1999): Hydrops fetalis: lysosomal storage disorders in extremis. *Adv. Pediatr.* **46**, 409–440.

Thomas, G.H. 'Pseudodeficiencies' of lysosomal hydrolases. (1994): *Am. J. Hum. Genet.* **54**, 934–940.

Tylki-Szymańska, A., Czartoryska, B., Vanier, M.T., Poorthuis, B.J., Groener, J.A., Ługowska, A., Millat, G., Vaccaro, A.M. & Jurkiewicz, E. (2007): Non-neuronopathic Gaucher disease due to saposin C deficiency. *Clin. Genet.* **72**, 538–542.

Vallance, H. & Ford, J. (2003): Carrier testing for autosomal-recessive disorders. *Crit. Rev. Clin. Lab. Sci.* **40**, 473–497.

Vellodi, A. (2004): Lysosomal storage disorders. *Br. J. Haematol.* **128**, 413–431.

Venkat-Raman, N., Sebire, N.J. & Murphy, K.W. (2006): Recurrent fetal hydrops due to mucopolysaccharidoses type VII. *Fetal Diagn. Ther.* **21**, 250-254.

Vervoort, R., Islam, M.R., Sly, W., Chabas, A., Wevers, R., de Jong, J., Liebaers, I. & Lissens, W. (1995): A pseudodeficiency allele (D152N) of the human beta-glucuronidase gene. *Am. J. Hum. Genet.* **57**, 798–804.

Waheed, A., Hasilik, A. & von Figura, K. (1981): Processing of the phosphorylated recognition marker in lysosomal enzymes. Characterization and partial purification of a microsomal alpha-N-acetylglucosaminyl phosphodiesterase. *J. Biol. Chem.* **256**, 5717–5721.

Wauters, J.G., Stuer, K.L., Elsen, A.V. & Willems, P.J. (1992): α-L-fucosidase in human fibroblasts. I. The enzyme activity polymorphism. *Biochem. Genet.* **30**, 131–141.

Wenger, D.A., De Gala, G., Williams, C., Taylor, H.A., Stevenson, R.E., Pruitt, J.R., Miller, J., Garen, P.D. & Balentine, J.D. (1989): Clinical, pathological, and biochemical studies on an infantile case of sulphatide/GM1 activator protein deficiency. *Am. J. Med. Genet.* **33**, 255–265.

Wraith, J.E. (2002): Lysosomal disorders. *Semin. Neonatol.* **7**, 75–83.

Zanetti, A., Ferraresi, E., Picci, L., Filocamo, M., Parini, R., Rosano, C., Tomanin, R. & Scarpa, M. (2009): Segregation analysis in a family at risk for the Maroteaux-Lamy syndrome conclusively reveals c.1151G>A (p.S384N) as to be a polymorphism. *Eur. J. Hum. Genet.* **17**, 1160–1164.

Zhang, X.K., Elbin, C.S., Chuang, W.L., Cooper, S.K., Marashio, C.A., Beauregard, C. & Keutzer, J.M. (2008): Multiplex enzyme assay screening of dried blood spots for lysosomal storage disorders by using tandem mass spectrometry. *Clin. Chem.* **54**, 1725–1728.

Chapter 3

Organizational and ethical aspects of newborn screening for lysosomal storage diseases

Carlo Corbetta and Luisella Alberti

UOC Laboratorio di Riferimento Regionale per lo Screening Neonatale,
Ospedale dei Bambini 'V. Buzzi', A.O. Istituti Clinici di Perfezionamento, via Castelvetro 32, 20154 Milan, Italy
carlo.corbetta@icp.mi.it

Summary

Because of the development of new technologies, such as mass spectrometry, as well as new therapeutic approaches, certain rare genetic diseases, such as aminoacidopathies, organic acidaemias, and fatty-acid oxidation defects, have become an important target for modern, expanded newborn screening programs. Lysosomal storage diseases (LSDs) are just such an interesting group of more than 45 diseases that may be subject to screening. Despite the technical feasibility of such a project, doubts, primarily ethical and economic, remain about whether such newborn screening programs should be established for this specific group of diseases in the whole neonatal population.

Introduction

Newborn screening programs are essential initiatives, along with the prevention of malnutrition and infections, to ensure the best outcome, in terms of health, to the newborn population. There is a parallel between the importance of screening and changes in economic and social evolution: newborn screening is important as the family structure evolves from a large family model with high childhood morbidity and mortality (typical of less-advanced countries) to models of smaller size (low reproductive index) and improved child survival (Pollitt, 2007). Today, fewer than 25 per cent of the infants in the world have the advantage of this effective tool of preventive medicine as the dissemination of systematic screening programs is still largely limited to economically advanced geographic areas (North America, Europe, Japan, and Australia) (Loeber, 2008). In Italy, newborn screening programs were started in the early 1970s. In 1992, about 20 years after the first regional initiatives, National Law n.104 (February 5, 1992) 'Framework law for the assistance, social integration and rights of persons with disabilities' mandated newborn screening for phenylketonuria (PKU), congenital hypothyroidism (CH), and cystic fibrosis (CF), leaving the possibility for regional governments to initiate further screening programs for endocrinopathies and inborn errors of metabolism.

Review of the topic

The introduction of new technologies in neonatal screening introduced during the last 15 years – especially the so-called 'tandem mass' (MS/MS) technology – has been one of the fundamental cornerstones for the extension of newborn screening programs to diseases which, if taken individually, have a low prevalence (< 5 cases/10,000 births), but when viewed as a group or set of diseases have a significant impact on children. Furthermore, some treatment options exist and the outlook is significantly improved if the diagnosis is made early after birth, while the child is in an asymptomatic healthy state. Technically, it is now possible to detect a number of inborn errors of metabolism (*e.g.*, aminoacidopathies, defects in fatty acid metabolism, organic acidaemias) in a single analytical session and with a single biological sample ('Guthrie cards') (Millington *et al.*, 1990; Chace *et al.*, 2003; Chace, 2005; Rinaldo *et al.*, 2004).

By now, it is the usual procedure, at least in the better systems for population-based screening of newborns (*e.g.*, those in the United States, Canada, Western Europe, Australia, New Zealand, and Japan) to screen for the traditional diseases, such as CH (congenital hypothyroidism), PKU, galactosaemia (GAL), and congenital adrenal hyperplasia, as well as for a selection of such 'rare' diseases as the organic acidaemias (OA), the defects of fatty acids oxidation, (FAO), and other aminoacidopathies (AA). Furthermore, in line with new screening criteria developed by the American College of Medical Genetics (ACMG) and the American Academy of Pediatrics (AAP), it appears to be increasingly important to bring to the clinician's attention, for the follow-up phase, even subclinical disease conditions or carrier status, which may suggest therapeutic interventions or appropriate genetic counselling, even if only in terms of reproductive risk (American College of Medical Genetics Newborn Screening Expert Group, 2006).

In the last few years interest in lysosomal storage diseases (LSDs) has increased as these represent a number of disorders involving more than 45 distinct genetic defects, mainly of an autosomal recessive inheritance (someone with X-linked inheritance), brought about by malfunction of a specific lysosomal protein or, in some cases, of nonlysosomal proteins involved in lysosomal biogenesis or maturation. The clinical spectrum of presentation is broad; many have a severely progressive course and a high risk of mortality. The clinical diagnosis of LSD is complex, difficult, and sometimes takes a lot of time to be made (Meikle *et al.*, 2004).

Until a few years ago, LSDs had a low priority in the context of newborn screening. The above-mentioned joint AAP-ACMG document has selected, among the initial group of 84 diseases, four LSDs (Fabry disease, Pompe disease, mucopolysaccharidosis type I (MPS I), and Krabbe disease) that are candidates for the establishment of effective screening programs. At the time of evaluation (2006), the score achieved by each of these diseases was significantly lower than the minimum threshold of 1,200 points required for entry into the group of diseases (the 'Core Panel') to be included in screening; they were therefore classified as genetic diseases for which newborn screening did not seem to be appropriate at the time.

However, the progressive and continuing introduction of effective therapeutic interventions (particularly enzyme therapy and bone marrow transplantation), the availability of new postnatal screening tests for LSDs, and the increasingly widespread application of MS/MS have greatly increased interest in this group of congenital disorders, making them, in some cases, strong candidates for inclusion in future mandatory screening panels.

In the United States, local or pilot newborn screening programs for LSD using MS/MS have been launched: the state of New York has set up a program for Krabbe disease and the state of Washington for Fabry disease, and the state of Illinois has made it mandatory, with start-up planned for 2010, to screen newborns for five LSDs (Krabbe, Pompe, Fabry, Gaucher and

Niemann-Pick) (De Jesus, 2008). For a number of years a screening program has been carried out in South Australia for LSDs using immunoquantification technology and measures of enzymatic activity; this program is able to screen for 13 diseases (Fabry and Gaucher diseases, metachromatic leukodystrophy, mucolipidosis II and III, mucopolysaccharidosis I, II, IIIA, and VI, multiple sulphatase deficiency, Niemann-Pick diseases A and B, and Pompe disease). From a methodologic point of view, the two technical options (MS/MS and protein immunoquantification) have different characteristics of efficiency, cost, and complexity, which requires a careful comparative assessment (Matern, 2008).

Conclusions

It should be emphasized that, although an increasing number of technical solutions have been proposed and implemented to perform the newborn screening for LSDs, many organizational and management issues are still problematic, particularly the establishment of an efficient *ad hoc* multidisciplinary and systematic network for the screening, diagnosis, and treatment of these disorders. The critical aspects of newborn screening for LSDs share some aspects with the general expansion of newborn screening (The President's Council on Bioethics, 2008), but others are specific to these diseases. There is, in particular, a strong debate in terms of ethics and principles of health economics about the costs, opportunity, and affordability – yet very high – of treatment. The costs are also conditioned by the decision about the age at which therapy should be started.

Newborn screening for LSDs must therefore be subject to a careful assessment of sustainability and suitability with respect to the economic resources that are available. In particular, extending to all LSDs the observations (Kemper, 2007) specific for newborn screening of Pompe disease, and despite certain benefits of targeted and early therapeutic intervention for some LSDs, doubts and concerns still remain about the real sensitivity of the laboratory technologies applied to newborn screening, about clinical management of late-onset cases discovered by the screening program and about the comprehensibility of the information provided to parents in relation to risks and benefits of the diagnosis through neonatal screening.

Recently, in the United States (Knapp *et al.*, 2009), the Advisory Committee on Heritable Disorders in Newborns and Children – U.S. Department of Health and Human Services – Health Resources and Service Administration (HRSA), with respect to Krabbe disease, and despite the great screening experience acquired in the state of New York (Duffner *et al.*, 2009; Orsini, *et al.*, 2009), was unable to fully respond to some important questions about: *(a)* an appropriate method of identifying infants with reduced enzymatic activity who may benefit from bone marrow transplantation; *(b)* the risks associated with screening, particularly in the cohort of asymptomatic subjects with reduced enzymatic activity; *(c)* the long-term neurologic outcome of children who received the transplant; and *(d)* the true relationship of cost/efficacy of newborn screening for Krabbe disease. All these unanswered questions resulted in the persistence of a more negative opinion towards newborn screening for this disease, so it would be good to have a research program and pilot studies in place to answer them.

We must make a general ethical reflection here: throughout the world a large number of children do not even have access to the *minimal* newborn screening programs for such 'traditional' diseases such as CH or PKU because of the lack of resources in their countries. The introduction of screening programs aimed at rare diseases in advanced health systems of countries with higher living standards increases the gap of inequality between populations belonging to privileged nations and those living in economic poverty: the characteristics of *universality* and *uniformity* (the two integral parts of neonatal screening) should be extended to all countries in the world and not only the few that can afford it.

References

American College of Medical Genetics Newborn Screening Expert Group (2006): Newborn screening: toward a uniform screening panel and system. Executive summary. *Pediatrics* **117**, S296–S307.

Chace, D.H. & Kalas, T.A. (2005): A biochemical perspective on the use of tandem mass spectrometry for newborn screening and clinical testing. *Clin. Biochem.* **38**, 296–309.

Chace, D.H., Kalas, T.A. & Naylor, E.W. (2003): Use of tandem mass spectrometry for multianalyte screening of dried blood specimens from newborns. *Clin. Chem.* **49**, 1797–1817.

De Jesus, V.R. (2008): *Newborn screening for lysosomal storage disease by MSMS*. Presented at the AHPL 2008 Newborn Screening and Genetic Testing Symposium. San Antonio, Texas, Nov. 3–6, 2008.

Duffner, P.K., Caggana, M., Orsini, J.J., Wenger, D.A., Patterson, M.C., Crosley, C.J., Kurtzberg, J., Arnold, G.L., Escolar, M.L., Adams, D.J., Andriola, M.R., Aron, A.M., Ciafaloni, E., Djukic, A., Erbe, R.W., Galvin-Parton, P., Helton, L.E., Kolodny, E.H., Kosofsky, B.E., Kronn, D.F., Kwon, J.M., Levy, P.A., Miller-Horn, J., Naidich, T.P., Pellegrino, J.E., Provenzale, J.M., Rothman, S.J. & Wasserstein, M.P. (2009): Newborn screening for Krabbe disease: the New York State model. *Pediatr. Neurol.* **40**, 245–252.

Kemper, A.R. (2007): Newborn screening for Pompe disease: synthesis of the evidence and development of screening recommendations. *Pediatrics* **120**, e1327–e1334.

Knapp, A.A., Kemper, A.R. & Perrin, J.M. (2009): *Evidence (ACHDNC–HRSA) review: Krabbe disease*. www.hrsa.gov/heritabledisorderscommitte/reports.

Loeber, J.G. (2008): *Development of a global neonatal screening database*. Presented at the AHPL 2008 Newborn Screening and Genetic Testing Symposium. San Antonio, Texas, Nov. 3–6, 2008.

Matern, D. (2008): Newborn screening for lysosomal storage disorders. *Acta Paediatrica* **97**, 33–37.

Meikle, P.J., Fietz, M.J. & Hopwood, J.J. (2004): Diagnosis of lysosomal storage disorders: current techniques and future directions. *Exp. Rev. Mol. Diagn.* **4**, 677–691.

Millington, D.S., Kodo, N., Norwood, D.L. & Roe, C.R. (1990): Tandem mass spectrometry: a new method for acylcarnitine profiling with potential for neonatal screening for inborn errors of metabolism. *J. Inherit. Metab. Dis.* **13**, 321–324.

Orsini, J.J., Morrissey, M.A., Slavin, L.N., Wojcik, M., Biski, C., Martin, M., Keutzer, J., Zhang, X.K., Chuang, W.L., Elbin, C. & Caggana, M. (2009): Implementation of newborn screening for Krabbe disease: population study and cut-off determination. *Clin. Biochem.* **42**, 877–884.

Pollitt, R.J. (2007): Introducing new screens: why are we all doing different things? *J. Inherit. Metab. Dis.* **30**, 423–429.

Rinaldo, P., Tortorelli, S. & Matern, D. (2004): Recent developments and new applications of tandem mass spectrometry in newborn screening. *Curr. Opin. Pediatr.* **16**, 427–433.

The President's Council on Bioethics (2008): *The changing moral focus of newborn screening: an ethical analysis by the President's Council on Bioethics*. Washington DC, December 2008. www.bioethics.gov.

Chapter 4

Pathophysiologic aspects of lysosomal storage disorders

Cinzia Maria Bellettato, Rosella Tomanin and Maurizio Scarpa

Department of Paediatrics, University of Padova, via Giustiniani 3, 35128 Padova, Italy
maurizio.scarpa@unipd.it

Summary

Lysosomal storage diseases (LSDs) are a group of rare, genetically inherited metabolic disorders resulting from lysosomal dysfunction, usually as a consequence of deficiency of a single lysosomal enzyme or lysosomal component, thus preventing the complete degradation of macromolecules and the recycling of their components. The accumulation of intermediate degradation products affects the appropriate functioning of lysosomes and other cellular organelles. This accumulation starts immediately after birth and progressively worsens, frequently affecting several organs, as well as the central nervous system (CNS). The production of an anomalous enzyme is the primary event that induces a cascade of secondary events leading to LSD pathology. Affected neurons may die through apoptosis or necrosis, although neuronal loss usually does not occur before advanced stages of the disease. CNS pathology provokes mental retardation and progressive neurodegeneration that ultimately ends in the premature death of these young patients.
Several of these characteristics are also found in adult neurodegenerative disorders, such as Alzheimer, Parkinson, or Huntington diseases. However, the nature of the secondary events and their exact contribution to mental retardation and dementia is still largely unknown. Improved knowledge about these events may have impact on diagnosis, staging, and follow-up of affected children. Importantly, new insights may provide indications about possible disease reversal upon treatment. The aim of this paper is to discuss the pathophysiology of CNS involvement in LSDs.

Introduction

Lysosomal storage diseases (LSDs) are a group of more than 50 rare, inherited metabolic diseases that result from the lack or reduced activity of a specific lysosomal hydrolase or other proteins important for normal function of the endosomal/lysosomal (E/L) system (Platt & Walkley, 2004). Two-thirds of them involve the central nervous system (CNS) (Meikle *et al.*, 1999).

In the past two decades knowledge about LSDs has grown significantly. All identified LSDs have been characterized genetically, but the biochemical mechanisms by which a mutation causes deficiency have only been partially elucidated. That such multifaceted and serious disease conditions result from simple congenital errors of metabolism raises the persisting question of why these disorders are ultimately so clinically complex (Walkley, 2009).

According to the initial pathogenic concept, these diseases are supposed to be caused by individual lysosomal enzyme deficiencies, followed by accumulation of a single major substrate normally degraded by that enzyme (Hers, 1965; Hers & Van Hoof, 1973). Consequently, the undegraded substrate accumulates within the E/L system, determining cell enlargement, collapse of the normal cell functions, and eventually cell death. This effect has been called the 'cytotoxicity hypothesis' (Desnick et al., 1976). In accordance with this explanation a very simple relation between the enzyme protein defect and the clinical phenotype should exist; however, one single protein alteration can induce many different clinical phenotypes.

In relation to this last point of view, lysosomes are not 'end-organelles', but rather they work in concert with endosomal, autophagosomal, and salvage processes, and, in coordination with the ubiquitin–proteosomal system, they represent a extremely complex regulatory and recycling mechanism essential to normal cell function – a central metabolic coordinator – named the *greater lysosomal system* (Walkley, 2007).

It is now commonly accepted that LSDs are not just a consequence of pure storage. In fact, the wide variety of enzyme and nonenzyme proteins constituting the lysosomal system produces a pathogenic cascade responsible for disease progression and clinical manifestations (Wraith, 2004). Other forms of lysosomal dysfunction, possibly leading to storage, include defects in post-translational processing of lysosomal enzymes, errors in enzyme trafficking/targeting, and defective function of nonenzymatic lysosomal transmembrane and soluble proteins (Platt & Walkley, 2004).

Classification of lysosomal storage disorders

LSDs can be grouped on the basis of the biochemical nature of the storage material or by the underlying mechanism causing the disease (Ballabio & Gieselmann, 2009; Platt & Walkley, 2004). The first classification might be very helpful, but runs into problems when multiple substrates are accumulated in a single disorder, which is not an uncommon scenario (Walkley et al., 2005). The second classification is based on the underlying mechanism causing disease (Platt & Walkley, 2004), irrespective of the type of macromolecule that is stored. This constitutes a theoretically useful scheme when we attempt to comprehend the basic mechanisms of pathogenesis and is fundamental for the rational design of new therapies (Platt & Lachmann, 2009). Although LSDs are frequently classified according to the major storage compound, perhaps the most useful classification is the one taking into account the defective enzyme or protein (Futerman & van Meer, 2004).

Lysosomal storage and cell function: what happens?

Over the past two decades remarkable progress has been made in understanding the mechanism responsible for lysosomal storage and today it is commonly held to be evident that the process is not so homogeneous. Conversely the process is much more complex than initially suspected, as it often does not consist of a one enzyme–one substrate relationship, but rather involves more concomitant and different storage products. Furthermore, multiple storage products are not just the result of different compounds sensitive to the same enzyme defect, but often they represent secondary storage unconnected to the primary protein defect as in the case of GM2 and GM3 secondary co-accumulation in Niemann-Pick type C (NPC) disease, mucopolysaccharidosis I (MPS) types I, III A, III B, and VII, and mucolipidosis type IV (ML IV) (Walkley & Vanier, 2009). These secondary storage compounds may in turn contribute to disease pathogenesis and neurologic decline (Walkley, 2004a). On the basis of the different cell types in which it is accumulated, storage material itself might have different effects. In particular the majority of LSDs have marked CNS manifestations, although the storage material concentration is lower in the brain than in other organs. In particular, neurons seem particularly vulnerable, most likely because of a limited cell regeneration potential in the CNS and also by a lack of compensatory cellular metabolic pathways (Futerman & van Meer, 2004; Tardy et al., 2004). For most LSDs, the pathology mainly involves neuronal dysfunction rather than loss.

What is the mechanism of neurodegeneration?

Statistical data show that more than 60 per cent of LSDs affecting children cause various grades of neurodegeneration, depending on their disease phenotype. Additional data indicate that neurodegeneration is not just a simple and isolated phenomenon; in fact, more events are associated with neurodegeneration as secondary changes in neurons, altered axonal transport (Coleman, 2005), and dysfunction of intracellular protein degradation and macroautophagy pathways (Rubinsztein, 2006; Settembre et al., 2007, Settembre et al., 2008), mitochondrial dysfunction (Lin & Beal, 2006), and altered calcium storage and endoplasmic reticulum (ER) function (Mattson, 2007). Moreover, the possible association between inflammation and neurodegeneration could also play a role, although the exact relationship is far from clear (Ausseil et al., 2008).

Secondary changes in neurons

As previously mentioned, most lysosomal disorders affect the central nervous system by having a direct impact on the neurons. Detailed morphologic study showed that affected neurons display storage of primary substrate. The neurons may stay alive for years while continuing to store material and to exhibit slowly accumulating changes in structure, including a variety of other structural and possibly functional modifications (Walkley, 2007).

Neurons mainly exhibit two kind of morphologic changes or dendritogenetic processes: meganeurites and axonal spheroids together with somatic swelling.

Meganeurites

Meganeurites are huge axon hillock enlargements containing characteristic storage bodies, which often exceed the volume of adjacent perikarya. It is possible to identify two categories of meganeurites: (a) spiny and covered with dendritic-like spines, neurite expansions, and synapses, and (b) aspiny or smooth, without any evidence of dendritic spines or new synaptic formations. Meganeurites are related to an increased expression of GM2 ganglioside (irrespective of whether it is induced by primary or secondary storage), and this has been shown to play a fundamental role in the regulation of dendritogenesis in cortical pyramidal neurons, probably acting as neurite growth-promoting factors or as acceptor molecules for growth factors which contact the cells (Roisen et al., 1981).

Axonal spheroids

Axonal spheroids consist of swellings located distal to the axon initial segment region. Whereas meganeurites contain storage material consistent with the specific defective lysosomal hydrolase (and their morphology is therefore considered disease-specific), axonal spheroids contain a specifically dissimilar assortment of materials with ultrastructural characteristics that are not substantially different across many types of storage disorders (Walkley, 1998).

In addition, in lysosomal diseases characterized by ganglioside storage, cortical pyramidal neurons also exhibit abnormal sprouting of new dendrites at the axon hillock (called ectopic dendritogenesis). These new dendrites are, in turn, contacted by axons that form new excitatory synaptic connections. Results from ultrastructural studies showed that these enlargements consist of collections of tubulovesicular profiles, mitochondria, and dense and multi-vesicular-type bodies (Walkley, 2004b). Today, although there is clear knowledge of possible mechanisms underlying the genesis of ectopic dendrites on cortical pyramidal neurons in LSDs, little is known concerning the functional consequences of this event. Asymmetrical synapses are known to occur on these dendrites, and this input is likely to be deleterious to neuronal function (Walkley & March, 1993). Even the proximal to the axonal initial segment location could contribute to neuronal dysfunction, increasing the defects in axoplasmic anterograde and retrograde transport. Spheroids can significantly interfere with the efficacy or timing of wave action potential propagation with profound effect on neuronal activity and brain function.

Endocytic events in lysosomal disease: a source of signaling errors? Retrograde axonal transport defect?

As previously revealed, GM2 gangliosides play a key role in the phenomenon of ectopic dendritogenesis and ganglioside synthesis, and trafficking may be the crucial event. Gangliosides are glycosphingolipids (GSLs) containing one or more sialic acid residues that are synthesized in the Golgi/trans-Golgi network (TGN); then, by vesicular transport, they are carried to functional sites in the plasmalemma, from whence they are eventually eliminated via endocytosis, and re-enter the neuron through the E/L system, where they are degraded.

Recent studies indicate that some simple gangliosides, such as GM2 or GM3, can exit the E/L system intact and be recycled to the Golgi/TGN, where they can be reglycosylated and delivered again to the plasmalemma. This retroendocytic trafficking represents a second metabolic route (Walkley, 2009). In particular this is true for GM1 gangliosides in GM1 gangliosidosis. GM1 in fact might 'leak' into membrane domains that normally do not contain it, inducing calcium storage depletion and ER stress response activation, including apoptosis and neurone cell death (d'Azzo et al., 2006). In the same way GM2 gangliosides in GM2 gangliosidosis might accumulate in microsomal membranes and be responsible for the inactivation of the sarco/ER calcium ATPase (SERCA) transporter, which pumps calcium from the cytoplasm back into the ER, with consequent ER stress response and apoptosis (Ginzburg et al., 2004). Similarly, an analogous mechanism could be at work in Gaucher or Niemann-Pick A diseases.

Morphologic studies have revealed that in healthy neurons, the late E/L compartment is primarily confined to the cell body, while in cultured neurons, lysosomes have also been reported in the axon (Overly & Hollenbeck, 1996). It is possible that lysosomes in the axon fuse with endosomes derived from axon terminals, and that some catabolism occurs whilst these organelles are en route to the neuronal cell body.

Differently, in affected neurons, the storage bodies are primarily confined to the perikarya, which might impair the retrograde transport of lysosomes, preventing the acidification of endosomes derived from the axon terminal. Moreover, it is also possible that storage in the cell body disrupts normal retrograde transport of components along the axon (Jeyakumar et al., 2005). As a result of all of the above-described reasons, many normal cell functions might be altered, possibly provoking a series of downstream consequences, such as the growth of ectopic dendrites, the formation of axonal spheroids, the neuronal death, and so forth.

Incapacity of recycling materials out of the E/L system in lysosomal disease may also lead to lack of precursor pools of metabolites, consequently altering cellular homeostatic functions. Moreover, recycling failure may also lead to changes in synthetic pathways and/or to autophagy in an effort to overcome these deficits (Walkley, 2009).

Lysosomal diseases: rediscovering autophagy

Even though LSDs are an extremely diverse group of diseases having different etiologies, the mechanisms of neurodegeneration may be similar, including a major role for autophagy.

Autophagy is a nonselective process in which cellular components are degraded within the lysosomes. Because degradation and recycling of cytoplasmatic cellular components are required for the maintenance of cell homeostasis, a possible impairment of autophagy can, in turn, contribute to and even worsen the accumulation in neurodegenerative diseases (Fortun *et al.*, 2003). Activation of autophagy might facilitate the elimination of intracellular protein aggregates (Larsen & Sulzer, 2002). It is important to note that the study of autophagy in LSDs represents a new field of investigation that needs to be extended. Anyway it is already clear that autophagy is implicated in the abnormal storage accumulation in LSDs, including the neuronal ceroid lipofuscinoses (NCLs) (Cao *et al.*, 2006; Koike *et al.*, 2005; Tardy *et al.*, 2004). Moreover it is commonly accepted that neuropathologic features such as the accumulation of autophagosomes and the subsequent induction of autophagic and apoptotic neurone death in NCL and LSDs are strictly related to apoptosis and autophagy. Therefore, despite the initiating biochemical event(s), neurodegenerative disease in its broadest scope may involve activation of both autophagic and apoptotic cell death pathways (Koike *et al.*, 2005; Shacka & Roth, 2005). Lysosomal storage may have an effect on fusion efficiency between autophagosomes and lysosomes, leading to a partial block of autophagy. This may in turn activate a compensatory feedback mechanism through which autophagy is induced (most likely by beclin-1-mediated activation) (Ballabio & Gieselmann, 2009). Considering that postmitotic cells, such as neurons or muscle cells, cannot dilute the accumulated material by cell division, it is consequently quite easy to understand how dangerous the effect of the accumulation of undegraded material may be (Raben *et al.*, 2009). In fact, as a consequence of the induced complete or partial block of autophagy, polyubiquitinated proteins aggregate and dysfunctional mitochondria accumulate, leading to overproduction of reactive oxygen species, inflammation, and cell death (Boya *et al.*, 2005; Tessitore *et al.*, 2009).

Mitochondria: autophagy and lysosomal storage disorders

Current knowledge of mechanisms driving the degenerative processes in LSDs supports the hypothesis of a lysosomal–mitochondrial connection defined as the mitochondrial–lysosomal axis. The mitochondrial–lysosomal axis theory of aging postulates that oxidized material accumulates in lysosomes as cells age, which results in decreased degradative capacity of lysosomes (Terman *et al.*, 2006). The autophagic/lysosomal pathway is the major route of destruction for damaged mitochondria (potent generators of reactive oxygen species); therefore, in case of unpaired autophagy, dysfunctional mitochondria accumulate and subject cells to increasing oxidative and autophagic stress (Kiselyov *et al.*, 2007). Again, considering the mitochondrion's ability to take up cytoplasmic calcium and its function as a cellular buffer shielding the cells from calcium pro-apoptotic effects, lysosomal dysfunction can promote cell death through accumulation of mitochondria with impaired abilities to buffer pro-death stresses (Jennings *et al.*, 2006; Kiselyov & Muallem, 2008).

The fact that mitochondrial abnormalities have been shown in many LSDs (Kiselyov *et al.*, 2007), together with the commonality of mitochondrial abnormalities across the spectrum of LSDs, constitutes proof of the above-mentioned theory. Since mitochondria are crucial in energy production via adenosine triphosphate (ATP) and lipid biosynthesis, alteration in their function induces activation of an ER stress response, mitochondrial apoptotic signaling, or both, triggering cell death under physiologic or pathologic conditions (D'Azzo *et al.*, 2006).

In particular, taking into account the pathologic manifestations and neurodegeneration in some forms of ceroid lipofuscinoses, there is clear confirmation of the presence of mitochondrial dysfunction. Many studies, in fact, have reported the presence of enlarged mitochondria and accumulation of subunit c of mitochondrial ATP synthase: these are common features of almost all neuronal ceroid lipofuscinosis disease forms. Importantly, autophagy appears to be a common factor in these diseases, even though the mechanisms by which it contributes to pathology and pathogenesis are variable. To date autophagy has been studied in many LSDs including multiple sulphatase deficiency (MSD), MPS Type IIIA, GM1 gangliosidosis, Pompe disease, NPC, NCL, ML type IV and Danon disease (Dierks *et al.*, 2009; Raben *et al.*, 2009).

Iron homeostasis and lysosomal storage disorders

Iron is an essential trace metal required by all living organisms in tissue and brain cells; however, excess concentrations can be harmful to many tissues. Therefore iron management is a crucial issue for all living cells, where its presence is necessary for carrying out numerous vital biologic reactions. Nevertheless, because of its extremely reactive nature, iron is particularly toxic if its concentrations are not tightly regulated intracellularly. Iron toxicity is due to the possible rapid reaction of iron in a divalent state with hydrogen peroxide and molecular oxygen to produce free radicals. Formation of free radicals will promote lipid peroxidation, DNA strand breaks, and modification or degradation of biomolecules, eventually leading to cell death. As discussed above, the cells have evolved highly regulated and sophisticated mechanisms to prevent abnormal concentrations of iron accumulation. This homeostatic regulation is achieved by intricately co-ordinated regulation of numerous proteins involved in iron uptake, storage, and secretion. In particular these proteins provide a state of cellular balance whereby iron is readily available for all metabolic functions, but prevented from taking part in cytotoxic reactive oxygen species (ROS)–generating reactions (Papanikolaou & Pantopoulos, 2005; Lee *et al.*, 2006; Nadadur *et al.*, 2008).

In the brain, iron plays a particularly critical role in sustaining the brain's high respiratory activity. Moreover it is important for the formation of myelin by oligodendritocytes, and for the production of several neurotransmitters such as dopamine, norepinephrine, serotonin, and generation of γ-aminobutyric acid (GABA)ergic activity (Moos & Morgan, 2004). In addition iron is also essential because it constitutes a fundamental component of oxidative metabolism enzymes (Sipe *et al.*, 2002).

It has been reported that iron homeostasis is altered in gangliosidosis and in addition it appears to play a role in the pathogenesis of neurodegenerative disease, including Parkinson and Alzheimer diseases (Moos & Morgan, 2004). To date the precise mechanism by which iron causes this pathogenic consequence is still not well defined, but it has been hypothesized that diminishment in brain iron content may be related to an E/L system alteration that, in turn, determines an alteration in iron metabolism. The precise mechanism by which storage disrupts iron homeostasis is still not understood. Data from GM1 and GM2 mouse models indicate that the decreased brain iron content could have consequences on the main source of oxidative energy in mitochondria, with subsequent reduction of ATP production, thereby determining further neuronal dysfunction and degeneration (Jeyakumar *et al.*, 2009).

Intracellular calcium and lysosomal storage disorders

In view of the fact that mechanisms responsible for neuronal cell death in LSDs are still not well understood, in order to furnish a complete elucidation of the pathophysiologic pathways that lead to cellular death, researchers have focused their attention on the role of intracellular calcium. Calcium is an essential and ubiquitous constituent of eukaryotic cells and plays a key role in cell homeostasis as an intracellular mediator (Berridge *et al.*, 2003).

It has been reported that calcium is involved in both immediate and long-term responses in neurons through alterations in cell-signaling pathways (Jeyakumar *et al.*, 2005). Because high calcium concentration is toxic to neurons, the cytosolic calcium concentration of resting cells is maintained at low levels by the concerted action of specialized channels, a calcium pump, calcium-dependent enzymes, and calcium-binding proteins. These mechanisms for balancing calcium homeostasis are localized in the cytosol, ER, and mitochondria: the three compartments that control the traffic of calcium across the plasma membrane or into intracellular stores (Berridge *et al.*, 2003). In neurons, calcium is pumped from the cytosol by the SERCA (Misquitta *et al.*, 1999) in the ER, where it is mainly stored (Vellodi, 2004). Calcium is then released back into the cytosol through two types of channels, one of which is a ryanodine receptor (Fill & Copello, 2002). Unbalanced calcium homeostasis is one of the most common pathologic features of lysosomal storage in LSDs. It has been described in several LSDs, including Gaucher disease (Korkotian *et al.*, 1999; Lloyd-Evans *et al.*, 2003), and Sandhoff disease (Pelled *et al.*, 2003; Pelled *et al.*, 2005), Niemann-Pick type A disease (Ginzburg & Futerman, 2005), NPC type I (Lloyd-Evans *et al.*, 2008), and ML IV (Jennings *et al.*, 2006). More information concerning calcium homeostasis alteration has been obtained by the use of a ryanodine receptor agonist in Gaucher mice cells, where it provoked an enhanced calcium release from the ER internal stores. In addition, glutamate-mediated neurotoxicity was augmented in these neurons, and the effect was repressed in the presence of ryanodine. There are suggestions for a potential functional link between altered calcium homeostasis and neuronal dysfunction or loss (Jeyakumar *et al.*, 2005).

It is important to note that cytoplasmic calcium levels control the ryanodine receptor so an increase in cytosolic calcium opens the receptor and leads to a further calcium release from the ER (Ballabio & Gieselmann, 2009).

Extralysosomal accumulation in plasma membranes and perturbation of lipid rafts

As already asserted, the role of lysosomes in cell biology is much more complex than initially suspected, and now there is growing evidence of lysosomal involvement in plasma membrane lipid raft-mediated pathobiology.

The plasma membrane is composed of a lipid bilayer. Contrary to what was initially supposed, the distribution of lipids is not uniform and gangliosides at the cell surface are not randomly dispersed and diffusely distributed, but rather are co-localized with cholesterol in specialized patches of membrane named *rafts* (Brown & London, 1998; Kasahara & Sanai, 2000). These microdomains represent signaling platforms that link receptor–ligand interactions at the cell surface with signal transduction events inside the cell. Data from the literature showed that these structures are not localized exclusively to the plasma membrane, but are also found in the endocytic system and mature lysosomes (Bagshaw et al., 2005; Dermine et al., 2001; Gruenberg, 2001; Sharma et al., 2003). There is evidence that in many GSL storage diseases sphingolipid accumulation is associated with increased levels of free cholesterol. Extralysosomal accumulation of substrates may thus be deleterious to the cell-signaling function. In fact alteration in cholesterol intracellular distribution in membrane composition results in defective sorting and transport of sphingolipids and to their accumulation in the late endosomal compartment (Pagano et al., 2000; Pagano, 2003). These events may in turn disrupt the function of key cell components, such as ion channels and transporters (Futerman & van Meer, 2004).

Neuroinflammation and neurodegeneration

In view of the fact that CNS dysfunction and degeneration represent the principal causes of mortality in neuroinflammatory and neurodegenerative diseases, a common pathogenetic model for brain pathology in LSDs has been proposed whereby a severe inflammatory response triggers acute neurodegeneration and/or dysmyelination (Visigalli et al., 2009). The mechanism responsible for activation of the inflammatory response follows several steps that are still not completely clear: it has been proposed that initially primary storage consequent to the metabolic defect activates blood monocytes and resident microglia (also called globoid cells in globoid cell leukodystrophy) and that then these activated cells trigger activation of the inflammatory response (German et al., 2002; Ohmi et al., 2003; Visigalli et al., 2009; Wada et al., 2000). Macrophages and microglia in particular are common findings in many LSDs, but it is still not clear how they are initially activated. They probably could be the result of disrupted signaling due to mislocalization of key proteins to the lysosomes.

Microglia, are the main immune cells of the brain and as macrophages they possess hydrolases. They are derived from circulating blood monocytes that invade the brain early in postnatal life and become amoeboid microglia. In many circumstances microglia cannot be distinguished from blood-derived macrophages (Ling & Wong, 1993; Streit et al., 1988). Postnatally, they are continuously replaced by blood-borne monocytes that cross the blood–brain barrier into the brain parenchyma.

When activated, microglia can play an important role in pathogenesis of LSDs as reported in mouse models of MPS I (Hurler syndrome) and MPS IIIB (Sanfilippo syndrome type B) (Ohmi et al., 2003). In fact, as a consequence of their activation following storage, macrophages are responsible for an increased amount of cytokines or chemokines, as seen in patients with Gaucher disease (Barak et al., 1999; Boot et al., 2004; Hollak et al., 1997).

These data indicate that activation of macrophages/microglia can trigger cell death by cytotoxic, inflammatory mediators, as has been suggested for other neurodegenerative conditions like Alzheimer disease (Proia & Wu, 2004).

Conclusions

The aim of this review is to demonstrate the complexity of the pathophysiology of LSDs, which represent a continuously evolving field in which biochemical input plays a relevant and very important role. This chapter shows the pathologic features of storage diseases and makes more clear the concept of an overlap between the pathology of storage disorders and that of other neurodegenerative conditions. Knowledge gained by studying the pathogenesis of storage diseases may also be of benefit in the understanding of various other neurodegenerative diseases. Amongst neurodegenerative diseases, LSDs are particularly suitable for investigation that may lead to the development and monitoring of restorative/disease-modifying therapies. A unique hallmark of LSDs is the fact that amongst all neurodegenerative diseases they are the only group for which therapy (enzyme replacement) is available that can reverse the natural history of the disease in peripheral organs. Unfortunately, enzyme replacement therapy has limited efficacy because it is still unable to effectively reach the CNS and consequently stop the progress of neurodegeneration. Currently, thanks to the availability of excellent animal models of these diseases and the growing knowledge of the genetic and biochemical features of neurodegenerative development, it is possible to better understand the cascade of pathologic events leading to loss of brain plasticity and mental retardation. Insights thus gained in paediatric neurodegeneration may help to explain these processes in the neurodegenerative diseases of the aged (*e.g.*, Alzheimer and Parkinson diseases). The potential for suppressing the primary cause of neurodegeneration in a young brain by supplementing the missing enzyme holds promise for maximizing benefit to a developing brain, which retains considerable plasticity. And because both paediatric and adult neurodegenerative diseases manifest common secondary events (*e.g.*, brain inflammation, alteration of intracellular trafficking, impairment of autophagy, or oxidative stress) that lead to neurodegeneration, at least some of the observations relative to loss and recovery of brain plasticity in paediatric neurodegeneration can be extrapolated to adult disorders, thereby providing unique insights into the pathophysiology of neurodegenerative diseases in general and, it is hoped, also provide ways to invoke the restorative capacities of the adult brain as well.

Acknowledgments: We would like to thank Professor Ed Wraith of the Manchester Children's Hospital, Manchester, UK, for critically reading this manuscript. Maurizio Scarpa has recently co-founded the pan-European consortium, Brains for Brain, designed to foster and improve research on, and treatment of, lysosomal storage disorders throughout Europe (www. brains4brain.eu).

References

Ausseil, J., Desmaris, N., Bigou, S., Attali, R., Corbineau, S., Vitry, S., Parent, M., Cheillan, D., Fuller, M., Maire, I., Vanier, M.T. & Heard, J.M. (2008): Early neurodegeneration progresses independently of microglial activation by heparan sulphate in the brain of mucopolysaccharidosis IIIB mice. *PLoS ONE* **3**, e2296.

Bagshaw, R.D., Mahuran, D.J. & Callahan, J.W. (2005): A proteomic analysis of lysosomal integral membrane proteins reveals the diverse composition of the organelle. *Mol. Cell. Proteomics* **4**, 133–143.

Ballabio, A. & Gieselmann, V. (2009): Lysosomal disorders: from storage to cellular damage. *Biochim. Biophys. Acta* **1793**, 684–696.

Barak, V., Acker, M., Nisman, B., Kalickman, I., Abrahamov, A., Zimran, A. & Yatziv, S. (1999): Cytokines in Gaucher's disease. *Eur. Cytokine Netw.* **10**, 205–210.

Berridge, M.J., Bootman, M.D. & Roderick, H.L. (2003): Calcium signalling: dynamics, homeostasis and remodelling. *Nature Rev. Mol. Cell Biol.* **4**, 517–529.

Boot, R.G., Verhoek, M., de Fost, M., Hollak, C.E., Maas, M., Bleijlevens, B., van Breemen, M.J., van Meurs, M., Boven, L.A., Laman, J.D., Moran, M.T., Cox, T.M. & Aerts, J.M. (2004): Marked elevation of the chemokine CCL18/PARC in Gaucher disease: a novel surrogate marker for assessing therapeutic intervention. *Blood* **103**, 33–39.

Boya, P., Gonzalez-Polo, R.A., Casares, N., Perfettini, J.L., Dessen, P., Larochette, N., Métivier, D., Meley, D., Souquere, S., Yoshimori, T., Pierron, G., Codogno, P. & Kroemer, G. (2005): Inhibition of macroautophagy triggers apoptosis. *Mol. Cell Biol.* **25**, 1025–1040.

Brown, D.A. & London, E. (1998): Functions of lipid rafts in biological membranes. *Rev. Cell Dev. Biol.* **14**, 111–136.

Cao, Y., Espinola, J.A., Fossale, E., Massey, A.C., Cuervo, A.M., MacDonald, M.E. & Cotman, S.L. (2006): Autophagy is disrupted in a knock-in mouse model of juvenile neuronal ceroid lipofuscinosis. *J. Biol. Chem.* **281**, 20483–20493.

Coleman, M. (2005): Axon degeneration mechanisms: commonality amid diversity. *Nat. Rev. Neurosci.* **6**, 889–898.

D'Azzo, A., Tessitore, A. & Sano, R. (2006): Gangliosides as apoptotic signals in ER stress response. *Cell Death Differ.* **13**, 404–413.

Dermine, J.F., Duclos, S., Garin, J., St-Louis, F., Rea, S., Parton, R.G. & Desjardins, M. (2001): Flotillin-1-enriched lipid raft domains accumulate on maturing phagosomes. *J. Biol. Chem.* **276**, 18507–18512.

Desnick, R.J., Thorpe, S.R. & Fiddler, M. (1976): Toward enzyme therapy for lysosomal storage diseases. *Physiol. Rev.* **56**, 57–99.

Dierks, T., Schlotawa, L., Frese, M.A., Radhakrishnan, K., Figura, K. & Schmidt, B. (2009): Molecular basis of multiple sulphatase deficiency, mucolipidosis II/III and Niemann–Pick C1 disease: lysosomal storage disorders caused by defects of non-lysosomal proteins. *Biochim. Biophys. Acta* **1793**, 710–725.

Fill, M. & Copello, J.A. (2002): Ryanodine receptor calcium release channels. *Physiol. Rev.* **82**, 893–922.

Fortun, J., Dunn, W.A. Jr, Joy, S., Li, J. & Notterpek, L. (2003): Emerging role for autophagy in the removal of aggresomes in Schwann cells. *J. Neurosci.* **23**, 10672–10680.

Futerman, A.H. & van Meer, G. (2004): The cell biology of lysosomal storage disorders. *Nat. Rev. Mol. Cell Biol.* **5**, 554–565.

German, D.C., Liang, C.L., Song, T., Yazdani, U., Xie, C. & Dietschy, J.M. (2002): Neurodegeneration in the Niemann–Pick C mouse: glial involvement. *Neuroscience* **109**, 437–450.

Ginzburg, L. & Futerman, A.H. (2005): Defective calcium homeostasis in the cerebellum in a mouse model of Niemann–Pick A disease. *J. Neurochem.* **95**, 1619–1628.

Ginzburg, L., Kacher, Y. & Futerman, A.H. (2004): The pathogenesis of glycosphingolipid storage disorders. *Semin. Cell Dev. Biol.* **15**, 417–431.

Gruenberg, J. (2001): The endocytic pathway: a mosaic of domains. *Nature Rev. Mol. Cell Biol.* **2**, 721–730.

Hers, H.G. (1965): Progress in gastroenterology: inborn lysosomal diseases. *Gastroenterology* **48**, 625–633.

Hers, H.G. & Van Hoof, F. (1973): *Lysosomes and storage diseases.* New York: Academic Press.

Hollak, C.E., Evers, L., Aerts, J.M. & van Oers, M.H. (1997): Elevated levels of M-CSF, sCD14 and IL8 in type 1 Gaucher disease. *Blood Cells Mol. Dis.* **23**, 201–212.

Jennings, J.J., Zhu, J.H. Jr., Rbaibi, Y., Luo, X., Chu, C.T. & Kiselyov, K. (2006): Mitochondrial aberrations in mucolipidosis t-Type IV. *J. Biol. Chem.* **281**, 39041–39050.

Jeyakumar, M., Dwek, R.A., Butters, T.D., & Platt, F.M. (2005): Storage solutions: treating lysosomal disorders of the brain. *Nat. Rev. Neurosci.* **6**, 713–725.

Jeyakumar, M., Williams, I., Smith, D.A., Cox, T.M. & Platt, F.M. (2009): Critical role of iron in the pathogenesis of the murine gangliosidoses. *Neurobiol. Dis.* **34**, 406–416.

Kasahara, K. & Sanai, Y. (2000): Functional roles of glycosphingolipids in signal transduction via lipid rafts. *Glycoconj. J.* **17**, 153–162.

Kiselyov, K. & Muallem, S. (2008): Mitochondrial Ca2+ homeostasis in lysosomal storage diseases. *Cell Calcium* **44**, 103–111.

Kiselyov, K., Jennings, J.J. Jr., Rbaibi, Y. & Chu, C.T. (2007): Autophagy, mitochondria and cell death in lysosomal storage diseases. *Autophagy* **3**, 259–262.

Koike, M., Shibata, M., Waguri, S., Yoshimura, K., Tanida, I., Kominami, E., Gotow, T., Peters, C., von Figura, K., Mizushima, N., Saftig, P. & Uchiyama, Y. (2005): Participation of autophagy in storage of lysosomes in neurons from mouse models of neuronal ceroid-lipofuscinoses (Batten disease). *Am. J. Pathol.* **167**, 1713–1728.

Korkotian, E., Schwarz, A., Pelled, D., Schwarzmann, G., Segal, M. & Futerman, A.H. (1999): Elevation of intracellular glucosylceramide levels results in an increase in endoplasmic reticulum density and in functional calcium stores in cultured neurons. *J. Biol. Chem.* **274**, 21673–21678.

Larsen, K.E. & Sulzer, D. (2002): Autophagy in neurons: a review. *Histol. Histopathol.* **17**, 897–908.

Lee, D.W., Andersen, J.K. & Kaur, D. (2006): Iron dysregulation and neurodegeneration: the molecular connection. *Mol. Intervent.* **6**, 89–97.

Lin, M.T. & Beal, M.F. (2006): Mitochondrial dysfunction and oxidative stress in neurodegenerative diseases. *Nature* **443**, 787–795.

Ling, E.A. & Wong, W.C. (1993): The origin and nature of ramified and amoeboid microglia: a historical review and current concepts. *Glia* **7**, 9–18.

Lloyd-Evans, E., Pelled, D., Riebeling, C., Bodennec, J., de-Morgan, A., Waller, H., Schiffmann, R. & Futerman, A.H. (2003): Glucosylceramide and glucosylsphingosine modulate calcium mobilization from brain microsomes via different mechanisms. *J. Biol. Chem.* **278**, 23594–23599.

Lloyd-Evans, E., Morgan, A.J., He, X., Smith, D.A., Elliot-Smith, E., Sillence, D.J., Churchill, G.C., Schuchman, E.H., Galione, A. & Platt, F.M. (2008): Niemann-Pick disease type C1 is a sphingosine storage disease that causes deregulation of lysosomal calcium. *Nat. Med.* **14,** 1247–1255.

March, P.A., Thrall, M.A., Wurzelmann, S., Brown, D. & Walkley, S.U. (1997): Dendritic and axonal abnormalities in feline Niemann-Pick disease type C. *Acta Neuropathol.* **94,** 164–172.

Mattson, M.P. (2007): Calcium and neurodegeneration. *Aging Cell* **6,** 337–350.

Meikle, P.J., Hopwood, J.J., Clague, A.E. & Carey, W.F. (1999): Prevalence of lysosomal storage disorders. *JAMA* **281,** 249–254.

Misquitta, C.M., Mack, D.P. & Grover, A.K. (1999): Sarco/endoplasmic reticulum Ca2+ (SERCA)-pumps: link to heart beats and calcium waves. *Cell Calcium* **25,** 277–290.

Moos, T. & Morgan, E.H. (2004): The metabolism of neuronal iron and its pathogenic role in neurological disease: Review. *Ann. N.Y. Acad. Sci.* **1012,** 14–26.

Nadadur, S.S., Srirama, K. & Mudipalli, A. (2008): Iron transport & homeostasis mechanisms: their role in health & disease. *Indian J. Med. Res.* **128,** 533–544.

Ohmi, K., Greenberg, D.S., Rajavel, K.S., Ryazantsev, S., Li, H.H. & Neufeld, E.F. (2003): Activated microglia in cortex of mouse models of mucopolysaccharidoses I and IIIB. *Proc. Natl. Acad. Sci. USA* **100,** 1902–1907.

Overly, C.C. & Hollenbeck, P.J. (1996): Dynamic organization of endocytic pathways in axons of cultured sympathetic neurons. *J. Neurosci.* **16,** 6056–6064.

Pagano, R.E. (2003): Endocytic trafficking of glycosphingolipids in sphingolipid storage diseases. *Phil. Trans R. Soc. Lond. B. Biol. Sci.* **358,** 885–891.

Pagano, R.E., Puri, V., Dominguez, M. & Marks, D.L. (2000): Membrane traffic in sphingolipid storage diseases. *Traffic* **1,** 807–815.

Papanikolaou, G. & Pantopoulos, K. (2005): Iron metabolism and toxicity. *Toxicol. Appl. Pharmacol.* **202,** 199–211.

Pelled, D., Lloyd-Evans, E., Riebeling, C., Jeyakumar, M., Platt, F.M. & Futerman, A.H. (2003): Inhibition of calcium uptake via the sarco/endoplasmic reticulum Ca2+-ATPase in a mouse model of Sandhoff disease and prevention by treatment with N-butyldeoxynojirimycin. *J. Biol. Chem.* **278,** 29496–29501.

Pelled, D., Trajkovic-Bodennec, S., Lloyd-Evans, E., Sidransky, E., Schiffmann, R. & Futerman, A.H. (2005): Enhanced calcium release in the acute neuronopathic form of Gaucher disease. *Neurobiol. Dis.* **18,** 83–88.

Platt, F.M. & Lachmann, R.H. (2009): Treating lysosomal storage disorders: current practice and future prospects. *Biochim. Biophys. Acta* **1793,** 737–745.

Platt, F.M. & Walkley, S.U. (2004): Lysosomal defects and storage. In: *Lysosomal disorders of the brain: recent advances in molecular and cellular pathogenesis and treatment*, 1st ed., eds. F.M. Platt & S.U. Walkley, pp. 32–49. New York: Oxford University Press.

Proia, R. & Wu, Y.P. (2004): Blood to brain to the rescue. *J. Clinl. Invest.* **113,** 1108–1110.

Raben, R.N., Shea, L., Hill, V. & Plotz, P. (2009): Monitoring autophagy in lysosomal storage disorders. *Methods Enzymol.* **453,** 417–449.

Roisen, F.J., Bartfeld, H., Nagele, R. & Yorke, G. (1981): Ganglioside stimulation of axonal sprouting in vitro. *Science* **214,** 577–578.

Rubinsztein, D.C. (2006): The roles of intracellular protein-degradation pathways in neurodegeneration. *Nature* **443,** 780–786.

Settembre, C., Annunziata, I., Spampanato, C., Zarcone, D., Cobellis, G., Nusco, E., Zito, E., Tacchetti, C., Cosma, M.P. & Ballabio, A. (2007): Systemic inflammation and neurodegeneration in a mouse model of multiple sulphatase deficiency. *Proc. Natl. Acad. Sci. USA* **104,** 4506–4511.

Settembre, C., Fraldi, A., Jahreiss, L., Spampanato, C., Venturi, C., Medina, D., de Pablo, R., Tacchetti, C., Rubinsztein, D.C. & Ballabio A. (2008): A block of autophagy in lysosomal storage disorders. *Hum. Mol. Genet.* **17,** 119–129.

Shacka, J.J. & Roth, K.A. (2005): Regulation of neuronal cell death and neurodegeneration by members of the Bcl-2 family: therapeutic implications. *Curr. Drug Targets CNS Neurol. Disord.* **4,** 25–39.

Sharma, D.K., Choudhury, A., Singh, R.D., Wheatley, C.L., Marks, D.L. & Pagano, R.E. (2003): Glycosphingolipids internalized via caveolar-related endocytosis rapidly merge with the clathrin pathway in early endosomes and form microdomains for recycling. *J. Biol. Chem.* **278,** 7564–7572.

Sipe, J.C., Lee, P. & Beutler, E. (2002): Brain iron metabolism and neurodegenerative disorders. *Dev. Neurosci.* **24,** 188–196.

Streit, W.J., Graeber, M.B. & Kreutzberg, G.W. (1988): Functional plasticity of microglia: a review. *Glia* **1,** 301–307.

Tardy, C., Andrieu-Abadie, N., Salvayre, R. & Levade, T. (2004): Lysosomal storage diseases: is impaired apoptosis a pathogenic mechanism? *Neurochem. Res.* **29,** 871–880.

Terman, A., Gustafsson, B. & Brunk, U.T. (2006): The lysosomal-mitochondrial axis theory of postmitotic aging and cell death. *Chem. Biol. Interact.* **163,** 29–37.

Tessitore, A., Pirozzi, M. & Auricchio, A. (2009): Abnormal autophagy, ubiquitination, inflammation and apoptosis are dependent upon lysosomal storage and are useful biomarkers of mucopolysaccharidosis VI. *Pathogenetics* **2,** 4.

Vellodi, A. (2004): Lysosomal storage disorders. *Br. J. Haematol.* **128,** 413–431.

Visigalli, I. Moresco, R.M., Belloli, S., Politi, L.S., Gritti, A., Ungaro D., Matarrese, M., Turolla, E., Falini, A., Scotti, G., Naldini, L., Fazio, F. & Biffi, A. (2009): Monitoring disease evolution and treatment response in lysosomal disorders by the peripheral benzodiazepine receptor ligand PK11195. *Neurobiol. Dis.* **34,** 51–62.

Wada, R., Tifft, C.J. & Proia, R.L. (2000): Microglial activation precedes acute neurodegeneration in Sandhoff disease and is suppressed by bone marrow transplantation. *Proc. Natl. Acad. Sci. USA* **97,** 10954–10959.

Walkley, S.U. (1998): Cellular pathology of lysosomal storage disorders. *Brain Pathol.* **8,** 175–193.

Walkley, S.U. (2004a): Secondary accumulation of gangliosides in lysosomal storage disorders. *Semin. Cell Dev. Biol.* **15,** 433–444.

Walkley, S.U. (2004b): Pathogenic cascades and brain dysfunction. In: *Lysosomal disorders of the brain*, eds. F.M. Platt & S.U. Walkley, pp. 32–49. New York: Oxford University Press.

Walkley, S.U. (2007): Pathogenic mechanisms in lysosomal disease: a reappraisal of the role of the lysosomes. *Acta Pædiat.* **96,** 26–32.

Walkley, S.U. (2009): Pathogenic cascades in lysosomal disease: why so complex? *J. Inherit. Metab. Dis.* **32,** 181–189.

Walkley, S.U. & March, P.A. (1993): Biology of neuronal dysfunction in storage disorders. *J. Inher. Metab. Dis.* **16,** 284–287.

Walkley, S.U. & Vanier, M.T. (2009): Secondary lipid accumulation in lysosomal disease. *Biochim. Biophys. Acta* **1793,** 726–736.

Walkley, S.U., Baker, H.J., Rattazzi, M.C., Haskins, M.E. & Wu, J.-Y. (1991): Neuroaxonal dystrophy in neuronal storage disorders: Evidence for major GABAergic neuron involvement. *J. Neurol. Sci.* **104,** 1–8.

Walkley, S.U., Thrall, M.A., Haskins, M.E., Mitchell, T.W., Wenger, D.A., Brown, D.E., Dial, S. & Seim, H. (2005): Abnormal neuronal metabolism and storage in mucopolysaccharidosis type VI (Maroteaux–Lamy) disease. *Neuropathol. Appl. Neurobiol.* **31,** 536–544.

Wraith, J.E. (2004): Clinical aspects and diagnosis. In: *Lysosomal disorders of the brain*, eds. F.M. Platt & S.U. Walkley, pp. 50–77. Oxford: Oxford University Press.

Clinical presentations in detail: Mucopolysaccharidoses and Anderson-Fabry disease

Chapter 5

Early signs and symptoms for the timely diagnosis of mucopolysaccharidosis

Maria Luisa Melzi, Francesca Furlan and Rossella Parini

*UOS Malattie Metaboliche Rare, Centro 'Fondazione Mariani per le Malattie Metaboliche dell'Infanzia',
Department of Paediatrics, Azienda Ospedaliera San Gerardo,
University of Milano–Bicocca, via Pergolesi 33, 20052 Monza, Italy*
m.melzi@hsgerardo.org

Summary

The mucopolysaccharidoses (MPSs) are rare genetic diseases caused by a deficiency of enzymes catalyzing the degradation of glycosaminoglycans (GAGs), resulting in cell, tissue, and organ dysfunction, directly or by activation of secondary pathways. These disorders are more complex, more heterogeneous, and may be more frequent than it has been previously assumed. The clinical features involve many tissues and organs such as skin and mucosae, airways, hearing, eyes, heart, joints, and bones and become progressively worse on account of the continuous accumulation of GAGs, with the result that the patient progressively loses already acquired functions and skills. The fact that new specific treatments for MPSs have been recently developed, places the responsibility squarely on the clinician to identify the diagnosis early, when the first symptoms of the disease appear. In fact, the positive effect of the treatments is largely based on this early intervention. Here we focus on the precocious signs and symptoms that should alert clinicians to the possible diagnosis of these diseases, to improve awareness and to reduce the delay between onset of symptoms and diagnosis.

Introduction

The mucopolysaccharidoses (MPSs) are a heterogenous group of genetic lysosomal storage disorders caused by deficiency of enzymes catalyzing the degradation of glycosaminoglycans (GAGs) (previously called mucopolysaccharides) (Neufeld & Muenzer, 2001). These enzyme deficiencies lead to accumulation of GAGs in the lysosomes of most cells, resulting in cell, tissue, and organ dysfunction, directly or by activation of other secondary pathways, among which inflammation seems to play a relevant role (Simonaro *et al.*, 2001). The GAGs themselves are lysosomal degradation products derived by the proteolytic removal of the core of proteoglycans, the macromolecular forms in which these molecules exist at the cell surface or in the extracellular matrix (Vellodi, 2004).

The MPSs are rare diseases, with a reported incidence between 1:25,000 and 1:45,000 (Nelson *et al.*, 2003). They are inherited by autosomal recessive means, the only exception being MPS II (Hunter syndrome), which is X-linked (Hopwood *et al.*, 1993). There are 11 known enzyme deficiencies that give rise to 7 distinct MPSs (Table 1). Depending on the enzyme deficiency, the catabolism of dermatan sulphate, heparan sulphate, keratan sulphate, chondroitin sulphate, or hyaluronan may be impaired, singly or in combination.

Table 1. Classification of MPS based on enzyme involved and GAG storage

Diseases	Eponym	Enzyme	GAGs stored (sulphates)
MPS I H	Hurler (severe)	α-L-iduronidase	Dermatan, heparan
MPS I H/S	Hurler-Scheie	α-L-iduronidase	Dermatan, heparan
MPS I S	Scheie (attenuated)	α-L-iduronidase	Dermatan, heparan
MPS IIA	Hunter A (severe)	Iduronate sulphatase	Dermatan, heparan
MPS IIB	Hunter B (attenuated)	Iduronate sulphatase	Dermatan, heparan
MPS IIIA	Sanfilippo A	Heparan N-sulphatase	Heparan
MPS IIIB	Sanfilippo B	α-N-acetyl-glucosaminidase	Heparan
MPS IIIC	Sanfilippo C	Acetyl CoA alpha Glucosaminide-acetyltransferase	Heparan
MPS IIID	Sanfilippo D	N-acetylglucosamine 6-sulphatase	Heparan
MPS IVA	Morquio A	Galactose-6-sulphate sulphatase	Keratan, chondroitin 6-
MPS IVB	Morquio B	β-galactosidase	Keratan
MPS VI	Maroteaux-Lamy	N-acetylgalactosamine 4-sulphatase	Dermatan
MPS VII	Sly	β-glucuronidase	Dermatan, heparan chondroitin 4-6
MPS IX		Hyaluronidase	Hyaluronan

The clinical phenotype of the MPSs involves virtually all organs and systems characterized by a chronic, progressive course. The age of the onset, severity of symptoms, clinical presentation, and degree of central nervous system involvement may vary widely both within and amongst the seven major types of MPSs.

Individuals affected by MPS disorders are normal at birth, although some patients, mostly those with MPS VII, may present with hydrops foetalis. In the other cases, the clinical signs appear after months or years (Muenzer, 2004).

Organ involvement is different in the various types; for example, MPS VI patients may have severe skeletal and heart disease without cognitive impairment, those with MPS IV have especially severe skeletal involvement, and MPS III subjects have very mild somatic involvement with early, severe cognitive impairment. Furthermore, a wide phenotypic spectrum is observed within the same type of MPS. For example, in the first 2 years of life, an early involvement of many organs and functions (heart, bones, joints, hearing, vision, and cognition) is the rule in the severe form of MPS type I (so-called Hurler syndrome), whereas MPS I patients with the attenuated form (so-called Scheie syndrome) may present with one isolated sign or symptom later in life, in the second or third decade.

Many specific treatments are now available, such as haematopoietic stem cell transplantation (HSCT) in selected cases (severe MPS I) and enzyme replacement therapy (ERT) for those with MPS I, II, and VI. Because these treatments now exist, it is incumbent upon the clinician to recognize these diseases early so that treatment can be started before severe damage has a chance to occur. Although the awareness of MPS symptoms is now better than in the past, it still needs to be improved. The aim of this chapter is to discuss the signs and symptoms of MPSs, mainly focusing on those that should alert paediatricians and other clinicians to an early diagnosis of mucopolysaccharidosis. MPS VII and MPS IX are not specifically discussed because of their extreme rarity.

Mucopolysaccharidosis: signs and symptoms

Dysmorphisms and physical aspects

Progressive coarsening of facial appearance, consisting in prominent forehead, flat nasal bridge with broad nose, and macroglossia, becomes evident in the first year of life in the more severe forms of MPS I and MPS VI. In MPS II, facial coarsening is less evident in the first year of life, but becomes clearly apparent subsequently. MPS III and IV may have less or no typical physiognomic changes in the first years. Fig. 1 shows the progression of the physical characteristics at various ages of the facies of a patient affected by 'attenuated' MPS II.

Other early signs of MPSs modifying the physical aspect of these patients are *protruding abdomen* due to organomegaly, *umbilical and inguinal hernia*, which are much more frequent and severe than in the normal population and *hirsutism with low posterior hairline* (Fig. 2).

Umbilical and inguinal hernias are frequent in these patients and have been reported as the first manifestation of MPS I in a relevant number of patients from the MPS I Registry who underwent surgical repair (Arn *et al.*, 2009): in about 1/3 of cases the surgery had been performed before the diagnosis was known. Umbilical hernias in these patients, different from the case of umbilical hernias in normal children, rarely have spontaneous resolution in the first 2 years of life and need surgical treatment. Inguinal hernias are frequently bilateral and may relapse a few years after surgical intervention (Hinek & Wilson, 2000).

ENT and airway obstructions

Almost all the MPS patients have ear, nose and throat (ENT) problems (Simmons *et al.*, 2005): *noisy breathing, recurrent otitis, sinusitis, and upper airway infections* with persistent copious discharge are frequent in the first 1-2 years of life. These disturbances are very common in normal children as well, but the difference with MPS patients is that they have earlier and more severe manifestations. In fact, it is quite uncommon to see severe ENT disturbances among healthy children below 2 years of age. The main causes for these disturbances are enlarged tongue, redundant mucosal tissue, and hyperplasia of adenoids and tonsils, which together with a narrowed trachea and thickened vocal cord, lead to airway obstruction. Obstructive sleep apnea is also a frequent and sometimes early finding due to the foregoing causes.

Combined conductive and neurosensory hearing deficit commonly occurs in MPS: frequent middle ear infections, deformities of the ossicles, and probable abnormalities of the inner ear are together responsible for this problem. Auditory brain-stem responses are often abnormal in a nonspecific way, probably reflecting a mixture of middle ear, cochlear, eight nerve, and lower-brain-stem anomalies. Early treatment with hearing aids is advised (Simmons *et al.*, 2005).

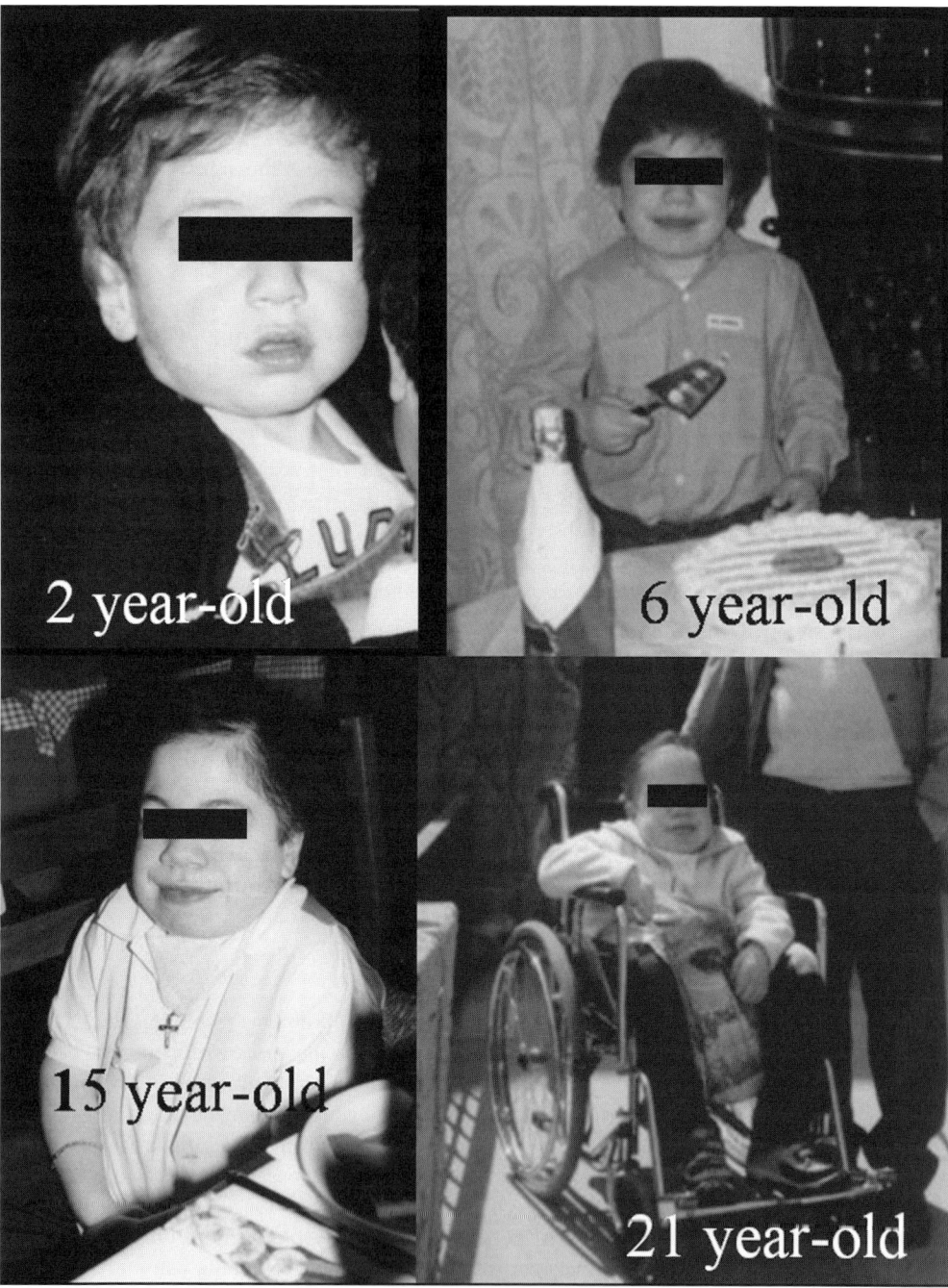

Fig. 1. Progression of the physical characteristics in MPS II.

Chapter 5   Early signs and symptoms for the timely diagnosis of mucopolysaccharidosis

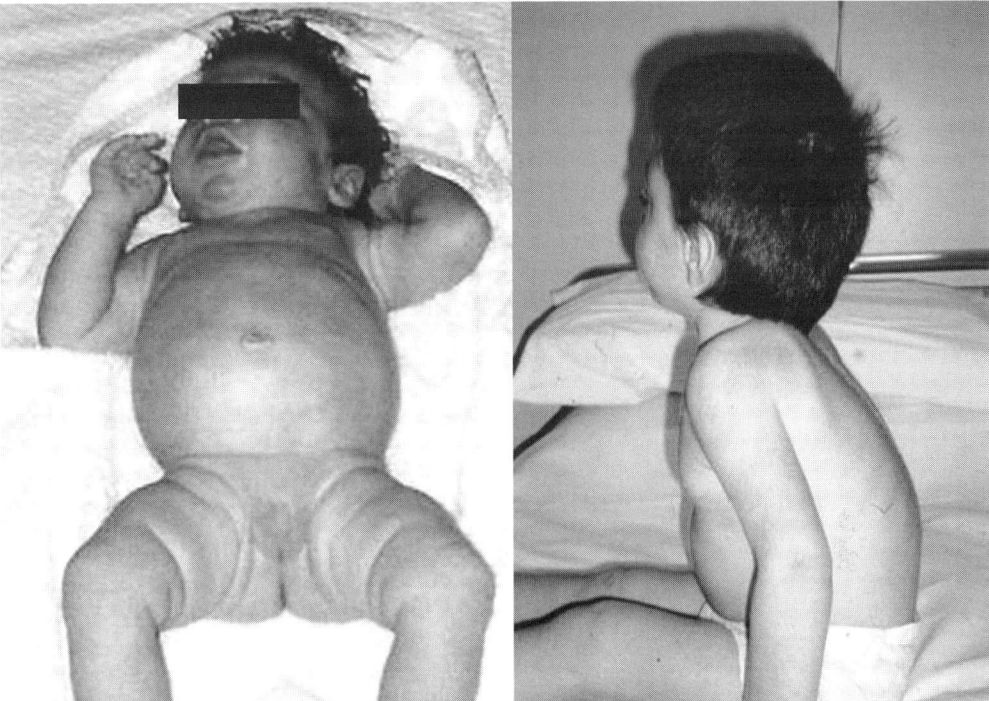

Fig. 2. *Protruding abdomen (left) and hirsutism with low posterior hairline and gibbus (right) in two patients with MPS I.*

While upper airways infections are very frequent in these patients, lower airway infections are not so common in MPSs (personal experience; Walker *et al.*, 2003). When lung infections develop, they can be attributed to the narrow trachea and larynx (see figure in the chapter by Marco Grimaldi *et al.* in this volume) and alterations in chest mobility.

Musculoskeletal findings

Dysostosis multiplex is the term used to collectively indicate the typical skeletal deformities of MPSs. It includes short stature, scaphocephalic head, odontoid hypoplasia, anterior hypoplasia of lumbar vertebrae with kyphosis, spade-like hands, enlarged diaphyses of the long bones with irregular appearance of the metaphyses, small femoral heads and coxa valga, short and thickened clavicles, oar-shaped ribs, tracheal deformities, and joint contractures (Weisstein *et al.*, 2004). *Hip dislocation* is a frequent early finding facilitated by radiologic screening that when seen in conjunction with other signs may help to point to the diagnosis of MPS. *Progressive lumbar gibbus with kyphosis* is commonly seen in all MPS disorders, except MPS III: this sign needs to be especially kept in mind because it is typical of MPSs and is never found in normal children. It is probably the earliest and most frequent sign of disease in the severe form of MPS I: it appears in the first months of life, frequently before the age of 6 months (Levin *et al.*, 1997). Figure 3 shows a mild and a severe early gibbus in two patients with MPS I at age 9 months and 6 years, respectively.

Other signs that may be early but are not so evident are claw-hand deformities secondary to flexion contractures of the fingers and in general joint stiffness and odontoid hypoplasia. Joint stiffness is a common, easily recognizable and typical feature of all the MPSs except for

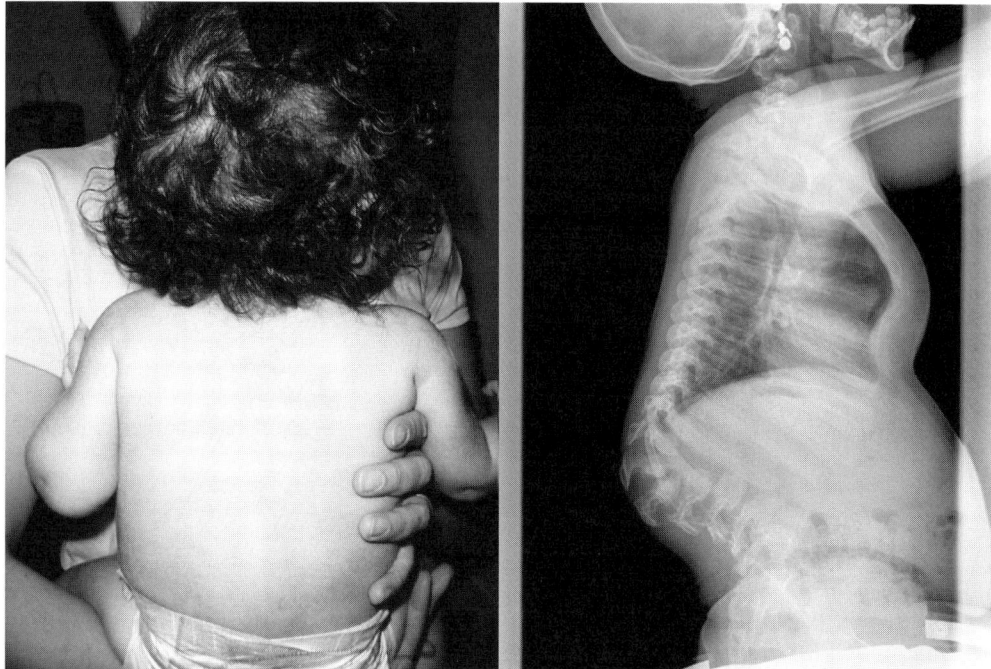

Fig. 3. Mild gibbus in a 9-month-old child (left) and a severe one in the X-ray of a 6-year-old chid (right), both with MPS I.

Morquio syndrome, in which the joints tend to be hypermobile secondary to ligamentous laxity. The abnormal joint function probably results from a combination of metaphyseal deformities and thickened joint capsules secondary to glycosaminoglycan accumulation and fibrosis. Limitations of motion and joint stiffness can cause significant disability because they hamper the everyday common actions of life, such as combing the hair, getting dressed, writing, eating, and drinking.

Odontoid hypoplasia is a characteristic radiologic finding that may have severe medical consequences: the instability of the hypoplastic odontoid process with ligamentous laxity can result in life-threatening atlanto-axial subluxation (Fig. 4). The major risk occurs in MPS IV and then, in descending order, by MPS I, VI, II, and III. It is an early sign and may easily be recognized, but needs a specific dynamic X-ray examination to be performed (Kachur & Del Maestro, 2000).

The clinical case shown in Box 1 is a good illustration of the difficult and lengthy progression to diagnosis for one of our patients who had many early orthopaedic problems.

Ocular problems

Vision problems are very common in MPS patients (Ashworth *et al.*, 2006): *Glaucoma and cataracts* are found in several types of the MPSs and may present very early. Glaucomas have been reported in MPS I and MPS VI and cataracts found in MPS III and IV (Ashworth *et al.*, 2006). We observed glaucoma and cataracts as the first sign of the disease in two of our patients with MPS I. Corneal clouding in MPS I, IV, VI and VII is the rule and may lead to significant visual disability (Ashworth *et al.*, 2006). Retinal degeneration commonly occurs later in life in MPS I, II, III, and IV, resulting in loss of peripheral vision and night blindness.

Box 2 illustrates a case where there was very early eye involvement.

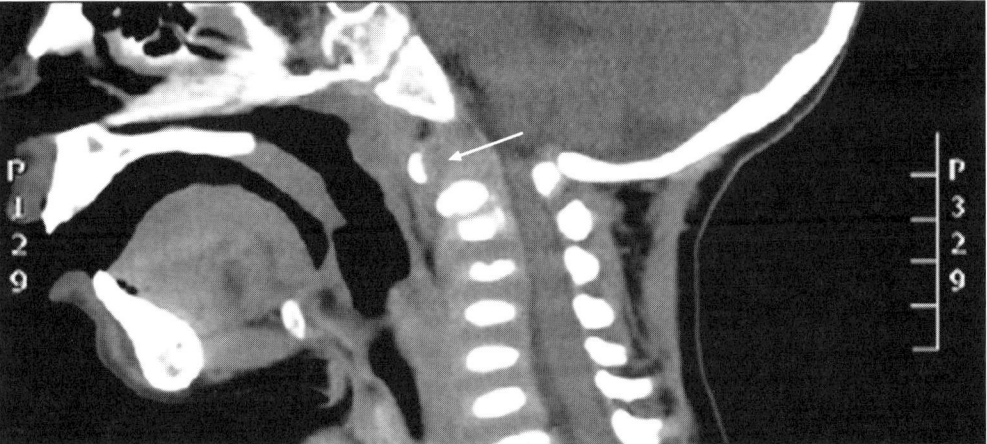

Fig. 4. Cervical CT scan of a 4-year-old patient with MPS IV hypo-/ -aplastic odontoid process.

Box 1. Delayed diagnosis, orthopaedic and heart problems: clinical case report

31-year-old male patient with the following history:
- *2 years of age:* joint stiffness of shoulders;
- *4 years of age:* claw-hand deformity;
- *6 years of age:* severe scoliosis requiring orthopaedic brace;
- *18 years of age:* severe mitral and aortic valvular disease → surgical substitution;
- *29 years of age:* epilepsy treated with valproic acid;
- *31 years of age:* cerebellar atrophy and altered signal in thalamic and periventricular area at cerebral MRI;
- *31 years of age:* diagnosis of MPS I (so-called attenuated type-Scheie syndrome).

Box 2. Orthopaedic and eye problems: clinical case report

Female patient born at term:
- *3 months of age:* bilateral congenital hip dysplasia at ultrasound screening;
- *4 months of age:* right cataract and corneal clouding;
- *9 months of age:* facies suggestive for lysosomal storage disorder, mild hypotonia of the lower limbs, and hepatomegaly;
- *10 months of age:* diagnosis of MPS I through the measurement of urinary GAGs and enzymatic activity.

Cardiac problems

Cardiac involvement is very frequent in all MPS patients and *valve damage* may be the first manifestation of the disease. In our experience, among 57 MPS patients, 34 had a valve disease at diagnosis, and 48 had valve disease at the last follow-up examination. In 6 patients the cardiologic diagnosis preceded that of MPS (Fesslovà *et al.*, 2009). The history of one of these patients is shown in Box 3.

> **Box 3. Early heart valve disease: clinical case report**
>
> *Female patient born at term:*
> - *8 months of age:* cardiac systolic murmur → ultrasound examination shows mild mitral valve dysplasia with regurgitation;
> - *15 months of age:* progression of valvular dysplasia and evidence of coarse facies. GAGs measured in the urine and enzymatic activity led to the diagnosis of MPS III.
> At the time of the patient's diagnosis, the mother was 6 months pregnant with a second child. This infant was found to be affected at birth, showing that early diagnosis is important not only for the affected subject, but also for family genetic counseling.

Mitral regurgitation is the most commonly found valve disease, followed by aortic regurgitation. We did not find any prevalence of one or the other valve damage among the various types of MPS, but found a faster progression of disease severity in MPS I and II compared to MPS III and IV (Fesslovà *et al.*, 2009). Other signs of cardiac involvement include left ventricular wall thickening, absolute or relative narrowing of the coronary arteries (leading to ischemia if not infarction), and systemic and pulmonary hypertension (Hayflick *et al.*, 1992; Braunlin *et al.*, 2001, Renteria *et al.*, 1976). These symptoms all contribute to the risk of congestive heart failure and sudden cardiovascular collapse (Fesslovà *et al.*, 2009).

Neurologic involvement

Both the central and the peripheral nervous systems are affected in MPS. *Carpal tunnel syndrome* may be the first sign of MPS in many patients with the attenuated form of MPS I, II, and VI. Occasionally *hydrocephalus* may be discovered in severely affected patients before the diagnosis of MPS has been made.

Ventricular enlargement may be due to the combination of cortical atrophy secondary to central nervous system degeneration and a defect in cerebrospinal fluid reabsorption (Sheridan & Johnston, 1994). The defective reabsorption of cerebrospinal fluid in MPS is presumably due to thickening of the meninges and dysfunction of the pacchionian granulation in the arachnoid villi. The communicating hydrocephalus that occurs in MPS is usually slowly progressive, with clinical symptoms that are difficult to distinguish from the primary neurologic disease. Acute symptoms such as vomiting and papilledema are uncommon. Ventricular enlargement is unsuspected in most patients at the time of initial evaluation, but most of the subjects with this sign have mental retardation, the degree of enlargement correlating with severity of retardation (Vedolin *et al.*, 2007).

Spinal cord compression more commonly occurs in MPS IV, but has been reported in all MPS disorders except MPS III and IX (Fig. 5). It can occur from subluxation due to atlanto-axial instability with odontoid hypoplasia and from increased soft tissue around the dens. The fibrous tissue around the dens may be secondary to the cervical instability. Reduced exercise tolerance may be the earliest symptom of a cervical myelopathy in MPS. To optimize the timing of surgical stabilization in MPS IV, an MRI of the cervical spine is recommended at the time of diagnosis and at regular intervals thereafter. Surgery to stabilize the spine by posterior fusion can be life saving. However, if cord compression is severe, with a significant anterior soft tissue mass, decompression followed by posterior fusion may be required. Progressive cord compression with resulting cervical myelopathy due to dura mater thickening is common in the mild forms of MPS I, II, and VI. Compression of the spinal cord at lower levels, dorsal or

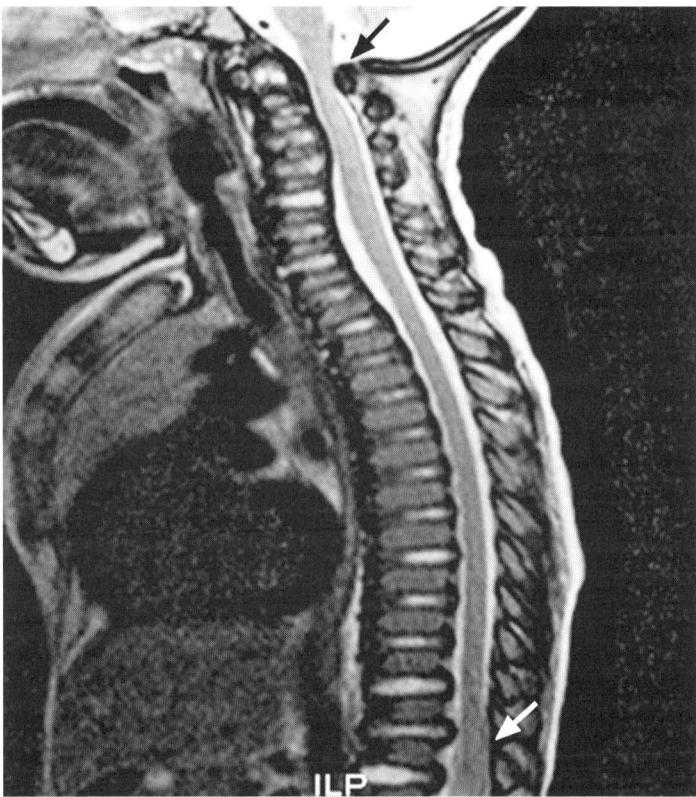

Fig. 5. Stenosis of the cervical spinal canal and mild signs of posterior spinal cord compression in a 4-year-old MPS IV patient.

lumbar, is less frequent, but may occur and may need surgical repair (Levin et al., 1997; Kachur & Del Maestro, 2000). Posterior spinal fusion is effective in stopping progressive spinal deformities and is mandatorily performed when progression is demonstrated and if neurologic deficits appear.

Nerve entrapment syndromes, particularly of the carpal tunnel, are common, but most patients lack typical symptoms (pain, tingling, or numbness) until severe compression occurs (Wraith & Alani, 1990). Because of the high incidence of carpal tunnel syndrome and the minimal subjective complaints, routine electromyographic/nerve conduction velocity testing is recommended. The loss of thumb function due to carpal tunnel syndrome can be a significant handicap in combination with skeletal dysplasia. Surgical decompression of the median nerve has resulted in complete restoration of motor hand activity in some patients and partial improvement in others (Yuen et al., 2007).

Seizures commonly occur in the oldest patients, but are usually easily controlled by monotherapy (see the paper by Daniele Grioni et al. in this volume).

Developmental delay

About half of the patients with MPS disorders show progressive developmental delay. It is found in the severe forms of MPS I and MPS II, and in MPS III (Sanfilippo syndrome). It is usually not found in the attenuated forms of MPS I and MPS II or in MPS IV and is rare in

MPS VI. No treatment is available to prevent cognitive delay, with the exception of very early stem cell transplantation in MPS I (see the chapter in this volume by Attilio Rovelli and his colleagues). As disease progresses, patients lose their previous skills, may become aggressive and hyperactive, and show sleep disturbances; in the last phase they can be very withdrawn and lose contact with the environment as a result of progressive dementia. Hyperactivity with developmental delay is often the first sign of disease in MPS III patients who, as already mentioned, have very few somatic signs of MPS. This is particularly true for MPS IIIB (Moog et al., 2007).

Anaesthesia problems

MPS patients have a major risk of complications when undergoing general anaesthesia and intubation. Mucosal tissue hypertrophy and inflammation, short neck, tonsil and adenoid hyperplasia, hypertrophic GAG-infiltrated tongue, high epiglottis, narrowing of larynx and trachea, vertebral malformations all combine to increase technical difficulties. These problems worsen with age. Consequently, these patients need to be treated by a well-informed anaesthesiologic team, aware of all the risks intrinsic in MPS and able to use fiberoptic endoscopy if necessary. For more details, see the chapter in this volume by Pablo Ingelmo et al.

Treatment options

Palliative treatment

Most of the signs and symptoms described above may be treated palliatively, in that such treatments do not provide a cure, but may help in improving the patient's quality of life. In the last 10 years, for many reasons (e.g., new specific treatment options, awareness of adverse events and how to avoid them, and easier approaches to surgical procedures in general), multiorgan periodic evaluation and palliative treatments have been offered more often to MPS patients, resulting in better control of the disease's effects. Examples of such beneficial effects follow.

Most MPS patients who have moderate to severe hearing loss may benefit from the placement of *hearing aids*. Aggressive audiologic management strategies help in maintaining the highest quality of life. *Adenotonsillectomy* may improve airway patency, while *ventilating tubes* can minimize the long-term sequelae of the frequent episodes of acute otitis media and chronic middle ear effusions that are commonplace in most MPS patients. *Continuous positive airway pressure* (CPAP) may be useful in treating sleep apnea while waiting for the surgical intervention of adenotonsillectomy. *Laser excision of laryngeal mucosal hypertrophy* has also been helpful in some selected patients with airway obstruction (Simmons et al., 2005). Tracheal stenting in cases of tracheal collapse has also been used (Davitt et al., 2002). *Respiratory physiotherapy* can improve the break-up of mucous secretions and lower the risk of infection (Savci et al., 2006). *Physical therapy*, such as range-of-motion exercises, appears to offer some benefits in preserving joint function and should be started early. Early surgery for carpal tunnel syndrome avoids peripheral nerve damage and improves fine-motor abilities (Yuen et al., 2007). Cervical decompression and vertebral fusion may avoid spinal cord damage and maintain motor function of the limbs or may even allow a recovery from previous neurological disturbances (Kachur & Del Maestro, 2000; Vijay & Wraith, 2005; Giussani et al., 2009).

Cardiac evaluation at regular intervals with ultrasound and judicious use of drugs in these patients has probably, in the last 10 years, allowed a reduction in the number of acute events such as acute heart failure and collapse (Fesslovà *et al.*, 2009). *Prophylactic treatment for bacterial endocarditis* should be advised for all the MPS patients with valve abnormalities. Successful *valve replacement* has been reported in MPS IH/S, MPS IS, MPS II, and MPS VI (Tan *et al.*, 1992; Antoniou *et al.*, 2009; Fesslovà *et al.*, 2009).

Ocular problems are managed both by pharmacologic (glaucoma) and surgical treatments. In particular, corneal transplantation has been performed with good results, but the long-term outcome may be compromised by associated retinitis pigmentosa and/or optic nerve disease (Ashworth *et al.*, 2006).

Ventriculoperitoneal shunting in MPS patients with dilated ventricles may be performed when increased intracranial pressure may be documented or if symptoms of hypertension are observed (Giugliani *et al.*, 2007). Hyperactivity and sleep disturbances may also benefit from pharmacologic treatments, resulting in improvement of behavior in the patient and relief for the family (Kalkan Ucar *et al.*, 2009; Guerrero *et al.*, 2006).

Specific treatments

For a discussion of specific treatment with haematopoietic stem cell transplantation, see the chapters by Attilio Rovelli *et al.* and Jaap Jan Boelens and for treatment with enzyme replacement therapy see that of Michael Beck in this volume. For MPS III and MPS IV no specific treatment is available at present; for MPS III, gene therapy has been advised and experimental studies in animals have recently been conducted. In murine models the injection into the brain of vectors derived from adeno- or lentivirus, coding for alpha-acetylglucosaminidase, leads to a restoration of enzyme activity and significantly improves behavioural performance (Cressant *et al.*, 2004; Di Domenico *et al.*, 2009). For MPS IV, ERT has been developed and it is currently under evaluation in a Phase I/II clinical trial (<http://www.morquiobmrn.com/>).

Conclusions:
How to recognize a mucopolysaccharide disorder early

Mucopolysaccharidoses are rare genetic diseases whose diagnosis is still difficult, although clinicians probably now have a better awareness of it than in the past. A delay between the appearance of signs and symptoms and diagnosis is reported for all the MPSs and is well demonstrated by the data of the recently developed registries for some of these diseases (Arn *et al.*, 2009; Parini *et al.*, 2009). The availability of specific therapies (haematopoietic stem cell transplantation since the 1980s and ERT since the 1990s) now makes this gap unacceptable because the earlier the treatment is started, the better the outcome. The registries show that the time between the first signs of the disease and diagnosis is shorter in more severe forms than in milder forms; nevertheless, in cases such as MPS IH where HSCT may be planned, the delay of even a few months can change the prognosis for the patient.

All but MPS III patients show early somatic signs that may easily be recognized, mainly if they are not alone but present in association. Table 2 summarizes the early first signs that are observed in MPS and that are described in this chapter. They are divided into three groups: (a) severe MPS I, II, IV and VI; (b) attenuated MPS I, II, IV and VI; and (c) MPS III. For group (a), it must be emphasized that many of these signs and symptoms are frequently found in normal infants and so may not arouse the suspicion of a systemic rare disease. However, careful observation reveals the differences between MPS and normal children: these 'common' symptoms are earlier and more severe in those with MPS than they are in normal children. For example, the median age at adenoidectomy and tonsillectomy is earlier in those with MPS than in the normal population (Arn *et al.*, 2009). Some signs of the disease are clearly pathognomonic and should lead directly to a prompt diagnosis: these are mainly gibbus, claw-hands, and the ocular signs of glaucoma and cataracts.

Table 2. Summary of the early signs in MPS

Disease	Early signs
Severe MPS I, II, IV, and VI	Dysmorphic facies, hirsutism Hepatosplenomegaly Umbilical and inguinal hernias Frequent upper airway infections Adenoid and tonsil hypertrophy Hip dysplasia and gibbus Heart valve disease Cardiomyopathy Glaucoma and cataracts Early surgery for hernias, adenotonsillectomy
Attenuated MPS I, II, IV, and VI	Joint contractures Carpal tunnel disorder Heart valve disease Cardiomyopathy
MPS III	Mild dysmorphism Hyperactivity Cognitive delay

It must also be kept in mind that urinary GAGs are not always useful for diagnosis because of false-negative results in a certain number of patients with MPS II, III, and IV (Mahalingam *et al.*, 2004). MPS III is characterized by only mild somatic and radiographic features and severe central nervous system degeneration. Such disproportionate involvement of the central nervous system is unique in this form of MPS. The high prevalence of false-negative results in testing for GAGs in the urine (Mahalingam *et al.*, 2004) may also account for a significant delay in the diagnosis of MPS III after the onset of symptoms. If effective treatments are to become available in the future, it will make neonatal screening for this disease necessary because early clinical recognition is impossible. Identification of the milder forms of MPS I, II, IV, VI, and VII may also be very difficult and many of these patients have only had the correct diagnosis decades after the first appearance of symptoms. Often in such cases the patient had a specific complaint that was addressed by a specialist such as a hand surgeon for carpal tunnel disorder or a cardiologist for valve disease. The specialist frequently does not take into account the other milder problems of other organs and systems and thus the disease is not recognized as a multiorgan disease with need of comprehensive diagnosis, but rather only as an organ-specific disturbance. The suspicion of a mild MPS in a child or an adult should always be aroused when the patient has valve abnormalities like mitral regurgitation and/or musculoskeletal problems like claw-hand or joint stiffness without inflammatory signs or limitation in joint motion, especially in the scapulo-humeral articulation.

Acknowledgments: The authors thank Fondazione Pierfranco e Luisa Mariani (Milan) for their generous economic support to the Centre for Metabolic Diseases of Infancy, and Vera Marchetti and Alessandro Baruzzo for their technical assistance in the preparation of this chapter.

References

Antoniou, T., Kirvassilis, G., Tsourelis, L., Ieromonachos, C., Zarkalis, D. & Alivizatos, P. (2009): Mitral valve replacement and Hunter syndrome: case report. *Heart Surg. Forum* **12**, E54–56.

Arn, P., Wraith, J.E. & Underhill, L. (2009): Characterization of surgical procedures in patients with mucopolysaccharidosis type I: findings from the MPS I Registry. *J. Pediatr.* **154**, 859–864.

Ashworth, J.L., Biswas, S., Wraith, J.E. & Lloyd, I.C. (2006): Mucopolysaccharidoses and the eye. *Surv. Ophthalmol.* **51**, 1–17.

Braunlin, E., Rose, A., Hopwood, J., Candel, R. & Krivit, W. (2001): Coronary artery patency following long-term successful engraftment 14 years after bone marrow transplantation in the Hurler syndrome. *Am. J. Cardiol.* **88**, 1075–1077.

Cressant, A., Desmaris, N., Verot, L., Bréjot, T., Froissart, R., Vanier, M.T., Maire, I. & Heard, J.M. (2004): Improved behavior and neuropathology in the mouse model of Sanfilippo type IIIB disease after adeno-associated virus-mediated gene transfer in the striatum. *J. Neurosci.* **24**, 10229–10239.

Davitt, S.M., Hatrick, A., Sabharwal, T., Pearce, A., Gleeson, M. & Adam, A. (2002): Tracheobronchial stent insertions in the management of major airway obstruction in a patient with Hunter syndrome (type-II mucopolysaccharidosis). *Eur. Radiol.* **12**, 458–462.

Di Domenico, C., Villani, G.R., Di Napoli, D., Nusco, E., Calì, G., Nitsch, L. & Di Natale, P. (2009): Intracranial gene delivery of LV-NAGLU vector corrects neuropathology in murine MPS IIIB. *Am. J. Med. Genet. A* **149**, 1209–1218.

Fesslovà, V., Corti, P., Sersale, G., Rovelli, A., Russo, P., Mandarino, S., Bufera, G. & Parini, R. (2009): The natural course and the impact of therapies of cardiac involvement in the mucopolysaccharidoses. *Cardiol. Young* **19**, 170–178.

Giugliani, R., Harmatz, P. & Wraith, J.E. (2007): Management guidelines for mucopolysaccharidosis VI. *Pediatrics* **120**, 405–418.

Giussani, C., Roux, F.E., Guerra, P., Pirillo, D., Grimaldi, M., Citerio, G. & Sganzerla, E.P. (2009): Severely symptomatic craniovertebral junction abnormalities in children: long-term reliability of aggressive management. *Pediatr. Neurosurg.* **45**, 29–36.

Guerrero, J.M., Pozo, D., Diaz-Rodriguez, J.L., Martinez-Cruz, F. & Vela-Campos, F. (2006): Impairment of the melatonin rhythm in children with Sanfilippo syndrome. *J. Pineal. Res.* **40**, 192–193.

Hayflick, S., Rowe, S., Kavanaugh-McHugh, A., Olson, J.L. & Valle, D. (1992): Acute infantile cardiomyopathy as a presenting feature of mucopolysaccharidosis VI. *J. Pediatr.* **120**, 269–272.

Hinek, A. & Wilson, S.E. (2000): Impaired elastogenesis in Hurler disease: dermatan sulphate accumulation linked to deficiency in elastin-binding protein and elastic fiber assembly. *Am. J. Pathol.* **156**, 925–938.

Hopwood, J.J., Bunge, S., Morris, C.P., Wilson, P.J., Steglich, C., Beck, M., Schwinger, E. & Gal, A. (1993): Molecular basis of mucopolysaccharidosis type II: mutations in the iduronate-2-sulphatase gene. *Hum. Mutat.* **2**, 435–442.

Kachur, E. & Del Maestro, R. (2000): Mucopolysaccharidoses and spinal cord compression: case report and review of the literature with implications of bone marrow transplantation. *Neurosurgery* **47**, 223–229.

Kalkan Ucar, S, Ozbaran, B., Demiral, N., Yuncu, Z., Erermis, S. & Coker, M. (2010): Clinical overview of children with mucopolysaccharidosis type III A and effect of risperidone treatment on children and their mothers psychological status. *Brain Dev.* **32**, 156–161.

Levin, T.L., Berdon, W.E., Lachman, R.S., Anyane-Yeboa, K., Ruzal-Shapiro, C. & Roye, D.P. (1997): Lumbar gibbus in storage diseases and bone dysplasias. *Pediatr. Radiol.* **27**, 289–294.

Mahalingam, K., Janani, S., Priya, S., Elango, E.M. & Sundari, R.M. (2004): Diagnosis of mucopolysaccharidoses: how to avoid false positives and false negatives. *Indian J. Pediat.* **71(1)**, 29–32.

Moog, U., van Mierlo, I., van Schrojenstein Lantman-deValk, H.M., Spaapen, L., Maaskant, M.A. & Curfs, L.M. (2007): Is Sanfilippo type B in your mind when you see adults with mental retardation and behavioral problems? *Am. J. Med. Genet. C Semin. Med. Genet.* **145C**, 293–301.

Muenzer, J. (2004): The mucopolysaccharidoses: a heterogeneous group of disorders with variable pediatric presentations. *J. Pediatr.* **144**, 527–534.

Nelson, J., Crowhurst, J., Carey, B. & Greed, L. (2003): Incidence of the mucopolysaccharidoses in Western Australia. *Am. J. Med. Genet.* **123A**, 310–313.

Neufeld, E.F. & Muenzer, J. (2001): The mucopolysaccharidoses. In: *The metabolic and molecular bases of inherited disease*, eds. C.R. Scriver *et al.*, pp. 3421–3452. New York: McGraw Hill.

Parini, R., Furlan, F., Wraith, J.E., Scarpa, M., Beck, M., Muenzer, J. & Giugliani, R. on behalf of the HOS Investigators (2009): The burden of surgery in Hunter syndrome: data from the Hunter Outcome Survey International Congress of Inborn Errors of Metabolism. August 29-September 2, San Diego, California, abstr. 753.

Piraud, M., Boyer, S., Mathieu, M. & Maire, I. (1993): Diagnosis of mucopolysaccharidoses in a clinically selected population by urinary glycosaminoglycan analysis: a study of 2,000 urine samples. *Clin. Chim. Acta* **221**, 171–181.

Renteria, V.G., Ferrans, V.J. & Roberts, W.C. (1976): The heart in the Hurler syndrome: gross, histologic and ultrastructural observations in five necropsy cases. *Am. J. Cardiol.* **38**, 487–501.

Savci, S., Ozturk, M., Inal-Ince, D., Gultekin, Z., Arikan, H. & Sivri, H.S. (2006): Inspiratory muscle training in Morquio's syndrome: a case study. *Pediatr. Pulmonol.* **41**, 1250–1253.

Sheridan, M. & Johnston, I. (1994): Hydrocephalus and pseudotumour cerebri in the mucopolysaccharidoses. *Childs Nerv. Syst.* **10**, 148–150.

Simmons, M.A., Bruce, I.A., Penney, S., Wraith, E. & Rothera, M.P. (2005): Otorhinolaryngological manifestations of the mucopolysaccharidoses. *Int. J. Pediat. Otorhinolaryngol.* **69**, 589–595.

Simonaro, C.M., Haskins, M.E. & Schuchman E.H. (2001): Articular chondrocytes from animals with a dermatan sulphate storage disease undergo a high rate of apoptosis and release nitric oxide and inflammatory cytochines: a possible mechanism underlyng degenerative joint disease in the mucolpolysaccharidoses. *Lab. Invest.* **81**, 1319–1328.

Tan, C.T., Schaff, H.V., Miller, F.A., Jr., Edwards, W.D. & Karnes, P.S. (1992): Valvular heart disease in four patients with Maroteaux-Lamy syndrome. *Circulation* **85**, 188–195.

Vedolin, L., Schwartz, I.V., Komlos, M., Schuch, A., Puga, A.C., Pinto, L.L., Pires, A.P. & Giugliani, R. (2007): Correlation of MR imaging and MR spectroscopy findings with cognitive impairment in mucopolysaccharidosis II. *A.J.N.R. Am. J. Neuroradiol.* **28**, 1029–1033.

Vellodi, A. (2004): Lysosomal storage disorders. *Br. J. Haematol.* **128**, 413–431.

Vijay, S. & Wraith, J.E. (2005): Clinical presentation and follow-up of patients with the attenuated phenotype of mucopolysaccharidosis type I. *Acta Paediat.* **94**, 872–877.

Walker, P.P., Rose, E. & Williams, J.G. (2003): Upper airways abnormalities and tracheal problems in Morquio's disease. *Thorax* **58**, 458–459.

Weisstein, J.S., Delgado, E., Steinbach, L.S., Hart, K. & Packman, S. (2004): Musculoskeletal manifestations of Hurler syndrome: long term follow-up after bone marrow transplantation. *J. Pediat. Orthop.* **24**, 97–101.

White, K.K., Steinman, S. & Mubarak, S.J. (2009): Cervical stenosis and spastic quadriparesis in Morquio disease (MPS IV): a case report with twenty-six-year follow-up. *J. Bone Joint Surg. Am.* **91**, 438–442.

Wraith, J.E. & Alani, S.M. (1990): Carpal tunnel syndrome in the mucopolysaccharidoses and related disorders. *Arch. Dis. Child.* **65**, 962–963.

Yuen, A., Dowling, G., Johnstone, B., Kornberg, A. & Coombs, C. (2007): Carpal tunnel syndrome in children with mucopolysaccaridoses. *J. Child. Neurol.* **22**, 260–263.

Chapter 6

Anderson-Fabry disease in children

Rossella Parini and Francesca Santus

UOS Malattie Metaboliche Rare, Centro 'Fondazione Mariani per le Malattie Metaboliche dell'Infanzia',
Department of Paediatrics, Azienda Ospedaliera San Gerardo,
University of Milano-Bicocca, via Pergolesi 33, 20052 Monza, Italy
rossella.parini@unimib.it

Summary

Anderson-Fabry disease is a rare genetic X-linked disease, caused by deficiency of lysosomal alpha-galactosidase A, an enzyme that is needed to degrade several glycosphingolipids and primarily globotriaosylceramide (Gb3). The lysosomal storage of Gb3 in many organs and tissues is responsible for the onset of the damage, eventually leading to functional insufficiency or failure of the organs involved. The disease has a subtle onset in infancy, with frequently overlooked symptoms such as neuropathic pain, gastrointestinal disturbances, heat and cold intolerance, vertigo, fatigue, headache and hypohydrosis, and is thus often undiagnosed or misdiagnosed for years until functional damage to vital organs (renal insufficiency, cardiac hypertrophy, or strokes) is recognized. Enzyme replacement therapy for this disease has been available since 2001 and is known to improve quality of life and reduce clinical signs and symptoms and complications. It is important that the treatment be started before severe organ damage is established. In this chapter we focus on the early signs and symptoms of the disease in order to help family paediatricians and general practitioners, as well as other medical professionals who are not familiar with rare diseases, to recognize the disease early in order to provide early access to treatment for their patients.

Introduction

Anderson-Fabry (AF) disease is the second most prevalent lysosomal storage disorder after Gaucher disease (Desnick *et al.*, 2001). It was first described independently in 1898 by two dermatologists, Dr. William Anderson and Dr. Johannes Fabry, who published a case report on one male patient each (13 and 39 years old, respectively) with angiokeratoma corporis diffusum and proteinuria (Anderson, 1898; Fabry, 1898).

More than 50 years later the disease was characterized as an X-linked, progressive, and multisystem disorder resulting from a deficiency of alpha-galactosidase, leading to lysosomal storage of glycosphingolipids (Opitz *et al.*, 1965; Brady *et al.*, 1967). It was learned only recently that females are frequently affected, even though the disease is X-linked (MacDermot *et al.*, 2001b; Whybra *et al.*, 2001; Deegan *et al.*, 2006; Wilcox *et al.*, 2008). The estimated incidence of the disease classically is 1:117,000 live male births (Meikle *et al.*, 1999). Spada *et al.* (2006) recently reported a much higher incidence (1:3,100) in a screening study in newborns that may reflect a high prevalence in the population of mild phenotypes that went undiagnosed in the past. AF disease is mainly known as a genetic disorder affecting heart, kidney, and brain, but skin, eye, hearing, bowel, lungs, endocrine glands, sweat glands, autonomic system, joints and other organs are also progressively affected (MacDermot *et al.*, 2001a and 2001b; Mehta *et al.*, 2004; Eng *et al.*, 2007; Waldeck *et al.*, 2009). Tissue and organ damage is triggered by glycosphingolipid (mainly Gb3) storage in the lysosomes of virtually all kind of cells. The sequence of events leading to tissue damage is not completely understood. The lysosomal storage is evident since birth in the tissues (Vedder *et al.*, 2006) and leads to progressive damage, becoming clinically evident after years.

The diagnosis of AF disease in children may be not easy because they present with mainly subjective symptoms and very few or no objective signs. Our aim is to describe the clinical picture of AF disease, with particular emphasis to its manifestations in children, in order to help paediatricians, paediatric neurologists, and rheumatologists to make an early diagnosis. Enzymatic replacement therapy (ERT) has been available for this disease since 2001, and recent evidence suggests that the earlier the treatment is started, the better is its efficacy (Germain *et al.*, 2007; Weidemann *et al.*, 2009; West *et al.*, 2009).

Genetic transmission and the female mystery

AF disease is an X-linked disease: heterozygous females pass their affected X chromosome to 50 per cent of their male and female children; affected males who are hemozygous pass their affected X chromosome to 100 per cent of their daughters. In most X-linked diseases, heterozygous females are asymptomatic. For many years it was believed that AF females were carriers, with minor symptoms and signs of the disease, and only in exceptional cases were there severe manifestations. In recent years, because of the more systematic observation of a relevant number of females, it has become clear that females show all signs of the disease, with a wide range of severity and a mean later presentation (approximately 10 years) compared to that in males (MacDermot *et al.*, 2001b; Whybra *et al.*, 2001; Deegan *et al.*, 2006; Wilcox *et al.*, 2008). The signs and symptoms of disease in females increase in number and severity with age as they do in males: this is well demonstrated by the worsening of the severity score index with years (Whybra *et al.*, 2004). Females' mean survival is higher than that of AF males, but lower than that of normal females (MacDermot *et al.*, 2001b). It is not clear why the majority of females have relevant symptoms during their life. It has been demonstrated that X-inactivation in females is random (Maier *et al.*, 2006) and not preferentially unfavourably skewed, as was previously hypothesized (Mehta *et al.*, 2004; Maier *et al.*, 2006). Also, the envisaged correlation between clinical severity and the pattern of X-inactivation (Morrone *et al.*, 2003) has not been confirmed (Maier *et al.*, 2006).

Recently other possible explanations for this mystery have been proposed. The recent demonstration of increased concentrations of deacylated Gb3 (lysoglobotriaosylsphingosine, lysoGb3) in the plasma of AF patients, both male and female, may partly clarify this issue (Aerts *et al.*, 2008). LysoGb3 seems to inhibit alpha-galactosidase A activity and when it is taken up into cells, it is probably reacylated to Gb3, thus increasing the extralysosomal pool of Gb3, which is not accessible to endogenous or exogenous (ERT) alpha-galactosidase A. In heterozygous females, then, circulating lysoGb3 may ultimately nullify the effects of alpha-galactosidase produced by enzyme-competent cells. Very recently, Marchesan *et al.* (2009) and Deegan *et al.* (2009) showed that human serum contains a substance inhibiting the uptake of alpha-galactosidase to cells; it is probably an alkaline phosphatase, which dephosphorylates the enzyme. This may be another reason explaining why females are affected.

Clinical picture

AF disease affects virtually all organs and systems, resulting in a proteiform disease that frequently manifests itself quite differently even within the same family.

Childhood and adolescence

Male patients with the classic form of disease typically show the first symptoms in childhood, starting at a very early age with acroparaesthesia, gastrointestinal symptoms (abdominal pain, nausea, vomiting, diarrhoea, constipation), tinnitus, vertigo, fatigue, heat and cold intolerance, and hypohydrosis (or less frequently anhydrosis) as the most frequent symptoms reported by children (Ries *et al.*, 2003, 2005; Ramaswami *et al.*, 2006; Hopkin *et al.*, 2008; Orteu *et al.*, 2007; Lidove *et al.*, 2006). Acroparaesthesia consists of chronic or acute neuropathic pain at the palms and the soles of the feet, with a typical burning sensation, sometimes severe enough to be compared to an iron burn. It may be triggered by changes in environment or body temperature or by emotional stress. Patients often say that as far as they can remember they always had this sort of pain, going back to 2–3 years of age. Hypohydrosis or anhydrosis are frequent, reported in up to 93 per cent of males and 25 per cent of females (Ries *et al.*, 2003; Orteu *et al.*, 2007); there is also a small percentage of patients with hyperhydrosis. This parameter could be quantified (Schiffmann *et al.*, 2003; Ries *et al.*, 2006), but these techniques are not part of routine clinical practice and most often the abnormalities of sweating are reported as subjective evaluation. Gastrointestinal problems consisting of recurrent abdominal pain, attacks of diarrhoea alternating with constipation, nausea, vomiting, and flatulence are often misdiagnosed as irritable bowel (Feriozzi *et al.*, 2007). Some patients have repeated trips to the emergency room for attacks of abdominal pain mimicking appendicitis. Aural symptoms such as tinnitus and vertigo are frequent, mainly in females, but rarely do the children spontaneously refer to these symptoms unless prompted by a precise question. Because of the recurrent pain and the frequent hypohydrosis, these children do not like sports and prefer sedentary activities.

Although it may appear as early as 5 years of age, angiokeratoma is most frequently evident at the end of the first decade and represents the first objective sign of the disease (Ries *et al.*, 2003, 2005; Ramaswami *et al.*, 2006; Orteu *et al.*, 2007; Hopkin *et al.*, 2008) (Fig. 1). Angiokeratoma is defined as a small dark red to purple skin spot with a scaly rough surface, originating from surface dilated capillaries. It may become dark purple or dark overnight if a clot develops in the lesion. The typical regions of distribution are mainly the bathing trunk area, followed by proximal limbs, palms and soles, around the nails, and the border of the lips. Angiokeratomas are found in two-thirds of males and one-third of females with AF disease and its presence seems to correlate with the severity of the disease (Orteu *et al.*, 2007).

Adulthood

Between 20 and 40 years of age, damage to the vital organs – kidney, heart, and brain – may often become clinically evident as renal insufficiency as well as hypertrophic cardiomyopathy, with rhythm disturbances, valve disease, and cerebrovascular damage. Renal insufficiency frequently progresses to failure and the need for dialysis; complications of heart disease include infarctions, arrhythmias, which require pacemaker implantation, and severe cardiac insufficiency; repeated strokes cause progressively severe handicaps and eventually premature death (Buechner *et al.*, 2008). The patients may also suffer from obstructive pulmonary disease, hearing impairment, endocrine deficits, and depression. Virtually all organs and systems may be affected by AF disease. Quality of life was tested before therapeutic intervention with ERT was undertaken, and a decreased quality of life for men and women was reported as comparable

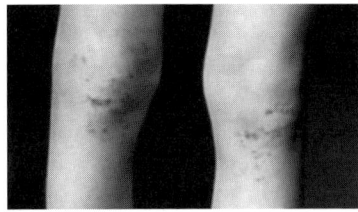

Fig. 1. Typical aspect of angiokeratoma in an 8-year-old patient.

to that of HIV patients (Gold et al., 2002; Miners et al., 2002). There are also milder variants of the disease, skipping infancy and adolescence, and presenting in adulthood as kidney or heart disease. As already noted, females show the whole spectrum of signs and symptoms presenting later in life. The difference from the males is that females less frequently have angiokeratoma, usually do not progress to dialysis or renal transplantation, and have fewer cerebrovascular events. The details of the clinical picture of AF disease have been better delineated in the last 8 years. In 2001 MacDermot et al. (2001a and 2001b) retrospectively studied a population of 98 males and 60 females with AF disease in the UK and showed the typical progression of the disease, with worsening of signs and symptoms and the appearance of new ones as age advances. They also showed that diagnosis was reached around 8–10 years after the onset of symptoms, that many patients with less severe disease were probably undiagnosed, and that the median cumulative survival of males was 50 years (that is, approximately 20 years less than that of the general population). More recent papers (Mehta et al., 2004; Eng et al., 2007; Waldeck et al., 2009) presenting data from patient databases substantially confirm the observations of MacDermot and colleagues (2001a and b).

Fig. 2 shows the prevalence of different signs and symptoms found in a group of 69 Italian patients, 37 males and 32 females, aged 4–74 years (mean age 35.5 years, median age 39 years). Most frequent signs and symptoms were cornea verticillata, angiokeratoma, and hypo/anhydrosis in males. In this group of patients, females also had the whole phenotypic spectrum of the disease with differences in prevalence as, for example, for angiokeratoma. Fig. 3 shows the increase of severity of the disease, measured with the Mainz severity score index (Whybra et al., 2004) in the same group of Italian patients (Parini et al., 2005); the progression with age is evident, as is the different slope in the two genders.

The clinical diagnosis in children

All the first symptoms presented in childhood are neurologic in origin and can all be attributed to a disturbance of the autonomic innervation of various organs. Since children for years may only have subjective symptoms, the diagnosis at this age may be extremely difficult, unless the disease is already known in the family because of the existence of affected adult relatives. Four studies are available in the literature on the expression of AF disease in children and adolescents (Ries et al., 2003, 2005; Ramaswami et al., 2006; Hopkin et al., 2008). The most frequent signs and symptoms were acroparaesthesia (from 58 to 88 per cent in males and 40 to 65 per cent in females), hypohydrosis (from 22 to 93 per cent in males and 11 to 25 per cent in females), gastrointestinal problems (from 23 to 80 per cent in males and 11 to 52 per cent in females) and angiokeratoma (from 20 to 53 per cent in males and 8 per cent to 38 per cent in females). The diagnosis of AF disease in male patients presenting with angiokeratoma is usually easily reached by the dermatologist. If angiokeratoma is not evident, the diagnosis becomes more difficult, especially when there is no family history, and it is probably the association of

Chapter 6   Anderson-Fabry disease in children

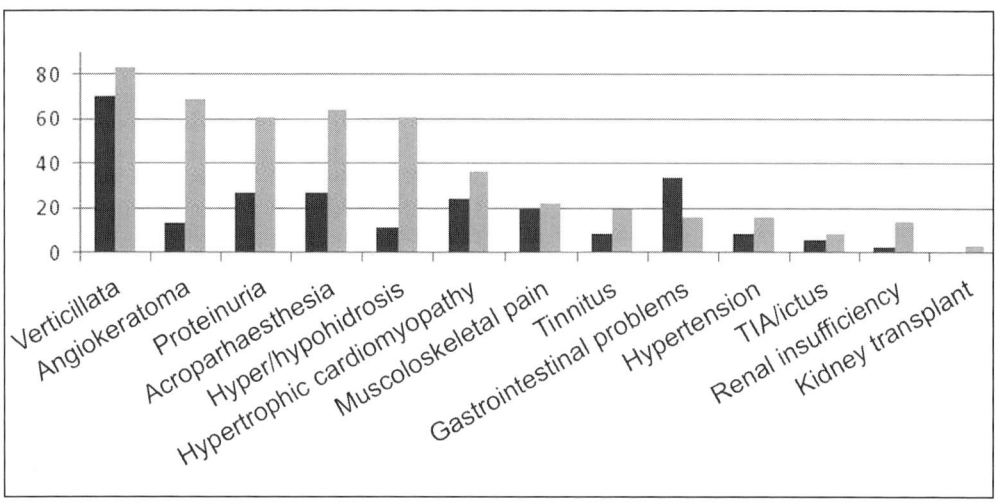

Fig. 2. Prevalence of different signs and symptoms found in 69 Italian patients, 37 males and 32 females (mean age 35.5 years, median age 39 years). Bars show the percentage of patients with particular sign/symptom (black bars show incidence in females, and shaded bars show that in males). Note that angiokeratoma and sweat disturbances are more frequent in males. Kidney transplantation was done only in males.

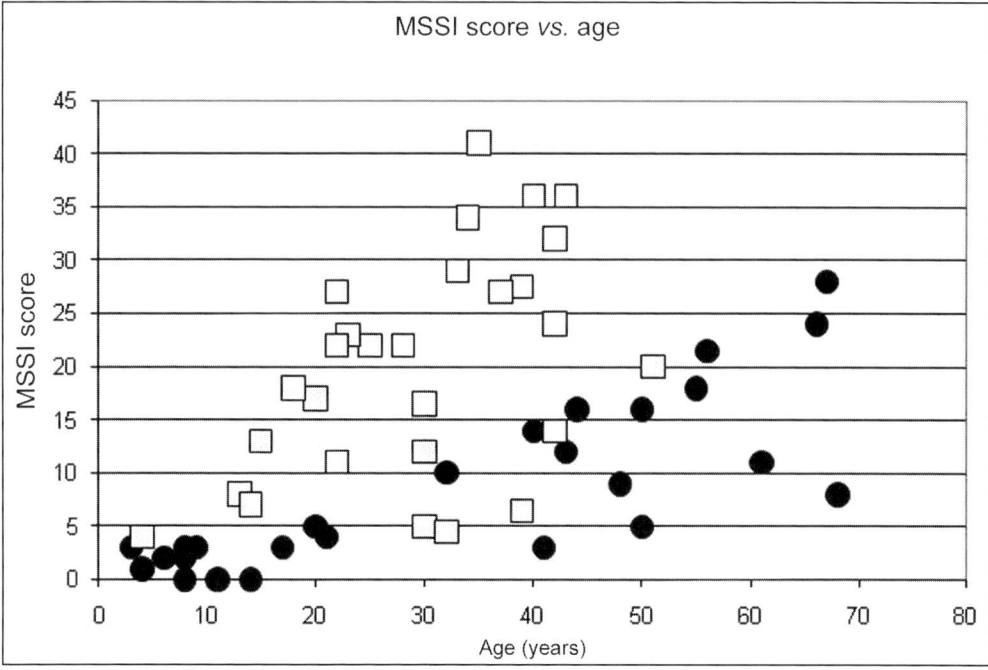

Fig. 3. Progression of Mainz severity score index with age in a group of 69 Italian patients, 37 males and 32 females (mean age 35.5 years, median age 39 years). White boxes represent males and black circles represent females. Note that in females the disease progresses at a slower rate than in males.

63

more symptoms that may help in arousing the suspicion of AF disease; this in turn triggers the request for further examination, such as searching for cornea verticillata. Prevalence of cornea verticillata in the young child is 66 to 90 per cent (Ries *et al.*, 2003, 2005; Ramaswami *et al.*, 2006). So, while the presence of cornea verticillata confirms the suspicion, its absence does not exclude it. Considering that treatment is available that could protect against further worsening, a mild suspicion should be followed by a complete work-up for exclusion of AF disease. In this situation, an accurate clinical history plays a primary role in detecting patients and sometimes entire families with AF disease. The pedigree needs to be well assessed, with specific questions, and with a very critical evaluation of previous diagnoses in the various members of the family. However, the proteiform nature of AF disease makes things more complicated, as shown by the pedigrees reported in Fig. 4. In these pedigrees, the patients of the three different families that are shown have very different signs and symptoms within the same family, making it difficult, when collecting the history, to relate all of them to a hypothetical familiar genetic disease.

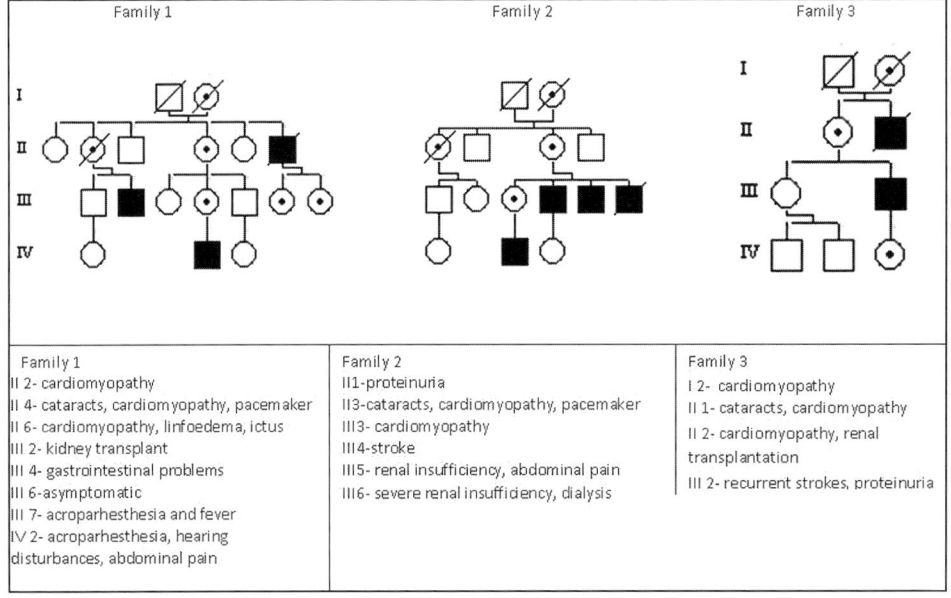

Fig. 4. Pedigrees of three families with many affected members. The proteiform nature of AF disease is evident even in the same family.

The laboratory diagnosis

The assay of enzymatic activity in the leukocytes or the fibroblasts will probably identify all affected males. Gb3 concentrations in plasma and urine may help in confirming the diagnosis. Identification of the mutation in the alpha-Gal gene is the last step of diagnosis in males. Females, on the contrary, both with and without symptoms, may express enzymatic activity at levels not much different from those of the normal population. Therefore the exclusion of the suspicion of AF disease in females depends on the results of the molecular analysis of the gene.

How do we measure the severity of the disease?

Biochemical markers, such as chitotriosidase in Gaucher disease, are very useful for stadiation of the disease, provide an objective parameter for comparing different patients and choosing between different therapeutic strategies, and may be helpful, together with the clinical parameters, for evaluating the efficacy of the treatment and taking decisions about its modulation. Unfortunately no satisfactory biochemical markers are available up to now for the follow-up of AF disease. Another way of evaluating progressive diseases in a possibly objective way is that of creating severity score indexes. This has recently been done, for example, for Gaucher disease (Di Rocco *et al.*, 2008) and metachromatic leukodystrophy (Krägeloh-Mann *et al.*, 2009). The Mainz group some years ago developed a scoring system for AF disease that was both simple and sensitive enough to be easily applied, reproducible and sensitive enough to detect improvement of phenotype after treatment (Whybra *et al.*, 2004, Parini *et al.*, 2008).

Can we say when the disease begins in the children?

Differently from other lysosomal storage disorders clinically presenting in early childhood, the signs of AF disease are subtle in the first years of life and apparent clinical damage to vital organs only shows in the adult age. This might lead one to think that the evidence of the storage in the tissues may be delayed in comparison with the other lysosomal storage disorders. However, this is not the case because it has been well demonstrated that the storage material can be found in significant amounts already in the kidney, cardiomyocytes, cornea, and placenta of affected fetuses (Elleder *et al.*, 1998; Tsutsumi *et al.*, 1985; Vedder *et al.*, 2006). Moreover, both kidney and heart, if accurately examined, show signs of disease very early in life in many patients. Tøndel *et al.* (2008) performed renal biopsies in nine symptomatic patients with minimal albuminuria and they demonstrated that glomerular and vascular changes were present before progression to overt proteinuria and decreased glomerular filtration rate. In the study by Hopkin *et al.* (2008), 9 of 86 children had some renal dysfunction and one 4-year-old boy had substantial decrease of glomerular filtration rate. In a study by Ries *et al.* (2005) 28 per cent of the patients had left ventricular hypertrophy. All of the 20 patients examined by Kampmann *et al.* (2008) had left ventricular mass indexed to height > 75th percentile of healthy controls. In the same study, males, but not females, had lower than normal heart rate variability. Few cases of stroke have been reported as early as 14 and 16 years of age (Ries *et al.*, 2006; Grewal *et al.*, 1994) and radiologic evidence of cerebral microvascular disease in children was reported by Cabrera-Salazar and colleagues in 2005. In conclusion, these data clearly demonstrate that although the life-threatening complications of AF disease occur almost exclusively in adulthood, the disease starts with the lysosomal storage in major organs during fetal life, and vital organs are histologically and functionally affected earlier and more frequently than was believed in the past.

When should children and females be treated?

Enzyme replacement therapy (ERT) with alpha-galactosidase A has been commercially available in Europe since 2001 in two different preparations: agalsidase alpha (Replagal, Shire Human Genetic Therapies, Inc., Cambridge, MA, USA) (Schiffmann *et al.*, 2000, 2001) and agalsidase beta (Fabrazyme, Genzyme Corp, Cambridge, MA, USA) (Eng *et al.*, 2001a, 2001b). The infused enzyme is taken up by endothelial and parenchymal cells into lysosomes through the mannose-6 phosphate, mannose, and asialoglycoprotein receptors. The two forms have the same amino acid sequence but a different glycosylation pattern (Lee *et al.*, 2003). Agalsidase alpha is produced by gene activation in a human cell line and is infused at a dosage of 0.2 mg/kg every other week, over a 40-minute period without routine premedication. Agalsidase beta is produced in Chinese hamster ovary cells and is infused at a dose of 1 mg/kg every other week, over a recommended period of 4 hours, with routine premedication. Both preparations have proved evidence of safety and efficacy (Ries *et al.*, 2006, 2007, Wraith *et al.*, 2008).

The question of when to treat children and females has been frequently asked at scientific meetings, and no clear answer has been given. Most available guidelines (Hughes *et al.*, 2005, Clarke *et al.*, 2005, Eng *et al.*, 2006) show a general agreement in starting treatment in children with relevant symptoms, but, for females and very young males (before 10–13 years of age) with very few or no symptoms we do not actually know at present what the better decision would be. On the one hand there are the apparently few symptoms in a child or woman otherwise looking healthy, the treatment that needs to be intravenously administered every other week may cause such unpleasant common adverse events as chills, fever, and bronchospasm and the increased costs of the treatment must be considered as well. On the other hand there is the possibility that not only doctors but also the family may underestimate many symptoms, the fact that the storage is definitely advancing and that a cascade of secondary mechanisms, not yet well understood, will eventually affect the clinical picture. As stated by Eng *et al.* (2006), proteinuria may remit with treatment, but it is clear that the loss of kidney function may not be recovered. It would be useful to be able to test objectively the severity of the disease in children, but no biochemical tests have yet been developed for this purpose. The MSSI score (Whybra *et al.*, 2004) is not very sensitive in young children and as such it is not useful to predict the future evolution of the disease. The decision to treat or not needs to be informed by the present symptoms and signs and the patient's gender, pedigree, and the nature of gene mutation–in all cases this should be a collective decision taken by the doctors, the patient, and the family itself.

Conclusions

Anderson-Fabry disease is a rare X-linked disorder affecting virtually all organs and tissues. It is caused by lysosomal storage of glycosphingolipids (mainly Gb3), priming a cascade of incompletely understood, secondary events in the tissues, ultimately producing progressive damage. It has an insidious onset in childhood with subjective, fastidious symptoms that may be easily overlooked both by the family and the doctors, evolving in adulthood to functional impairment of vital organs (heart, kidney, and brain) and other disturbances such as hearing loss and endocrinologic deficiencies. Patients have a reduced quality of life, suffer from depression, and die prematurely. Because of the subtle nature of the first signs of the disease, the diagnosis may be delayed for years, reached only when the patient already has severe organ damage such as renal insufficiency. In view of the fact that a specific treatment for this disease has been available since 2001, a treatment that is likely to reduce serious complications and improve the quality of life, it is imperative that the medical community be aware of this disorder and become able to diagnose it early in its course.

References

Aerts, J.M., Groener, J.E., Kuiper, S., Donker-Koopman, W.E., Strijland, A., Ottenhoff, R., van Roomen, C., Mirzaian, M., Wijburg, F.A., Linthorst, G.E., Vedder, A.C, Rombach S.M., Cox-Brinkman, J., Somerharju, P., Boot, R.G., Hollak, C.E., Brady, R.O. & Poorthuis B.J. (2008): Elevated globotriaosylsphingosine is a hallmark of Fabry disease. *Proc. Natl. Acad. Sci. USA* **105**, 812–2817.

Anderson, W. (1898): A case of angiokeratoma. *Br. J. Dermatol.* **1**, 113–117.

Brady, R.O., Gal, A.E., Bradley, R.M., Martenson, E., Warshaw, A.L. & Laster, L. (1967): Enzymatic defect in Fabry's disease: ceramidetrihexosidase deficiency. *N. Engl. J. Med.* **276**, 1163–1167.

Buechner, S., Moretti, M., Burlina, A.P., Cei, G., Manara, R., Ricci, R., Mignani, R., Parini, R., Di Vito, R., Giordano, G.P., Simonelli, P., Siciliano, G. & Borsini, W. (2008): Central nervous system involvement in Anderson Fabry disease: a clinical and MRI retrospective study. *J. Neurol. Neurosurg. Psychiatry* **79**, 1249–1254.

Cabrera-Salazar, M.A., O'Rourke, E., Charria-Ortiz, G. & Barranger, J.A. (2005): Radiological evidence of early cerebral microvascular disease in young children with Fabry disease. *J. Pediatr.* **147**, 102–105.

Clarke, L.A., Clarke, J.T.R., Sirrs, S., West, M.L, Iwanochko, R.M., Wherrett, J.R., Greenberg, C.R., Chan, A.K.J. & Casey, R. (2005): *Fabry disease: recommendations for diagnosis, management, and enzyme replacement therapy in Canada.* [Revision November 2005] <http://www.garrod.ca/>

Deegan, P.B., Baehner, A.F., Barba Romero, M.A., Hughes, D.A., Kampmann, C., Beck, M. & European FOS Investigators (2006): Natural history of Fabry disease in females in the Fabry Outcome Survey. *J. Med. Genet.* **43**, 347–352.

Deegan, P.B., Marchesan, D. & Cox, T.M. (2009): *Studies on the serum phosphatase that abrogates uptake of mannose 6-phosphate-containing therapeutic lysosomal enzymes.* Abstract No. 100. Seventeenth Workshop of European Study Group on Lysosomal Diseases, Bad Honnef, Germany, Sept. 10–13.

Desnick, R.J., Ioannou, Y.A. & Eng, C.M. (2001): α-Galactosidase A deficiency: Fabry disease. In: *The metabolic and molecular bases of inherited disease*, 8th ed., eds. C.R. Scriver, A.L. Beaudet, W.S. Sly & D. Valle, pp. 3733–3774. New York: McGraw-Hill.

Di Rocco, M., Giona, F., Carubbi, F., Linari, S., Minichilli, F., Brady, R.O., Mariani, G. & Cappellini, M.D. (2008): A new severity score index for phenotypic classification and evaluation of responses to treatment in type I Gaucher disease. *Haematologica* **93**, 1211–1218.

Elleder, M., Poupetova, H. & Kozich, V. (1998): Fetal pathology in Fabry's disease and mucopolysaccharidosis type I. *Ceskoslov. Patol.* **34**, 7–12.

Eng, C.M., Banikazemi, M., Gordon, R.E., Goldman, M., Phelps, R., Kim, L., Gass, A., Winston, J., Dikman, S., Fallon, J.T., Brodie, S., Stacy, C.B., Mehta, D., Parsons, R., Norton, K., O'Callaghan, M. & Desnick, R.J. (2001a): A phase 1/2 clinical trial of enzyme replacement in Fabry disease: pharmacokinetic, substrate clearance, and safety studies. *Am. J. Hum. Genet.* **68**, 711–722.

Eng, C.M., Guffon, N., Wilcox, W.R., Germain, D.P., Lee, P., Waldek, S., Caplan, L., Linthorst, G.E., Desnick, R.J. & International Collaborative Fabry Disease Study Group (2001b): Safety and efficacy of recombinant human alpha-galactosidase A: replacement therapy in Fabry's disease. *N. Engl. J. Med.* **345**, 9–16.

Eng, C.M., Fletcher, J., Wilcox, W.R., Waldek, S., Scott, C.R., Sillence, D.O., Breunig, F., Charrow, J., Germain, D.P., Nicholls, K. & Banikazemi, M. (2007): Fabry disease: baseline medical characteristics of a cohort of 1,765 males and females in the Fabry Registry. *J. Inherit. Metab. Dis.* **30**, 184–192.

Eng, C.M, Germain, D.P., Banikazemi, M., Warnock, D.G., Wanner, C., Hopkin, R.J., Bultas, J., Lee, P., Sims, K., Brodie, S.E., Pastores, G.M., Strotmann. J.M. & Wilcox, W.R. (2006): Fabry disease: guidelines for the evaluation and management of multi-organ system involvement. *Genet. Med.* **9**, 539–548.

Fabry, J. (1898): Ein Beitrag zur Kenntnis der Purpura haemorrhagica nodularis (*Purpura papulosa haemorrhagica* Hebrae). *Arch. Dermatol. Syph.* **43**, 187–200.

Feriozzi, S., Torre, E., Ranalli, T., Cardello, P., Morrone, A. & Ancarani, E. (2007): A diagnosis of Fabry gastrointestinal disease by chance: a case report. *Eur. J. Gastroenterol. Hepatol.* **19**, 163–165.

Germain, D.P., Waldek, S., Banikazemi, M., Bushinsky, D.A., Charrow, J., Desnick, R.J., Lee, P., Loew, T., Vedder, A.C, Abichandani, R., Wilcox, W.R. & Guffon, N. (2007): Sustained, long-term renal stabilization after 54 months of agalsidase beta therapy in patients with Fabry disease. *J. Am. Soc. Nephrol.* **18**, 1547–1557.

Gold, K.F., Pastores, G.M., Botteman, M.F., Yeh, J.M., Sweeney, S., Aliski, W. & Pashos, C.L. (2002): Quality of life of patients with Fabry disease. *Qual. Life Res.* **11**, 317–327.

Grewal, R.P. (1994): Stroke in Fabry's disease. *J. Neurol.* **241**, 153–156.

Hopkin, R.J., Bissler, J., Banikazemi, M., Clarke, L., Eng, C.M., Germain, D.P., Lemay, R., Tylki-Szymanska, A. & Wilcox, W.R. (2008): Characterization of Fabry disease in 352 pediatric patients in the Fabry Registry. *Pediatr. Res.* **64**, 550–555.

Hughes, D.A., Ramaswami, U., Elliott, P., Deegan, P., Lee, P., Waldek, S., Apperley, G., Cox, T. & Mehta, A.B. (2005): *Guidelines for the diagnosis and management of Anderson-Fabry disease.* <http://www.dh.gov.uk/>

Kampmann, C., Wiethoff, C.M., Whybra, C., Baehner, F.A., Mengel, E. & Beck, M. (2008): Cardiac manifestations of Anderson-Fabry disease in children and adolescents. *Acta Paediatr.* **97**, 463–469.

Krägeloh-Mann, I., Kehrer, C., Kustermann-Kuhn, B., Groeschel, S. & Grodd, W. (2009): *Clinical course description of metachromatic leukodystrophy (MLD) in children using standardized motor and neuroimaging scores.* Abstract No. 107. Seventeenth Workshop of European Study Group on Lysosomal Diseases, Bad Honnef, Germany, Sept 10–13.

Lee, K., Jin, X., Zhang, K., Copertino, L., Andrews, L., Baker-Malcolm, J., Geagan, L., Qiu, H., Seiger, K., Barngrover, D., McPherson, J.M. & Edmunds, T. (2003): A biochemical and pharmacological comparison of enzyme replacement therapies for the glycolipid storage disorder Fabry disease. *Glycobiology* **13**, 305–313.

Lidove, O., Ramaswami, U., Jaussaud, R., Barbey, F., Maisonobe, T., Caillaud, C., Beck, M., Sunder-Plassmann, G., Linhart, A., Mehta, A. & FOS European Investigators (2006): Hyperhydrosis: a new and often early symptom in Fabry disease: international experience and data from FOS–the Fabry Outcome Survey. *Int. J. Clin. Pract.* **60**, 1053–1059.

MacDermot, K.D., Holmes, A. & Miners, A.H. (2001a): Anderson-Fabry disease: clinical manifestations and impact of disease in a cohort of 98 hemozygous males. *J. Med. Genet.* **38**, 750–760.

MacDermot, K.D., Holmes, A. & Miners, A.H. (2001b): Anderson-Fabry disease: clinical manifestations and impact of disease in a cohort of 60 obligate carrier females. *J. Med. Gene.* **38**, 769–775.

Maier, E.M., Osterrieder, S., Whybra, C., Ries, M., Gal, A., Beck, M., Roscher, A.A. & Muntau, A.C. (2006): Disease manifestations and X inactivation in heterozygous females with Fabry disease. *Acta Paediatr.* (Suppl.) **451**, 30–38.

Marchesan, D., Deegan, P.B. & Cox, T.M. (2009): *Effect of serum and cell type on mannose 6-phosphate mediated delivery of enzyme therapy in cell models of Fabry disease.* Abstract No. 96. Seventeenth Workshop of European Study Group on Lysosomal Diseases, Bad Honnef, Germany, Sept 10–13.

Mehta, A., Ricci, R., Widmer, U., Dehout, F., Garcia de Lorenzo, A., Kampmann, C., Linhart, A., Sunder-Plassmann, G., Ries, M. & Beck, M. (2004): Fabry disease defined: baseline clinical manifestations of 366 patients in the Fabry Outcome Survey. *Eur. J. Clin. Invest.* **34**, 236–242.

Meikle, P.J., Hopwood, J.J., Clague, A.E. & Carey, W.F. (1999): Prevalence of lysosomal storage disorders. *JAMA* **281**, 249–254.

Miners, A.H., Holmes, A., Sherr, L., Jenkinson, C. & MacDermot, K.D. (2002): Assessment of health-related quality-of-life in males with Anderson Fabry disease before therapeutic intervention. *Qual. Life Res.* **11**, 127–133.

Morrone, A., Cavicchi, C., Bardelli, T., Antuzzi, D., Parini, R., Di Rocco, M., Feriozzi, S., Gabrielli, O., Barone, R., Pistone, G., Spisni, C., Ricci, R. & Zammarchi, E. (2003): Fabry disease: molecular studies in Italian patients and X inactivation analysis in manifesting carriers. *J. Med. Genet.* **40**, e103.

Opitz, J.M., Giles, F.C., Wise, D., Race, R.R., Sander, R., von Gemmingen, G.R., Kierland, R.R., Cross, E.G. & De Groot, W.P. (1965): The genetics of angiokeratoma corporis diffusum (Fabry's disease) and its linkage with Xg-locus. *Am. J. Hum. Genet.* **17**, 325–342.

Orteu, C.H., Jansen, T., Lidove, O., Jaussaud, R., Hughes, D.A., Pintos-Morell, G., Ramaswami, U., Parini, R., Sunder-Plassman, G., Beck, M., Mehta, A.B. & FOS Investigators (2007): Fabry disease and the skin: data from FOS, the Fabry Outcome Survey. *Br. J. Dermatol.* **157**, 331–337.

Parini, R., Rigoldi, M., Santus, F., Borsini, W., Burlina, A.B., Concolino, D., DiVito, R., Furlan, F., Ravaglia, R., Ricci, R. & Strisciuglio, P. (2005): *I pazienti italiani inseriti nel Fabry Outcome Survey (FOS): analisi dei dati clinici di base e di follow-up.* VII Congresso Nazionale SISMME (Società Italiana per lo Studio delle Malattie Metaboliche Ereditarie), Pollenzo-Bra (CN), 16–18 ottobre.

Parini, R., Rigoldi, M., Santus, F., Furlan, F., De Lorenzo, P., Valsecchi, G., Concolino, D., Strisciuglio, P., Feriozzi, S., Di Vito, R., Ravaglia, R., Ricci, R. & Morrone, A. (2008): Enzyme replacement therapy with agalsidase alfa in a cohort of Italian patients with Anderson-Fabry disease: testing the effects with the Mainz Severity Score Index. *Clin. Genet.* **74**, 260–266.

Ramaswami, U., Whybra, C., Parini, R., Pintos-Morell, G., Mehta, A., Sunder-Plassmann, G., Widmer, U., Beck, M. & FOS European Investigators (2006): Clinical manifestations of Fabry disease in children: data from the Fabry Outcome Survey. *Acta Paediatr.* **95**, 86–92.

Ries, M., Ramaswami, U., Parini, R., Lindblad, B., Whybra, C., Willers, I., Gal, A. & Beck, M. (2003): The early clinical phenotype of Fabry disease: a study on 35 European children and adolescents. *Eur. J. Pediatr.* **162**, 767–772.

Ries, M., Gupta, S., Moore, D.F., Sachdev, V., Quirk, J.M., Murray, G.J., Rosing, D.R., Robinson, C., Schaefer, E., Gal, A., Dambrosia, J.M., Garman, S.C., Brady, R.O. & Schiffmann, R. (2005): Pediatric Fabry disease. *Pediatrics* **115**, e344–355.

Ries, M., Clarke, J.T.R., Whybra, C., Timmons, M., Robinson, C., Schlaggar, B.L., Pastores, G., Lien, Y.H., Kampmann, C., Brady, R.O., Beck, M. & Schiffmann, R. (2006): Enzyme replacement therapy with agalsidase alfa in children with Fabry disease. *Pediatrics* **118**, 924–932.

Schiffmann, R., Murray, G.J., Treco, D., Daniel, P., Sellos-Moura, M., Myers, M., Quirk, J.M., Zirzow, G.C., Borowski, M., Loveday, K., Anderson, T., Gillespie, F., Oliver, K.L., Jeffries, N.O., Doo, E., Liang, T.J., Kreps, C., Gunter, K., Frei, K., Crutchfield, K., Selden, R.F. & Brady, R.O. (2000): Infusion of alpha-galactosidase A reduces tissue globotriaosylceramide storage in patients with Fabry disease. *Proc. Natl. Acad. Sci. USA* **97,** 365–370.

Schiffmann, R., Kopp, J.B., Austin, H.A., Sabnis, S., Moore, D.F., Weibel, T., Balow, J.E. & Brady, R.O. (2001): Enzyme replacement therapy in Fabry disease: a randomized controlled trial. *JAMA* **285,** 2743–2749.

Schiffmann, R., Floeter, M.K., Dambrosia, J.M., Gupta, S., Moore, D.F., Sharabi, Y., Khurana, R.K. & Brady, R.O. (2003): Enzyme replacement therapy improves peripheral nerve and sweat function in Fabry disease. *Muscle Nerve* **28,** 703–710.

Spada, M., Pagliardini, S., Yasuda, M., Tukel, T., Thiagarajan, G., Sakuraba, H., Ponzone, A. & Desnick, R.J. (2006): High incidence of later onset Fabry disease revealed by newborn screening. *Am. J. Hum. Genet.* **79,** 31–40.

Tøndel, C., Bostad, L., Hirth, A. & Svarstad, E. (2008): Renal biopsy findings in children and adolescents with Fabry disease and minimal albuminuria. *Am. J. Kidney Dis.* **51,** 767–776.

Tsutsumi, O., Sato, M., Sato, K., Mizuno, M. & Sakamoto, S. (1985): Early prenatal diagnosis of inborn error of metabolism: a case report of a fetus affected with Fabry's disease. *Asia Oceania J. Obstet. Gynaecol.* **11,** 39–45.

Vedder, A.C., Strijland, A., vd Bergh Weerman, M.A., Florquin, S., Aerts, J.M. & Hollak, C.E. (2006): Manifestations of Fabry disease in placental tissue. *J. Inherit. Metab. Dis.* **29,** 106–111.

Waldek, S., Patel, M.R., Banikazemi, M., Lemay, R. & Lee, P. (2009): Life expectancy and cause of death in males and females with Fabry disease: findings from the Fabry registry. *Genet. Med.* **11,** 790–796.

Weidemann, F., Niemann, M., Breunig, F., Herrmann, S., Beer, M., Stork, S., Voelker, W., Ertl, G., Wanner, C. & Strotmann, J. (2009): Long term effects of enzyme replacement therapy on Fabry cardiomyopathy: evidence for a better outcome with early treatment. *Circulation* **119,** 524–529.

West, M., Nicholls, K., Mehta, A., Clarke, J.T., Steiner, R., Beck, M., Barshop, B.A., Rhead, W., Mensah, R., Ries, M. & Schiffmann, R. (2009): Agalsidase alfa and kidney dysfunction in Fabry disease. *J. Am. Soc. Nephrol.* **20,** 1132–1139.

Wraith, J.E., Tylki-Szymanska, A., Guffon, N., Lien, Y.H., Tsimaratos, M., Vellodi, A. & Germain, D.P. (2008): Safety and efficacy of enzyme replacement therapy with agalsidase beta: an international, open-label study in pediatric patients with Fabry disease. *J. Pediatr.* **152,** 563–570.

Whybra, C., Kampmann, C., Willers, I., Davies, J., Winchester, B., Kriegsmann, J., Brühl, K., Gal, A., Bunge, S. & Beck, M. (2001): Anderson-Fabry disease: clinical manifestations of disease in female heterozygotes. *J. Inherit. Metab. Dis.* **24,** 715–724.

Whybra, C., Kampmann, C., Krummenauer, F., Ries, M., Mengel, E., Miebach, E., Baehner, F., Kim, K., Bajbouj, M., Schwarting, A., Gal, A. & Beck, M. (2004): The Mainz Severity Score Index: a new instrument for quantifying the Anderson-Fabry disease phenotype, and the response of patients to enzyme replacement therapy. *Clin. Genet.* **65,** 299–307.

Wilcox, W.R., Oliveira, J.P., Hopkin, R.J., Ortiz, A., Banikazemi, M., Feldt-Rasmussen, U., Sims, K., Waldek, S., Pastores, G.M., Lee, P., Eng, C.M., Marodi, L., Stanford. K.E., Breunig, F., Wanner, C., Warnock, D.G., Lemay, R.M., Germain, D.P. & Fabry Registry (2008): Females with Fabry disease frequently have major organ involvement: lessons from the Fabry Registry. *Mol. Genet. Metab.* **93,** 112–128.

Mucopolysaccharidoses
from the specialists' point of view

Chapter 7

Epilepsy in mucopolysaccharidosis: clinical features and outcome

Daniele Grioni*, Margherita Contri*, Francesca Furlan°, Miriam Rigoldi°, Attilio Rovelli^ and Rossella Parini°

Paediatric Neurophysiological Unit, ° Rare Metabolic Disease Unit,
and ^ Paediatric BMT Unit, San Gerardo Hospital and the 'Monza e Brianza per il Bambino e la sua Mamma' Foundation, via Pergolesi 33, 20052 Monza, Italy
neuroped@hsgerardo.org

Summary

Mucopolysaccharidoses (MPSs) are a group of inherited diseases with central nervous system (CNS) involvement in approximately 50 per cent of the patients. The aim of this study is to describe our clinical experience in a group of 61 MPS patients followed at the Rare Metabolic Diseases Unit of San Gerardo Hospital, Monza, Italy. In our cohort, epilepsy occurred in 2/7 MPS I patients not undergoing haematopoietic stem cell transplantation (HSCT), 5/16 MPS II patients, and 6/13 MPS III patients. Overall the prevalence of epilepsy was 13 of 61 patients (21 per cent). The seizures were most frequently partial. Differentiating between a partial or generalized onset of seizure in these patients might be difficult since they are often unable to speak, so prolonged video EEG became the principal tool for correctly evaluating the onset of epileptic discharge. However, MPS patients do not always tolerate prolonged neurophysiologic studies. Although epilepsy is a common event during the lifetime of MPS patients, seizures can be easily controlled by conventional medical treatment without significant adverse effects. We suggest a slow initial titration of antiepileptic drugs at low dose. All the epileptic patients underwent medical therapy with anticonvulsant drugs and nine of them are currently free of seizures. Furthermore, we would like to highlight that some 'critical' episodes are nonepileptic and that neurologic networks other than the cerebral cortex, such as the extrapyramidal system, may be involved.

Introduction

Mucopolysaccharidoses (MPSs) are rare inherited metabolic diseases with progressive multiorgan involvement. About 50 per cent of MPS patients develop mental retardation on account of central nervous system damage. Many of them also have peripheral nerve abnormalities resulting from compression.

Epilepsy is considered a common neurologic complication in MPS, usually presenting when deterioration of neurocognitive function is already advanced. Literature in the field is scanty, and only limited data are available about prevalence, phenotype, course, and treatment of epilepsy in these patients. Schwartz *et al.* (2007) reported a prevalence of 27.7 per cent in MPS

II patients with severe phenotype and Ruijter et al. (2008) observed epilepsy in 43 per cent of MPS III C patients. Epilepsy is much less frequent in its attenuated forms, with no or minimal cognitive involvement (Schwartz et al., 2007).

The 61 MPS patients followed at our hospital have been retrospectively and prospectively analysed. Our aims were to evaluate: (1) the age of onset and prevalence of epilepsy in MPS patients; (2) the clinical features of seizures; and (3) the response to treatment.

Material and methods

We collected data on 61 MPS patients: 10 children with MPS Type IH who previously underwent haematopoietic stem cell transplantation (HSCT) (current mean age, 8 years; range, 5–11 years); two with MPS Type IH who had not been allografted (current age 10 and 17 years old), and five with the attenuated form (Hurler/Scheie or Scheie) of MPS type I (current mean age, 28 years: range 29–42); 16 with MPS type II (current mean age, 17 years; range, 8–49 years), 13 with MPS type III (current mean age, 18 years; range, 9–23 years), 11 with MPS type IV (current mean age, 18 years; range 8–34), and four with MPS type VI (current mean age, 6 years; range 3–8 years) (Table 1). Patients with MPS types II and VI and those with type I who did not undergo transplantation have been treated with enzyme replacement therapy (ERT) since the time when it was commercially available.

All patients underwent neurologic evaluation, including an accurate physical examination and an awakening or sleeping electroencephalogram (EEG) at different time points during the course of the disease and every year or more often after the onset of epilepsy. We collected data about the development of any critical neurologic events and reviewed neurophysiologic data obtained at any time during the course of disease (awakening EEG, sleeping EEG, and video EEG).

Table 1. Overall prevalence of epilepsy

Disease	No. of patients	Mean age (± SD) (years)	Epilepsy	Mean age at onset of seizures (years)
HSCT MPS I	10	8 (± 3.5)	0	
No HSCT MPS I (severe and attenuated)	7	28	2 (29%)	14–31
MPS II	16	16 (± 10)	5 (31%)	10
MPS III	13	17 (± 4)	6 (46%)	13
MPS IV	11	18 (± 9)	0	
MPS VI	4	6 (± 2)	0	

Results

Age of onset and prevalence of epilepsy

None of the MPS IH patients who underwent HSCT has developed epilepsy up to now. On the contrary, 2/7 patients with MPS I who had not undergone allografting presented with epilepsy at the age of 14 and 31 years, respectively. The first one is a male patient who has been affected by severe cognitive delay since the age of 10 years; the second patient is a 42-year-old man with the attenuated form and adequate cognitive function, but presently severely depressed, who developed epilepsy late in life, at 31 years of age. Epilepsy occurred in 5/16 patients (38 per cent) with MPS II (mean age at onset, 10 years; range, 9–12) and in 6/13 (46 per cent) patients with MPS III (mean age at onset, 13 years: range 10–15). Seizures were not recorded in patients with MPS types IV and VI. The overall prevalence of epilepsy was 13/61 patients (21 per cent) (Table 1).

Clinical features

We observed both partial and generalized or secondarily generalized seizures (mainly tonic-clonic).

Partial seizures occurred in eight patients: in four of them epilepsy presented like complex partial seizures with impairment of consciousness or autonomic signs, which can be difficult to recognize as critical epileptic events in MPS patients, who are often unable to speak and to refer to their symptoms. Five patients had generalized or secondarily generalized seizures.

In the event of generalized seizures, partial onset may not be recognized if the clinical manifestations are only subtle. Two patients affected by MPS II (case 5) and MPS III (case 10) had status epilepticus, which occurred at onset of epilepsy in case 5 and later during the course of epilepsy in case 10.

A 20-year-old patient with MPS III (case 11) whose epilepsy was well-controlled since 10 years of age presented at the age of 17 with a 'pseudocrisis' with repetitive movement of the arm, impairment of consciousness, and autonomic signs such as tachycardia and sweating. In this case, the video EEG recordings showed a lack of correlation between the clinical features and bioelectrical activity on the scalp, allowing us to conclude that these features were not epileptic (Table 2).

Response to treatment

All 13 epileptic patients underwent medical therapy. Nine (70 per cent) patients are at this time seizure-free, four patients (cases 2, 4, 9, and 10) achieved a decrease in seizure frequency (*i.e.*, the generalized tonic-clonic seizures disappeared, but the complex partial seizures were only partially responsive to treatment). Patients achieved good responses with conventional antiepileptic drugs. (monotherapy in 13 cases and polytherapy in one case). No side effects have been recorded. In the patients with the 'pseudocrisis' (case 11), a response was obtained with antipsychotic (risperidone) and antispasmodic (baclofen) drugs (Table 2).

Discussion

In our sample the prevalence of epilepsy is 2/7 (in patients with MPS I without transplant), 5/16 (in MPS II), and 6/13 (in MPS III). The mean age at onset of epilepsy ranges between 9.5 (MPS II) and 22.5 (MPS I) years. Very little is known from the literature about epilepsy in MPS. It was reported as an exceptional finding in 1 of 29 patients with the attenuated form of MPSI (Suresh *et al.*, 2005). In MPS II Schwartz *et al.* (2007) found an overall prevalence of 10 of 77 (13 per cent), with a higher prevalence in the severe phenotype. Rujter *et al.* (2008) described in MPS IIIC a prevalence of epilepsy (10/22 patients) similar to our sample, but the mean age at onset of epilepsy was higher (23 years, with a range of 16–33) than that of our cases. On the contrary, Nidiffer and Kelly (1983) reported a lower age at onset in 30 children with Sanfilippo disease, which was closer to our findings. It is possible that this difference of

Table 2. Outcome in patients with epilepsy

Case No.	Type of seizure	Drugs	Seizure-free	Side effects
1	Complex partial seizures (Fig. 1)	VPA	Yes	No
2	Generalized tonic-clonic seizures	CBZ	No	No
3	Autonomic signs (Fig. 2)	VPA	Yes	No
4	Clonic seizures (partial?)	LTG	No	No
5	Generalized epileptic status	TPM + PHT	Yes	No
6	Generalized tonic-clonic seizures	OXC	Yes	No
7	Generalized tonic-clonic seizures	VPA	Yes	No
8	Complex partial seizures evolving to generalized	VPA	Yes	No
9	Generalized tonic during sleep + complex partial with automatism	OXC	No	No
10	Epileptic status + partial seizures	PB	No	No
11	Seizures and pseudoseizures	CBZ	Yes	No
12	Simple partial motor	PB	Yes	No
13	Generalized tonic-clonic seizures	LEV	Yes	No

VPA, valproic acid; CBZ, carbamazepine; LTG, lamotrigine; TPM, topiramate; PHT, phenytoin; OXC, oxcarbamazepine; PB, phenobarbital; LEV, levetiracetam.

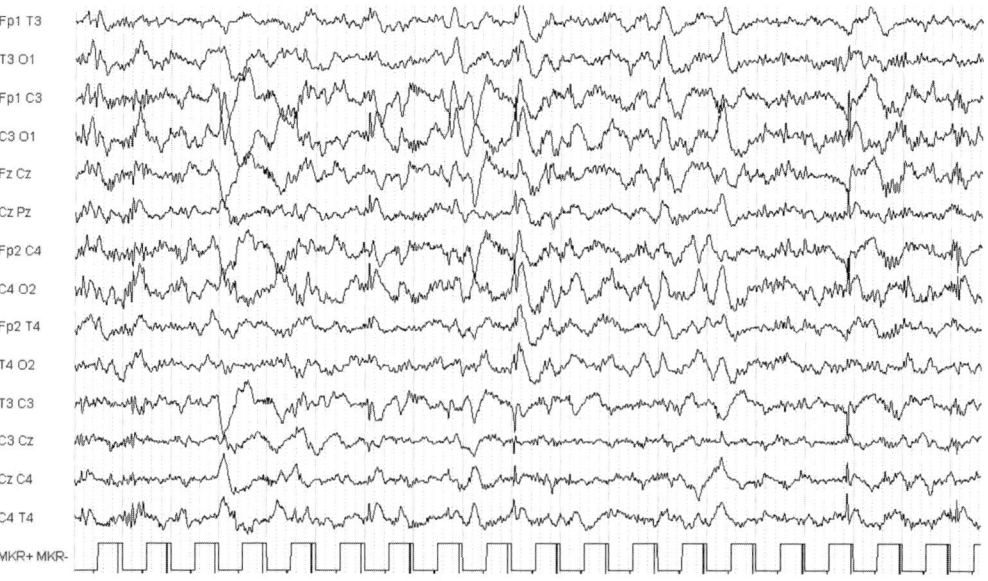

Fig. 1. Left temporal partial spikes on sleep EEG in patient with MPS II.

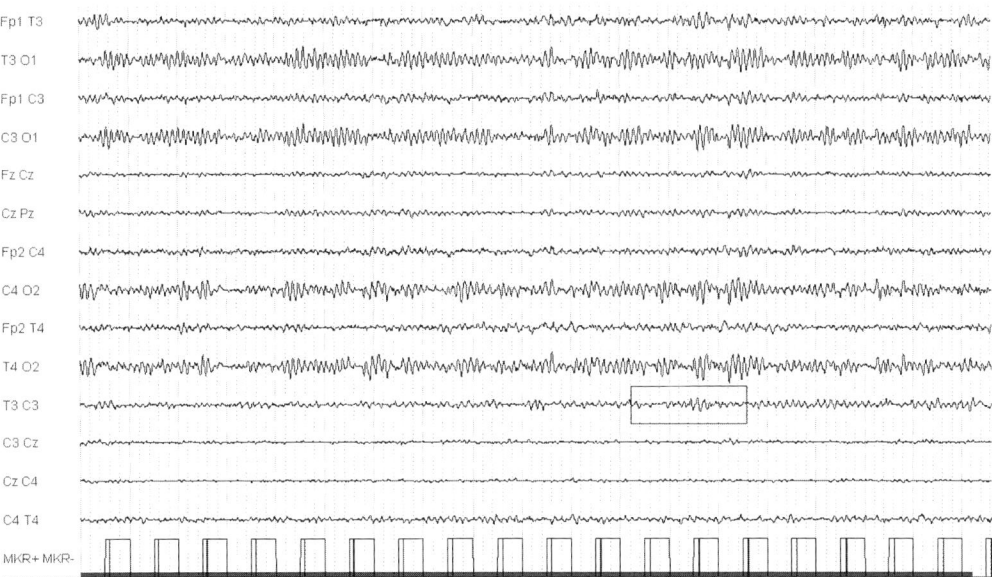

Fig. 2. Normal background activity and left temporal partial 'theta pointu' on the awake EEG in a patient with MPS IS.

age at onset is due to the fact that while our MPS III patients are mostly affected with MPS IIIA, all the patients described by Ruijter *et al.* had MPS IIIC, which is heterogeneous in its clinical severity, but probably less severe than MPS IIIA (Valstar *et al.*, 2008). Azevedo *et al.* (2004) reported the occurrence of epilepsy in 5/28 MPS VI patients with a mean age of 8 years (range 4–15) The lack of epilepsy in our group of patients with MPS VI may be occasional or may depend on the lower age of our patients in comparison to the mean age of the group studied by these authors. Similarly, the mean age of 8 years in the MPS I patients with transplants is too low to rule out the risk of epileptic seizures in these patients.

Partial seizures (8/13) are the predominant clinical types in our sample, whereas generalized seizures occurred only in five cases. Few reports describe the clinical type of the seizures in MPS patients. Wraith *et al.* (2008) reported both generalized and partial seizures in MPS II, in concordance with our observations. In this group of patients with frequent severe impairment of cognitive function, the type of the crisis may be difficult to recognize. The detailed information about signs and symptoms related to the crisis, useful to determine the partial or generalized nature of the seizures, most frequently may only be obtained from witnesses (*e.g.*, parents or teachers), but rarely from the patients themselves, thereby missing the whole report of subjective symptoms. Complex partial seizures with impairment of consciousness only or simple partial seizures with autonomic signs or symptoms such as flushing or pallor are most often missed in these patients. Moreover, in the event of generalized seizures, their partial onset may not be recognized if the clinical manifestations are only subjective symptoms.

It is important to recognize the epileptic nature of these subtle episodes in order to diagnose the epilepsy at its onset and establish appropriate pharmacologic therapy to treat the seizures and prevent the occurrence of generalized tonic–clonic seizures or status epilepticus in the course of disease. In fact, in our sample complex partial seizures anticipated the occurrence of generalized seizures in 2 patients (cases 8 and 9) and a generalized status epilepticus in one patient (case 10). The lower mean age at onset of epilepsy in our cohort compared with reports in the literature may depend on the earliest recognition of the epileptic nature of subtle seizures.

Additionally, also recognizing that some 'crises' are nonepileptic in nature, even in epileptic patients, is the key for planning appropriate therapy: 'Pseudoseizures' may occur and can mimic epileptic seizures, probably involving a neurologic network different from that of cortical neurons (*e.g.*, the extrapyramidal system). We suggest that attention be brought to bear on differentiating epileptic seizures from nonepileptic crises so that the appropriate therapy may be instituted.

We were unable to find any report in the literature about the occurrence of status epilepticus in MPS patients, although it was quite a common event (15 per cent) in our epileptic patients. In 8/13 patients (73 per cent) the epileptic seizures were totally responsive to conventional treatment at prevalently low dose, with no adverse events, showing that, unlike the case with other genetic disorders, there is no need for special drugs or complex treatments in most patients with MPS.

We emphasize the practice of prescribing low-dosage medication, preferably as monotherapy, in order to prevent adverse effects, mainly on wakefulness and cognitive function, considering that these patients are affected by progressive cerebral damage and may suffer from an impairment of drug metabolism due to liver involvement of the disease. In the two patients with status epilepticus good results were obtained with intravenous diazepam (DZP).

Conclusions

Epilepsy is a frequent event during the lifetime of MPS patients. Approximately more than one-third of patients in our cohort developed seizures at a mean age of 14 years (range 13–20). Affected patients were those with MPS II and III and those with MPS I who did not undergo HSCT. Seizures were most frequently partial or secondarily generalized. All patients showed good response to treatment and 9/13 are actually seizure-free and without adverse effects on low-dose treatment. Status epilepticus occurred in two patients and was easily treated with benzodiazepines.

We stress the importance of early recognition of subtle seizures as epileptic in MPS patients in order to establish the proper diagnosis and the appropriate treatment. We also would like to highlight the relevance of differentiating seizures from pseudoseizures so that each disorder can be treated appropriately.

Acknowledgments: We gratefully acknowledge the Fondazione Pierfranco e Luisa Mariani for its generous economic support to the Rare Metabolic Disease Unit.

References

Azevedo, A.C., Schwartz, I.V., Kalakun, L., Brustolin, S., Burin, M.G., Beheregaray, A.P., Leistner, S., Giugliani, C., Rosa, M., Barrios, P., Marinho, D., Esteves, P., Valadares, E., Boy, R., Horovitz, D., Mabe, P., da Silva, L.C., de Souza, I.C., Ribeiro, M., Martins, A.M., Palhares, D., Kim, C.A. & Giugliani, R. (2004): Clinical and biochemical study of 28 patients with mucopolysaccharidosis type VI. *Clin. Genet.* **66,** 208–213.

Nidiffer, F.D. & Kelly, T.E. (1983): Developmental and degenerative patterns associated with cognitive, behavioural and motor difficulties in the Sanfilippo syndrome: an epidemiological study. *J. Ment. Defic. Res.* **2,** 185–203.

Ruijter, G.J.G., Valstar, M.J., van de Kamp, J.M., van der Helm, R.M., Durand, S., Diggelen, O.P., Wevers, R.A., Porthuis, B.J., Pshezhetsky, A.V. & Wijburg, F.A. (2008): Clinical spectrum of Sanfilippo type C (MPS IIIC) disease in the Netherlands. *Mol. Genet. Metab.* **93,** 104–111.

Schwartz, I.V., Ribeiro, M.G., Mota, J.G., Toralles, M.B., Correia, P., Horovitz, D., Santos, E.S., Monlleo, I.L., Fett-Conte, A.C., Sobrinho, R.P., Norato. D.Y., Paula, A.C., Kim, C.A., Duarte, A.R., Boy, R., Valadares, E., De Michelena, M., Mabe, P., Martinhago, C.D., Pina-Neto, J.M., Kok, F., Leistner-Segal, S., Burin, M.G. & Giugliani, R., *et al.* (2007): A clinical study of 77 patients with mucopolysaccharidosis type II. *Acta Paediatr. Suppl.* **96,** 63–70.

Vijay, S. & Wraith, J.E. (2005): Clinical presentation and follow-up of patients with the attenuated phenotype of mucopolysaccharidosis type I. *Acta Paediat.* **94,** 872–877.

Valstar, M.J., Ruijter, G.J.G., van Diggelen, O.P., Poorthuis, B.J. & Wijburg, F.A. (2008): Sanfilippo syndrome: a mini review. *J. Inherit. Metab. Dis.* **31,** 240–252.

Wraith, J.E., Scarpa, M., Beck, M., Bodamer, O.A., De Meirleir, L., Guffon, N., Meldgaard Lund, A., Malm, G., van der Ploeg, A.T. & Zeman, J. (2008): Mucopolysaccharidosis type II (Hunter syndrome): a clinical review and recommendations for treatment in the era of enzyme replacement therapy. *Eur. J. Pediatr.* **167,** 267–277.

Chapter 8

Psychological assessment and support for patients with mucopolysaccharidosis

Milena Marini and Alessio Gamba*

Centre for Metabolic Diseases, Fondazione MBBM, San Gerardo Hospital, via Pergolesi 33, 20052 Monza (MB), Italy
* *Developmental Psychology Unit, San Gerardo Hospital, 20052 Monza, Italy*
milena.marini@libero.it

Summary

Treatment of patients with mucopolysaccharidosis (MPS) needs a multidisciplinary team in order to most effectively manage all the different aspects of this complex of diseases. In this chapter, we will present our experience with MPS patients in which a clinical psychologist is part of the MPS care team with the remit of providing psychological assessment and support for these patients. We describe here the procedures used in our centre. First, a psychological assessment is scheduled to monitor disease progression and the well-being of the patient in order to recommend specific interventions. This assessment is multidimensional, encompassing cognitive, communicative, and relational abilities, regulation of affect, and evaluation of daily living skills. Psychological interventions are planned to help patients and their family to cope with the disease, providing functional strategies and modifying dysfunctional ones. Starting from the assessment sessions, we organize specific programs and interventions for each patient, in which we also consider the wellness of the entire family. Counselling and psychological support may help parents to cope with their child's behavioural problems as well as with their own anxieties and distress. Psychological intervention also fosters good communication between parents, school, and rehabilitation and health care providers in order to create the atmosphere of trust and support that is necessary to deal with these disorders.

Introduction

The mucopolysaccharidoses (MPSs) are complex diseases whose consequences affect many bodily systems and may lead to organ damage. There is a great deal of variation in the severity of clinical features and different levels of disability involving physical, cognitive, and psychological development. About 50 per cent of MPS patients show cognitive impairment. For those patients, we generally observe slow progress in development at the beginning of the disease, followed later by a regression, with the loss of previously acquired skills (autonomy, language, and motor and cognitive abilities) up to the point of early death in cases of severe multi-organ disease. The other patients, without cognitive impairment, are facing the progressive loss of motor or sensory functions during their lifetime, which gradually reduces their day-to-day autonomy and their ability to interact with other people.

To effectively care for these patients and their families a multi-dimensional and multi-professional patient-tailored approach is required. Additionally, particular attention must be paid to the psychological dimensions of the disease (Bax & Coville, 1995), both for these patients and for their families, in which the evolution of the disease is taken into account and the most appropriate treatments carried out. For such a complex disease it is important to involve a clinical psychologist amongst those taking care of these patients.

Assessment session: the need for evaluation

Which is the real meaning of psychological assessment? What does 'to assess' mean in this context? What do we want to assess?

Psychological assessment is a process that usually involves the integration of information from multiple sources – objective measures with subjective perceptions – in order to obtain a complete picture of the individual we meet. (Kaplan & Saccuzzo, 2005). In MPS, this assessment is an important element in understanding the natural history of the disease as manifested in a specific individual as well as a way to observe the effects of treatment. It is a tool to understand how patients and parents live and how they feel about their life with MPS.

What is the real meaning of MPS for patients and their family? The main critical issues for both the patient and his or her family are shown in Table 1.

Table 1. The main critical issues for patients with MPS and their parents

For patient	For parents
Altered cognitive development	Heavy care demands
Sensory and motor deficits	Disease evolution anxiety
Lack of autonomy	Narcissistic wound
Damaged body image	Collapse of parents' expectations
Diminished expectations of life	Sense of genetic fault
	Sense of social isolation and loneliness

Procedures for psychological assessment must necessarily involve a multidimensional evaluation of different aspects of the disease as it affects the patient: cognitive, communicative, and relational abilities, the affect regulation, the attainment of daily living skills, and the patient's perception of his or her well-being. Because of the rapid regression in skills and behaviour experienced in the severe form of the disorder, frequent monitoring is required so that necessary changes in the individualized educational plan can quickly be made to support the child whose skills are deteriorating.

We use a scheduled assessment of cognitive, affective and communicative abilities with observational procedures, standardized and adapted tests, and clinical interviews with parents to obtain a regular, comprehensive evaluation of the disease, the efficacy of treatment, and the state of family functioning. Table 2 lists the main assessment tools used in our centre

Assessment sessions are held during the routine clinical follow-up of the patients in order to have repeated measures of clinical conditions and psychological issues. Usually an assessment session is held at diagnosis in order to establish a baseline for each patient, and then scheduled for every six months (at the beginning) or once a year, depending on the patient's needs.

Particular attention is paid to the quality of life, which in the end is the real goal of our interventions, both psychological and medical. The World Health Organization (WHO) defines quality of life as 'physical, social and emotional aspects of a patient's well-being that are

Table 2. Assessment tools used in the centre in San Gerardo Hospital in Monza

	Assessment tools	Functional domains evaluated	Age range and notes
Developmental scales	Bayley scales of infant and toddler development	Cognitive abilities Motor abilities Behaviour observations	0–48 months
	Griffiths mental development scales	Personal-social skills Locomotor skills Understanding and speech Eye and hand coordination Performance	1–8 years
Cognitive function	Wechsler scales (Wechsler, 2008)	Verbal and performance cognitive domains General intellectual ability	WPPSI (children aged 2 years, 5 months–7 years, 3 months) WISC (children aged 6–16 years) WAIS (adults aged 16–89)
	Leiter–R (Roid & Miller, 1997)	Visualization and reasoning Attention and memory Nonverbal cognitive abilities	From 2 years old
Adaptive behaviour	Vineland adaptive behavior scales (Sparrow et al., 2005)	Communication Daily living skills Socialization Motor skills Maladaptive behaviour	From 6 years to adult (structured interview for caregivers of children and adult with disability)
Quality of life	Peds-QL (Varni, 1998)	Physical functioning Emotional functioning Social functioning School functioning	2–18 years
	EQ–5D (self-report form and proxy form)	Health status	Adult version
	MPS HAQ (Italian version, 2004)	Functional capabilities and performance in children and adults with MPS	From 14 years old: self-report form For child < 14, or for patient with severe disability: proxy form
Parental distress	Nonstructured clinical interview		

relevant and important to the individual' (WHO, 2004). But how can we understand how our patients really feel? Is it possible to know that in a patient with a very severe disability? We usually use a number of questionnaires and scales (*e.g.*, EQ-5d, PedsQl, MPS HAQ) to collect different kinds of information (physical indexes and emotional and psychosocial functioning) in order to have a more complete view. The gold standard should be to collect self-reported data, where possible, selecting, for example, the more simple questionnaires, and then to complete the picture with observational data and caregivers' observations or questionnaires by proxy.

Methodologic problems

Progressive regression of the patient's health in MPS and continuous decreases in abilities make assessment quite difficult. We often have only minimal existing abilities to measure in a patient with a severe disease burden, and again we have to ask 'How can we meet that individual beyond his or her disability?'.

Accuracy of instruments and *biases in setting* are the two main methodologic problems we encounter in this situation, and this has consequences on test validity. First, the most common psychological tests are not specific for this complex population, in which there are a wide range of physical, sensory, and motor deficits (Martin *et al.*, 2008), so often our patients show very poor results because of these deficits. Among biases due to the setting, we have to consider the emotional distress inherent in the hospital environment to which our patients have been admitted (Kaplan & Saccuzzo, 2005) and its role on the patient's responses.

Specific attention should also be paid when parents take part in the assessment session, and sometimes act as intermediaries, interpreting the patient's responses from their own points of view. In such situations, we have to learn to interpret their interference and attributions, and, while it is impossible to avoid these biases, we can use them in a diagnostic perspective, for example, in observing the quality of the parent–child relationship.

Thus, our first step in organizing a valid assessment session, with comparable measures, is to find appropriate instruments, or better yet, to adapt scales usually used in different contexts, (*e.g.* Wechsler scales, developmental scales, and so on) and to use them with these patients who have severe physical and sensory disabilities. A good knowledge of the patient, using information gathered from a previous observation as well as information from others who have attended to the child, as well as longitudinal observations with repeated measures, may help us in doing this (Martin *et al.*, 2008) as much as the specific experience of a psychologist in disability management.

Another thing that must be considered is the meaning of the testing session for the parents. Often they have a great deal of stress during testing, fearing that they are about to hear a 'sentence' pronounced about their child. It is very important to give them a synthesis about what happened during the testing, because the resulting information could reinforce a picture of a 'damaged child' or, on the other hand, it could give a picture of a child with serious difficulties, but who is nevertheless still functioning despite disability. This helps families to preserve a balance between an illness-affected experience of life with a healthy one; and this is important for the patient too: finding functional areas, beyond disability, may help the patient to preserve a notion of self-efficacy (Bandura, 1982).

Psychological intervention

In a holistic approach to MPS care, assessment work becomes the first step in setting up a personalized care plan for each patient. A good assessment is foundational in planning for interventions (*e.g.*, psychological, educational) and setting appropriate goals for (and with) each patient and his or her family.

The complexity of these rare diseases requires a corresponding, complex 'caring niche' (Axia, 2004) involving different 'players', including school personnel, health care providers, and persons working in rehabilitation centres. Psychological intervention has to promote communication and collaboration amongst all of them to create the atmosphere of trust and support that is so necessary to treat these patients.

Psychological support for the patient

Which kind of support should be given for patients with MPS?

First we have to identify the functional and dysfunctional personal resources of each patient – and assessment work makes this possible – in order to support or to modify them.

Psychological support means that we must talk about MPS with the MPS patient. In making a diagnosis it is first necessary to obtain an informed consent by the patient to therapy; this engenders better compliance and a better psychosocial response (Gamba & Saccomani, 2003), even when there is cognitive impairment. Psychological support also means encouraging the patient and family to take part in personalized rehabilitative programs; there are many such programs providing strategies, psychoeducational programs, or rehabilitative methods, such as the TEACCH approach (Schopler & Olley, 1982; Watson *et al.*, 1989), or Augmentative-Alternative Communication (Wheeler *et al.*, 1983) – all aimed at helping the child to achieve a good quality of life.

Psychological support for the family

We cannot forget the family, which is wholly and primarily involved in the heavy burden of daily care. Parents usually have many stressors coming from all directions, including the frequency of medical appointments, repeated hospital admissions, or trips to the emergency room (Macias *et al.*, 2006). Much parental distress is caused as their children have progressive cognitive impairment: often they lose language skills and become increasingly unable to communicate with their parents (Kratz *et al.*, 2009).

The diagnosis of MPS causes a wound in parental attitudes; after the diagnosis, the parents lose the 'idealized child' (and the idealized parents, too) and must instead accommodate the notion of a 'damaged child', without the future they had envisaged for the child. They find themselves in a very different and difficult situation that is very far from anything they might choose for themselves or their family.

Parents often feel guilty because of the genetic origin of MPS, and because they 'gave' abnormal chromosomes to their child. In the inner world of these parents, depression, overprotection, and angry and guilty feelings must be managed. (Seligman & Darling, 2007). So, in order to help parents to cope with this situation, we have to sustain their parental identity and buttress their coping resources, for example, by supporting the parent–child relationship. At the same time, we cannot forget the necessity of working through emotions to enable the expression and management of the parents' feelings (Winnicott, 1960).

Some critical moments in disease progression needs specific attention. The first point occurs at the time of diagnosis, which is sometimes made after the parents have endured a long and fraught course of seeing their child undergo a number of diagnostic procedures; this is accompanied by a high level of anxiety about prognosis. Other key moments are during treatment planning (*e.g.* by enzyme replacement therapy or bone marrow transplantation), when changes occur during therapy, when there is a regression in skill levels, and, of course, during palliative care.

All of the family, not only the parents, are affected by the stresses of daily care and the psychological needs of the other children in the family need to be considered as well: How do siblings live their experience? Siblings (Atkins, 1989) often have to cope with the heavy demands of the health problem of their brother or sister, with parental anxiety, and with parents who are less available to them as they are involved in the daily care of the sick child. Sometimes they find it difficult to talk with others about their sibling's disease and they do not always have complete comprehension of it. Therefore it is important to include them in communication sessions and to monitor their psychological well-being. Also, because of the genetic origin of these diseases, the siblings may feel some sense of burden and responsibility and fear for their own future as well. Specifically targeted genetic counselling (Brunger *et al.*, 2000) and appropriate support should be offered to them as well, according to their developmental age, to preserve or sustain a healthy self-image, mainly when they are immune carriers.

Conclusions

A psychological approach to MPS is necessary because MPS involves not only the patient, but also a complex interactional system including the school, peer group, family, and health care professionals, among others. Beyond the issues of disease progression, it is necessary to be aware of the severe psychological burden that MPS imposes, to differing degrees, on each member of this system. Medical and psychological approaches need to be fully integrated from the time of diagnosis as life goes on through all the stages of disease. Such assistance will help the patient and the persons he or she depends on and interacts with to live their lives as fully as possible. Facilitating communication, buttressing coping skills, and watching for signs of personal distress in all the involved parties are the key concepts of the personalized care that such a devastating disease demands.

References

Atkins, S. (1989): Siblings of handicapped children. *Child Adolesc. Social Work J.* **6**, 271–282.

Axia, V. (2004): *Psycho-oncology manual*. Roma: Carocci ed.

Bandura, A. (1982): Self-efficacy mechanism in human agency. *Am. Psychol.* **37**, 122–147.

Bax, M.C. & Colville, G.A. (1995): Behaviour in mucopolysaccharide disorders. *Arch. Dis. Child.* **73**, 77–81.

Bayley, N. (1993): *Bayley's scales of infant development*, 2nd ed. San Antonio, TX: The Psychological Corporation.

Brunger, J.W., Murray, G.S., O'Riordan, M., Matthews, A.L., Smith, R.J. & Robin, N.H. (2000): Parental attitudes toward genetic testing for pediatric deafness. *Am. J. Hum. Genet.* **67**, 1621–1625.

EuroQol Group.EQ-5D. www.euroqol.org.

Gamba, A. & Saccomani, R. (2003): *Oggi comando io: psicologia, etica ed economia sanitaria nella cura delle malattie oncologiche pediatriche*. Milano: Cortina.

Genzyme Corporation. MPS I Registry. www.lsdregistry.net

Kaplan, M. & Saccuzzo, D. (2005): *Psychological testing: principles, applications, and issues*, 6th ed. Belmont, CA: Wadsworth/Thomson.

Kratz, L., Uding, N., Trahms, C.M., Villareale, N. & Kieckhefer, G.M. (2009): Managing childhood chronic illness: parent perspectives and implications for parent-provider relationships. *Fam. Syst. Health* **27**, 303–313.

Macias, M.M., Roberts, K.M., Saylor, C.F. & Fussell, J.J. (2006): Toileting concerns, parenting stress, and behavior problems in children with special health care needs. *Clin. Pediatr. (Phila)* **45**, 415–422.

Martin, H.R., Poe, M.D., Reinhartsen, D., Pretzel, R.E., Roush, J., Rosenmberg, A., Dusing, S.C. & Escolar, M.L. (2008): Methods for assessing neurodevelopment in lysosomal storage disases and related disorders: a multidisciplinary perspective. *Acta Paediatr. Suppl.* **457**, 69–75.

Roid, G. & Miller, L. (1997): *Leiter international performance scale revised*, 2nd ed. Wood Dale, IL: Stoelting.

Schopler, E. & Olley, J. (1982): Comprehensive educational services for autistic children: the TEACCH model. In: *The handbook of school psychology*, eds. R Reynolds & T.B. Gutkin. New York, NY: Wiley.

Seligman, M. & Darling, R.B. (2007): *A systems approach to childhood disability*, 3rd ed., pp. 434. New York: Guilford Press.

Sparrow, S., Cicchetti, D.V. & Balla, D.A. (2005): *Vineland adaptive behaviour scales*, 2nd ed. San Antonio, TX: The Psychological Corporation.

Varni, J.W. (1998): The Peds-QL measurement model for pediatric quality of life. www.pedsql.org

Watson, L., Lord, C., Schaffer, B. & Schopler, E. (1989): *Teaching spontaneous communication to autistic and developmentally handicapped children*. New York: Irvingstone.

Wechsler, D. (2008): Wechsler Intelligence Scale for children, 4th ed. San Antonio, TX: The Psychological Corporation.

Wheeler, J., Kangas, K.A., Brankin, G., Cochran, P.R. & Freagon, S. (1983): Alternative communication systems for severely handicapped students. In: *Curricular processes for the school and community integration of severely handicapped students ages 6–21: Project replication guide*, eds. S. Freagon, J. Wheeler, G. Brankin, K. McDannel, D. Costello & W.M. Peters, pp. 168–196. Washington, DC: Government Printing Office.

Williams, P.D., Williams, A., Graff, J.C., Hanson, S., Stanton, A., Hafeman, C., Liebergen, S., Leuenberg, K., Setter, R., Ridder, L., Curry, L., Barnard, M. & Sanders, S. (2002): Interrelationships among variables affecting well siblings and mothers in families of children with a chronic illness or disability. *J. Behav. Med.* **25,** 411–424.

Winnicott, D.W. (1960): The theory of the parent–infant relationship, *Int. J. Psycho-Anal.* **41,** 585–595.

Chapter 9

Mucopolysaccharidosis: radiologic findings

Marco Grimaldi, Daniela Di Marco and Paolo Remida

UOS Neuroradiologia, Servizio di Radiodiagnostica, Risonanza Magnetica Nucleare, Azienda Ospedaliera San Gerardo, University of Milano–Bicocca, via Pergolesi 33, 20052 Monza, Italy
m.grimaldi@hsgerardo.org

Summary

With the development of new technologies, the role of the radiologist in the diagnosis and management of rare diseases is changing, gaining importance both at the time of diagnosis as well as during follow-up, particularly with regard to providing morphologic and functional information about lesion burden, related clinical risks, and response to therapy. The diagnosis of MPS is based on clinical, radiologic, and biochemical criteria, but after the clinician has raised the suspicion, the first evaluation often needs to be done by the radiologist, who aids in recognizing the most significant pictures of the disease and pointing out the most accurate means to prevent complications. Conventional radiology, CT, and MRI give data for an accurate study of morphologic modifications associated with MPS, but these modalities are now also considered useful in functional assessment, for example, airway evaluation with MDCT in planning surgical and other procedures requiring anaesthesia.

Introduction

One of the main features of the mucopolysaccharidoses (MPSs), as for other thesaurismoses, is multi-systemic involvement: for this reason the role of radiologic examination, not only in the study of the skeletal system, but also in morphofunctional evaluation of other organs and systems, is fundamental in developing a diagnostic and flow chart.

Imaging is particularly significant:
- at the time of diagnosis, directly indicating the etiology or establishing a correlation between the dysostotic picture and clinical suspicion;
- determining lesion burden;
- defining and dealing with complications;
- and evaluating the response to therapy at follow-up examination.

The diagnosis of MPS is based on clinical, radiologic, and biochemical criteria; although there are no direct pathognomonic radiologic signs to assign a dysmorphic picture to this group of diseases, many radiologic images can suggest the possibility of a particular disease or confirm the diagnosis.

The main radiologic feature in MPS is the presence of complex skeletal malformations, known as 'dysostosis multiplex', and multiple skeletal malformations are present even in other storage diseases such as mucolipidoses (II and III or pseudo-Hurler disease) (Robinson *et al.*, 2002), multiple sulphatase deficiency, and GM I gangliosidosis. The expression 'dysostosis multiplex' is used to describe a range of skeletal malformations, dysplasias, and dysmorphisms, whose presence and associations represent a picture suggestive of MPS or other storage diseases (Weisstein *et al.*, 2004).

In MPS the development of such skeletal malformations correlates with the pathogenesis of the disease and particularly with cellular dysfunction and reduced resistance of the bone matrix because of a deficit in metabolism of glycosaminoglycans (GAGs).

This is particularly evident in periods of fast development and growth, in which important modifications in bone and cartilage remodeling processes take place.

Although the basis of abnormalities in the development of bone and cartilage is not fully understood, investigations performed in animal models suggest that GAG accumulation promotes inflammation, with tumor necrosis factor (TNF-α) and other inflammatory cytokines released from chondrocytes, resulting in apoptosis. In addition, matrix metalloproteinases (MMPs) are released, contributing to the destruction of bone and joints (Pastores *et al.*, 2008).

Dysplasias and dysmorphisms with abnormalities in the shape of skeletal segments and growth retardation, which have consequences on static and dynamic functions, demonstrate the progressive, invalid-making osteoarthropathies developed by MPS patients during the course of the disease.

Because both the clinical presentation and the development of the disease may vary widely both within and between the seven major types of MPS, even the distribution and the extent of bone alterations are not always the same. This reflects both the different characteristics in the biochemical deficit (for example, there is a predominance of bone involvement in MPS IH, I, and VI) and the different expression of the disease's seriousness within the same group in the phenotype (for example, it is more severe in MPS IH than in MPS IH-S) (Giugliani *et al.*, 2007).

Nevertheless, a certain uniformity of signs can be recognized in radiologic images; these signs, regardless of their extent, are typical for this group of diseases.

Radiologic findings

The main manifestations of dysostosis are observed in the skull, vertebrae, ribs, clavicles, long bone diaphyses, hands, and hip.

Skull

Modifications in the skull are represented essentially by macrocephaly with dolicocephaly and presence of a vertical frontal crest (due to premature suture closure and metopic perisutural hyperostosis). The cortical bone of the skull is thickened; the sella turcica is usually wide with long clinoid apophyses and with horizontal orientation (so called 'J-shaped sella'); and platibasia can be found (Fig. 1).

Facial anomalies include bone dysplasias, lack of pneumatization of mastoid process cells and of paranasal cavities, and an obtuse mandibular angle with prognathism; the teeth are usually widely spaced.

Chapter 9 Mucopolysaccharidosis: radiologic findings

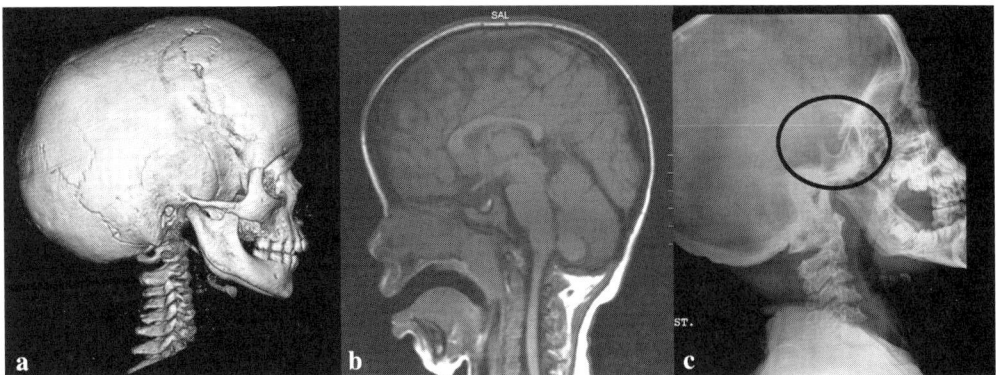

Fig. 1. (a) MDCT-3D reconstruction in patient with MPS IH; (b) MRI-T1W sagittal plane in patient with MPS VI; and (c) skull radiograph in patient with MPS II showing J-shaped sella.

Spine

Anomalies in the vertebral column are very frequent and are the basis of important complications due to the possible compressive effects on the spinal cord and emerging nerve roots.

Malformations involve the shape of vertebral bodies (growth retardation or absence of ossification nuclei), and hypoplasia of anterosuperior corners can be seen, especially at the thoracolumbar passage (D12, L1 and L2) and proximal thoracic tract. The vertebral bodies can show a typical aspect, with apparent prolongation of the anteroinferior corner, so called 'tongue-shaped' (Fig. 2), flattened vertebra with anterior beaking, conditioning a disalignment on the sagittal plane with thoracolumbar gibbus deformity associated with kyphoscoliosis, often one of the most important and early clinical signs in all forms of MPS except MPS III.

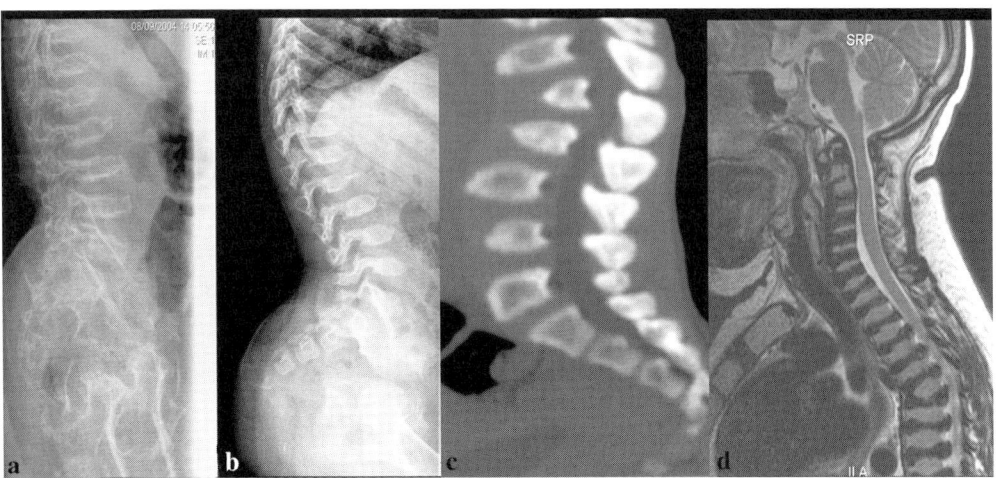

Fig. 2. MPS IV: (a) and (b) Lateral spine radiograph show typical middle or inferiorly beaked vertebral bodies; (c) MDCT/MIP reconstruction of lumbar spine; (d) T_2-weighted MRI midsagittal image of cervical-dorsal spine.

In some cases hypoplasia of both anterior corners gives the vertebral body a wedge shape. Odontoid hypoplasia is a characteristic radiologic finding particularly in MPS IV and then in descending order in MPS I, VI, II and III.

Modification at the craniovertebral junction includes thickening of periodontoid soft tissues and ligaments; these changes can produce stenosis of the spinal canal with risk of instability, causing spinal cord compression with severe neurologic deficits.

Cervical myelopathy may initially present as reduced activity or exercise intolerance; if it remains untreated, irreversible cord damage can occur. For this reason we recommend extensive neuroimaging evaluation, including flexion-extension cervical spine X-ray films, spinal CT scans with 3D reconstructions, MRI and dynamic MRI, with descriptions of the bone abnormalities, dimensions, and dynamic modifications of the spinal canal and measurement of atlantodens interval (ADI is the distance between the posterior surface of the anterior arch of C1 and the anterior surface of the dens, considered abnormal if more than 5 mm) (Giussani *et al.*, 2009; Nader-Sepahi *et al.*, 2005) (Fig. 3).

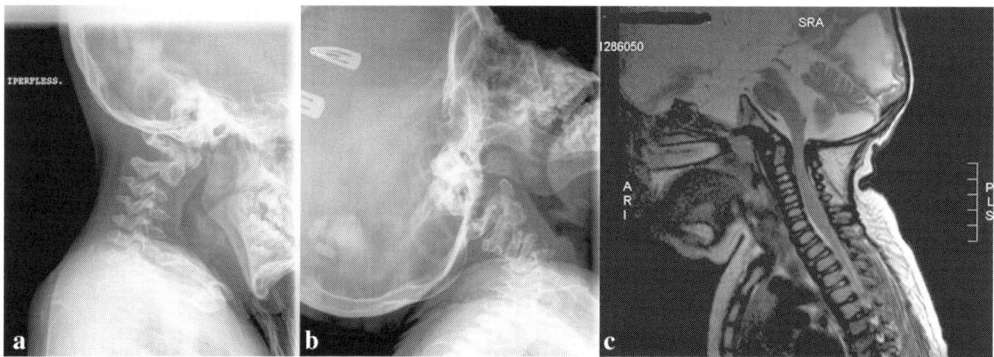

Fig. 3. (a) and (b) Flexion-extension cervical spine X-ray films; (c) T_2-weighted MRI midsagittal image shows narrowing of the arachnoid space at the level of the cranio-cervical junction.

Hands

Characteristic radiologic signs of the hand include wide, short metacarpal bones, with thin cortices and proximal pointing, short and trapezoidal phalanges, and irregular carpal bones. These signs are often associated with clinical syndromes such as carpal tunnel syndrome, and joint stiffness and progressive flexion contractures of the fingers, with claw-hand deformities (Fig. 4).

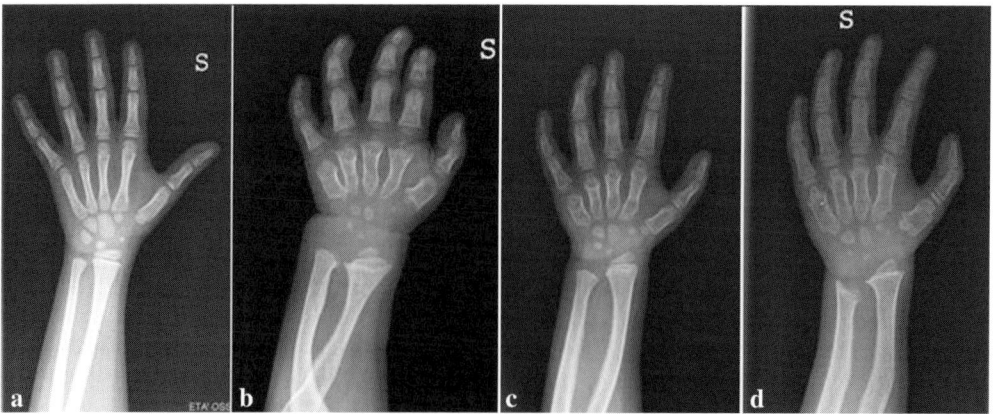

Fig. 4. (a) Healthy 5-year-old subject; (b) A 4-year-old child with MPS I; (c) A 5-year-old child with MPS IH; (d) A 6-year-old child with MPS IV. Wide, short metacarpal bones, proximal pointing, short and trapezoidal phalanges, and hypoplastic carpal bones are seen. Curved diaphyses were noted for the distal radius and ulna.

Thorax

The most common and significant modifications in the thorax affect the clavicles, which are short and thickened in the medium tract, and the ribs, which are horizontal and so-called 'paddle'- or 'oar'-shaped. The scapulae can be small, with flattened glenoid cavities, while the sternum is usually short in MPS IV (Fig. 5).

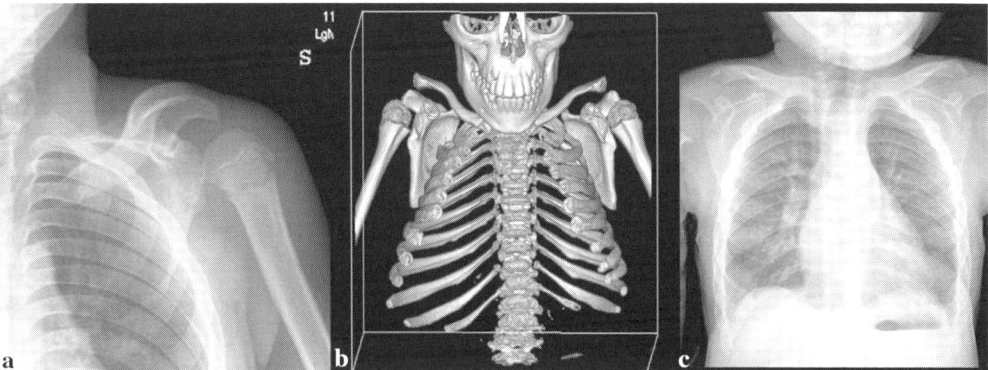

Fig. 5. (a) Short thick clavicles in MPS II; MDCT 3D reconstruction showing paddle-shaped ribs in MPS IV (b); (c) short thick clavicles in MPS VI.

Pelvis

The radiologic picture of the pelvis is characterized by tapered iliac bases with rounded iliac wings, hypoplastic acetabulum, wide cotilis, coxa valga, and small and flattened cephalic femoral nuclei. These alterations clinically determine progressive arthropathy and high frequency of hip subluxation (Fig. 6).

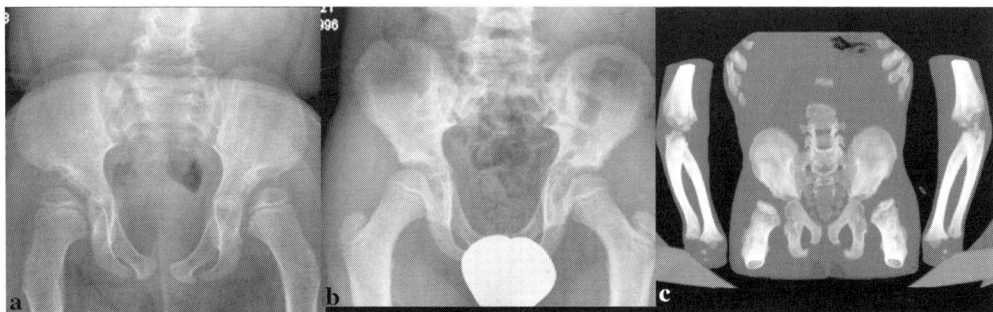

Fig. 6. Rounded iliac wings with inferior tapering, hypoplastic acetabulum, and bilateral coxa valga seen in (a) MPS I, (b) MPS II, and (c) MPS IV.

Long bones

Long bone diaphyses appear shortened, distally curved, wide and stick-shaped (except in MPS IV, in which they are thinner but present severe alterations of epiphyseal-metaphyseal junctures). The cortical bone is thin with moderate osteoporosis. Femoral findings show great diagnostic significance, with a small femoral head and narrow neck; the lateral tibial emiplate is hypoplastic and results in valgism of the knees (Fig. 7).

The skeletal age in always retarded compared to the recorded age (except for MPS III).

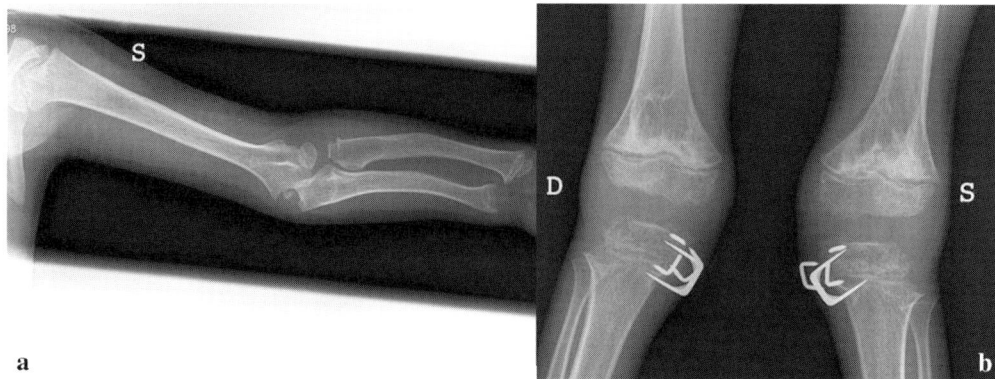

Fig. 7. (a) Radiograph of upper extremity shows curved diaphyses and hypoplastic distal ulna and radius; (b) valgism of the knees in MPS IV is shown.

MRI brain findings

Cerebral features and related MRI findings in MPS can be grouped in three main lesion patterns:
(1) dilated perivascular spaces (due to extra-cellular storage);
(2) dilated ventricular cavities; and
(3) demyelinated and gliotic areas (Fig. 8).

Perivascular space dilatation, the most characteristic modification in this group of diseases, appears as a variable number of small spot-like cystic lesions with CSF-like signal in all sequences. It is probably determined by GAG storage in large inclusions between vascular adventitial cells, typically at basal ganglia, subcortical parietal and occipital white matter, and in the corpus callosum, with radial orientation along the vascular developmental lines (van der Knaap & Valk, 1995).

Widening of liquoral spaces can be caused by hydrocephalus due to pathologic leptomeningeal thickening, with re-absorbition deficit at Pacchioni's granulations and liquoral circulation obstructions (in cases of severe neurologic compromission leading to derivation) or as a consequence of neuronal loss, reduction of associative fibres, and atrophy (Matheus et al., 2004).

Expression of dystrophy, probably on a microvascular basis, was observed in several other diseases that share the same vulnerable areas, such as peritrigonal white matter. Compared to

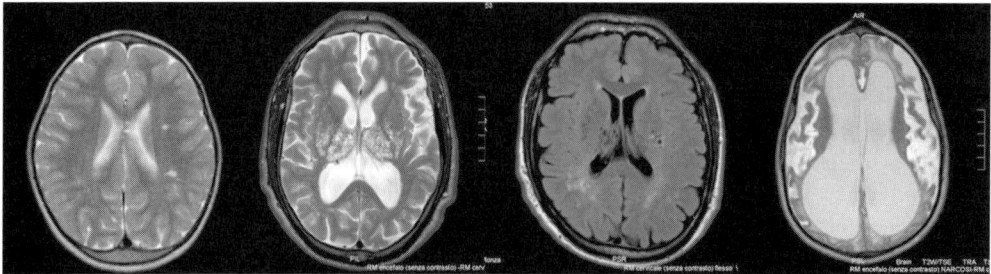

Fig. 8. MRI axial T_2-weighted and FLAIR images show small hyperintense spots, indicative of widened perivascular spaces, gliotic white matter areas, and dilated ventricular cavities.

dilated perivascular spaces, these lesions show hyperintense signals both in T_2-weighted and FLAIR images (Fig. 8).

The relationship between neuroimage findings and mental dysfunction is still controversial, however (Gabrielli et al., 2004; Matheus et al., 2004).

Airway imaging

The advent of multi-detector CT (MDCT) has revolutionized noninvasive imaging of anatomic structures, not only because it allows faster scan speed and better spatial resolution compared to standard helical CT scanners (Ames et al., 2007), but also because it provides the opportunity to reformat images acquired from the same data set.

This allows the rapid obtaining of high-quality two- or three-dimensional reconstruction images (Rydberg et al., 2000), which can be used for different purposes other than the initial aim of the examination.

In our institution patients affected by MPS undergo MDCT examinations to obtain the most accurate evaluation of lesion burden, especially concerning the spine: this fast technique allows us to avoid sedating the patient and to use the same data set for airway analysis.

Patients affected by MPS frequently undergo surgical procedures (otorhinolaryngologic, orthopedic, odontoiatric, neurosurgical, hematologic, and general surgical) and present considerable anaesthesiologic problems, such as difficult intubation, obstruction of upper airways, and thick secretions in the airways (King et al., 1984) For this reason pre-operative airway evaluation is mandatory in patients with MPS.

In view of these clinical demands and the fact that the previous techniques were conventional radiography (Bartz et al., 1999), conventional computerized axial tomography, and fibroendoscopy (which requires sedation, is invasive, and sometimes is unable to provide information about subglottic airways), multi-detector CT (MDCT) also has the advantage of providing a noninvasive airway evaluation (Boiselle et al., 2005).

In a recent clinical study, Shih et al. (2005) using MDCT showed airway modifications in patients affected by MPS. These authors noticed a significant tracheal narrowing and significant modifications in the shape of the tracheal lumen in the pathologic group compared to the 'normal' control group.

Our experience confirms this observation: the preliminary data of our studies (submitted for publication) point to a significant difference in the morphology and in the diameters of the trachea between patients with MPS and those of a control group, with narrowing of the subglottic tract seen in patients with MPS.

The quantification of tracheal stenosis has also been useful for planning anaesthetic procedures (Fig. 9). Although the number of examined patients is still limited, it seems possible to define the most frequent points of stenosis, such as the middle tracheal tract, and probably also non-homogeneous severity of the radiologic pictures in the different subtypes of illness (Fig. 10).

The origin of the tracheal alterations in MPS probably resides in the structure of tissues that compose the trachea, on the anterior side formed by C-shaped rings of hyaline cartilage, and on the posterior side by bundles of smooth muscle and a fibroelastic ligament attached to the perichondrium. Hyaline cartilage contains mainly type II collagen, which is rich in keratan sulphate, whereas the perichondrium possesses type I collagen, which is rich in dermatan sulphate, both glycosaminoglycans whose altered catabolism is considered an expression of illness in some MPSs.

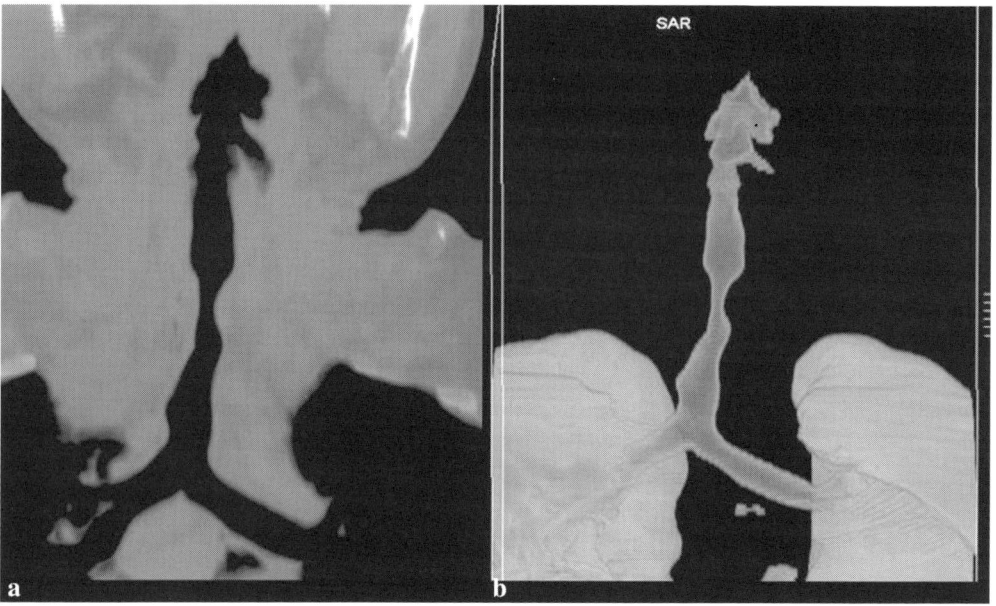

Fig. 9. (a) Coronal minimal intensity projection (MinIP) and (b) 3-dimensional external rendering of the trachea in a patient with MPS IH.

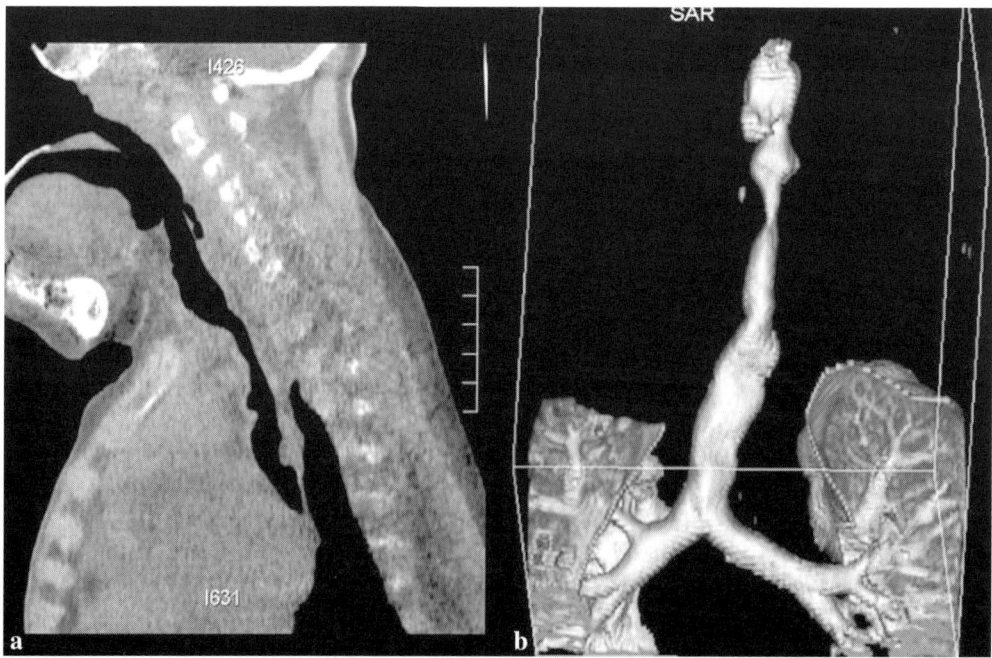

Fig. 10. (a) Sagittal multiplanar reformation image in a patient with MPS IH and (b) three-dimensional volume rendering of the trachea in a patient with MPS VI.

Conclusions

Mucopolysaccharidoses are a group of rare diseases whose early recognition can change the patient's prognosis. The role of the radiologist is important in confirming the diagnosis, even at first diagnostic steps, which are usually simple, conventional radiologic exams required on a clinical basis. There are still no pathognomonic radiologic signs to assign a dysmorphic picture to this group of diseases, but many radiologic pictures can suggest the diagnosis: the presence of 'dysostosis multiplex', a range of skeletal malformations with dysmorphisms and dysplasias that variably involve all skeletal areas, must point the radiologist to a systemic disease. In addition, some radiologic signs, if promptly recognized, are highly suggestive for a storage disease. Examples of these cranial malformations are the typical 'J-shaped sella', dysmorphisms of vertebral bodies (such as anterior corner hypoplasia, frequently found in the proximal thoracic and lumbar tract, leading to early gibbus deformity), dysmorphism of the clavicles, ribs, hip, and hands, and long bone diaphyses.

The knowledge of these alterations forms the basis for their early recognition.

As well, this group of diseases represents an example of how the evolution of technology provides new opportunities for radiologists to play an important role not only in diagnosis, but also in preventing complications and understanding the underlying pathogenetic mechanisms in evaluating the response to therapy.

Examples of these new technologies are CT scans with 3D reconstructions and MRIs for spinal static and dynamic evaluation, MDCT anatomic imaging of the central airways, and recent clinical functional studies with MR spectroscopy (Vedulin, 2007).

References

Ames, W., Macleod, D., Ross, A., Marcus, J. & Mukudan, S. (2007): The novel use of computer generated visual imaging to assess the difficult pediatric airway. *Anesth. Analg.* **104**, 1154–1156.

Bartz, H.J., Wiesner, L. & Wappler, F. (1999): Anaesthetic management of patients with mucopolysaccharidoses IV presenting for major orthopaedic surgery. *Acta Anaesthesiol. Scand.* **43**, 679–683.

Boiselle, P.M., Lee, K.S. & Ernst, A. (2005): Multidetector CT of the central airways. *J. Thorac. Imaging* **20**, 186–195.

Gabrielli, O., Polonara, G., Regnicolo, L., Petroni, V., Scarabino, T., Coppa, G.V. & Salvolini, U. (2004): Correlation between cerebral MRI abnormalities and mental retardation in patients with mucopolysaccharidoses. *Am. J. Med. Genet.* **125A**, 224–231.

Giussani, C., Roux, F.E., Guerra, P., Pirillo, D., Grimaldi, M., Citerio, G. & Sganzerla, E.P. (2009): Severely symptomatic craniovertebral junction abnormalities in children. *Pediatr. Neurosurg.* **45**, 29–36.

Giugliani, R., Harmatz, P. & Wraith, J.E. (2007): Management guidelines for mucopolysaccharidosis VI. *Pediatrics* **120**, 405–418.

King, D.H., Jones, R.M. & Barnett, M.B. (1984): Anhaesthetic considerations in the mucopolysaccharidoses. *Anaesthesia* **39**, 126–131.

Matheus, M.G., Castillo, M., Smith, J.K., Armao, D., Towle, D. & Muenzer, J. (2004): Brain MRI findings in patients with mucopolyssaccharidosis types I and II and mild clinical presentation. *Neuroradiology* **46**, 666–672.

Nader-Sepahi, A., Casey, A.T., Hayward, R., Crockard, H.A. & Thompson, D. (2005): Symptomatic atlantoaxial instability in Down syndrome. *J. Neurosurg.* **103**, 231–237.

Pastores, G.M. (2008): Muscoloskeletal complications encountered in the lysosomal storage disorders. *Best Pract. Res. Clin. Rheumatol.* **22**, 937–947.

Rydberg, J., Buckwalter, K.A., Caldemeyer K.S., Phillips, M.D, Conces, D.J. Jr, Alsen, A.M., Persohn, S.A. & Kopecky, K.K (2000): Multislice CT: scanning techniques applications. *Radiographics* **20**, 1787–1806.

Robinson, C., Baker, N., Noble, J., King, A., David, G., Sillence, D., Hofman, P. & Cundy, T. (2002): The osteodystrophy of mucolipidosis type III and the effects of intravenous pamidronate treatment. *J. Inherit. Metab. Dis.* **25**, 681–686.

Shih, S.L., Lee, Y.J., Sheu, C.Y. & Blickman, J.G. (2002): Airway changes in children with mucopolysaccharidoses. *Acta Radiol.* **43,** 40–43.

van der Knaap, M.S. & Walk, J. (1995): *Magnetic resonance of myelin, myelination, and myelin disorders*, pp. 97–105. Heidelberg: Springer Verlag.

Vedulin, L., Schwartz, I.V.D., Komios, M., Schuch, A., Puga, A.C., Pinto, L.L.C., Pires, A.P. & Giugliani, R. (2007): Correlation of MR imaging and MR spectroscopy findings with cognitive impairment in mucopolysaccharidosis II. *Am. J. Neuroradiol.* **28,** 1029–1033.

Weisstein, J.S., Delgado, E., Steinbach, L.S., Hart, K. & Packman, S. (2004): Musculoskeletal manifestations of Hurler syndrome: long term follow-up after bone marrow transplantation. *J. Pediatr. Orthop.* **24,** 97–101.

Chapter 10

Anaesthesia for children with mucopolysaccharidosis

Pablo Mauricio Ingelmo[*,o] and Emre Sahillioğlu[o,^]

[*] U.O. Anestesia e Rianimazione I, Azienda Ospedaliera San Gerardo, via Pergolesi 33, 20052 Monza, Italy;
[o] Department of Experimental Medicine, Milan Bicocca University, Milan, Italy;
[^] Department of Anesthesiology and Reanimation, Kocaeli University Medical Faculty, Kocaeli, Turkey
pabloingelmo@libero.it

Summary

Mucopolysaccharidoses are heterogeneous metabolic disorders characterized by lysosomal enzymatic defects, with accumulation of glycosaminoglycans in various tissues; they are a well-known cause of major difficulty in administering anaesthesia. It has been shown that an experienced surgical and anaesthetic team considerably decreases morbidity and mortality in young children or those presenting with complex disorders. Children with mucopolysaccharidoses who undergo anaesthesia must be managed by anaesthesiologists who have received the necessary training in pediatric anaesthesia and resuscitation. Paramount in the anaesthetic care of patients with mucopolysaccharidoses is a careful preoperative airway examination since many factors in such patients make airway management difficult. The association of cervical spine instability and difficult airway management may increase the risk of spinal cord damage. These patients are described as presenting the 'worst airway problem in pediatrics'. The primary goal of airway management in these children is to avoid the 'cannot intubate/cannot ventilate' scenario, maintaining whenever possible, spontaneous ventilation until the airway is secured. Regional anesthesia should be always kept in mind, with a backup plan for airway management. Postoperative measures include early extubation, trying to avoid the use of postoperative mechanical ventilation as much as possible, aggressive chest physiotherapy, and early investigation and treatment of respiratory infectious complications.

Introduction

Mucopolysaccharidoses (MPSs) are heterogeneous metabolic disorders characterized by lysosomal enzymatic deficits with accumulation of glycosaminoglycans in various tissues and are a well-known cause for major anaesthetic difficulties. Children suffering from MPS frequently need more and recurrent surgical treatments and sedation or anaesthesia is often required for diagnostic and therapeutic procedures (Baum & O'Flaherty, 2007). This paper discusses all the issues that must be taken into account when operating on these already compromised patients, including choice of the care team, preoperative evaluation, airway examination and management, the presence of cervical spine instability, and respiratory and cardiac function. Techniques for administering anaesthesia are also outlined, and postoperative measures are listed that must be carried out in order to avoid further complications of surgery.

Care team

The outcome of surgery and anaesthesia in children is closely related to the experience of the clinical team involved. It has been shown that an experienced surgical and anaesthetic team considerably decreases morbidity and mortality in young children or children with complex disorders (Campling, 1990). Anaesthesia for children with MPS demands properly trained and skilled staff with appropriate facilities. Thus, these patients should not be assisted where these conditions are not available; rather, they should be transferred to specialized centres. The decision to transfer should be based on the number of procedures performed per year and the experience of all the staff at the centre. Experienced paediatric departments with intensive care services should be available commensurate with the type of surgery to be undertaken.

Children with MPS who undergo anaesthesia must be managed by anaesthesiologists who have received the necessary training in paediatric anaesthesia and resuscitation. In children with MPS there is no such thing as 'minor' surgery or anaesthesia because even in lesser procedures the management of these patients can be difficult if the staff are not familiar with children with this type of disorder.

Preoperative evaluation

A thorough preoperative evaluation of the airway and the cardiac, pulmonary, and neurologic functions is of extreme importance in children with MPS. These patients should be examined by an ENT surgeon, a paediatrician, and by the anaesthesiologist as part of the team caring for these special children. Preoperative investigations should include ECG and echocardiography, routine laboratory tests, and chest X-ray examination. All this information should then be included in the routine follow-up of these children and should not be repeated unless a new clinical indication surfaces.

Airway evaluation

Paramount in the anaesthetic care of MPS patients is a careful preoperative airway examination. Many factors are present in these children to make airway management difficult. Intracellular accumulation of mucopolysaccharides with generalized soft tissue infiltration may produce macroglossia, tonsil enlargement, thickening and narrowing of the oral and nasal mucosa, adenoidal hypertrophy, and chronic congestion of the upper airway with production of copious secretions. A shaped overhanging epiglottis, thickened vocal cords, distortion of the larynx, and redundant tissue in the upper airway may also be present. The trachea is flattened and granulomatous tissue may exist everywhere from subglottic region to the main bronchus, producing multiple narrowing or deformation of the trachea, which could change and weaken the cartilage. A coarse facial appearance, prominent maxilla, a limited mouth opening due to involvement of the temporo-mandibular joint, and a short neck associated with various degrees of mental retardation complete the unfavourable scenario for the airway management of many children with MPS (Baum & O'Flaherty, 2007).

The standard clinical and radiologic evaluation may convey insufficient information about the airway. Upper airway imaging techniques including magnetic resonance imaging (MRI) and computer tomography (CT) play an important role in noninvasive evaluation of obstructive sleep apnoea syndrome (OSAS), which is commonly present in children with MPS. Computerized tomography (CT) has also been selected as a reliable measure of the efficacy of medical or nonmedical interventions in OSAS. CT scans avoid the use of sedation, but use high radiation doses. On the other hand, MRI allows multiple scanning planes, provides high-contrast resolution, and does not require radiation exposure, although many MPS children need sedation (Lerman, 2009; Santamaria et al., 2007).

In the last several years, multidetector computer tomography (MDCT) revolutionized noninvasive imaging. MDCT makes it possible to evaluate the airways in few seconds as well as to obtain a 3D reconstruction of the airway from previous studies of the spine and the thorax, thus avoiding new exposure to radiation. Compared to the standard CT scan, MDCT provides greater coverage and improved spatial resolution. The technique can also create images of thick and thin collimation from the same data set. The axial images can display complex anatomic relations in the thoracic structures. Finally, MDCT images with 3D reconstruction may predict difficult airway management in children with MPS and could be a useful tool in the evaluation and preoperative planning of the airway management of children with MPS (Mauri et al., 2009).

The association of cervical spine instability and difficult airway management may increase the risk of spinal cord damage in children with MPS. Cervical spine abnormalities are very common in children with the Morquio syndrome and have also been reported in children with Hurler syndrome (Walker et al., 1997). All MPS patients at risk of cervical spine instability should have preoperative radiologic screening of the cervical spine.

Cardiopulmonary function

Respiratory and cardiac functions can be compromised in patients with MPS. Chronic respiratory disease may be related to chronic hypoxaemia from upper airway obstruction/sleep apnoea, kyphoscoliosis, or recurrent pulmonary infections. Moreover, many children with MPS may present secondary pulmonary problems associated with cardiac dysfunction from either myocardial dysfunction or valvular lesions (Baum & O'Flaherty, 2007).

Kyphoscoliosis and pectus carinatum may lead to a reduction in vital capacity, functional residual capacity, and total lung capacity, indicating a pulmonary disorder of a restrictive nature (Bartz et al., 1999). Recurrent lower airway infections are common. Chest infections and sputum retention should be treated pre- and postoperatively with chest physiotherapy and frequent suctioning to reduce pulmonary complications. Moreover, chest deformities may cause complications associated with mechanical ventilation during or after anaesthesia; these complications involve elevated airway pressure, hypercapnia, and hypoxaemia. If the patient must be placed in prone position for posterior fusion, ventilation problems may worsen. Furthermore, when the patient is in a prone position, pressure areas should be carefully protected by padding as it is likely that the skeletal deformities can lead to a higher incidence of nerve or tissue damage.

Cardiac involvement is well recognized in most forms of mucopolysaccharidosis. The range of cardiac abnormalities varies from mild to severe valvular lesions and coronary artery infiltration and narrowing to pulmonary hypertension due to chronic hypoxaemia. Therefore, physical examination, preoperative chest X-ray, ECG, and echocardiography should rule out major organ dysfunction.

Cardiac infiltration leading to myocardial dysfunction, coronary artery lesions, and valvular dysfunction are well described in patients with Hurler syndrome and Hunter syndrome and may be an important problem in Morquio syndrome. Although coronary artery involvement is generally extensive, coronary thrombosis and myocardial infarction are uncommon (Baum & O'Flaherty, 2007). However, intraoperative deaths have been attributed to coronary artery involvement, and further preoperative evaluation by a paediatric cardiologist should be recommended for patients with direct or indirect symptoms of myocardial ischemia.

Patients with a history of significant upper airway obstruction or sleep apnoea may require echocardiogram and pulmonary function testing (only in children who are able to communicate easily) to exclude the presence of pulmonary hypertension or right ventricular dysfunction (Lerman, 2009).

Premedication

Premedication with benzodiazepines should be used only in patients without symptoms or signs of airway obstruction or pulmonary disease. In children with excessive airway secretions the use of anticholinergic drugs as premedication is recommended. Because glycopyrrolate has fewer chronotropic effects than atropine, it may be advantageous in patients with heart disease. In case of confirmed valvular stenosis or insufficiency, antibiotic prophylaxis is indicated in any surgical intervention.

Airway management

Inadequate oxygenation due to the difficult airway management, including tracheal intubation, is the most important cause of cardiac arrest during anaesthesia in the paediatric population. The management of the airway is a major problem in patients with mucopolysaccharidosis. Some authors describe these patients as presenting the 'worst airway problem in paediatrics'. Walker *et al.* analysed the data of 34 children with different types of mucopolysaccharidoses who underwent anaesthesia 89 times for 110 operations. Difficulty in tracheal intubation was encountered in seven of 13 patients with MPS IH (Hurler's syndrome) and two of four patients with MPS IV. Their results showed an almost uniform incidence of difficult intubations of 50 per cent across the spectrum of mucopolysaccharidoses (Walker *et al.*, 1994).

The primary goals of airway management in these children is to avoid the 'cannot intubate/ cannot ventilate' scenario, maintaining whenever possible spontaneous ventilation until the airway is secured.

Although the administration of neuromuscular blocking drugs may appear safe once adequate bag-mask ventilation is demonstrated, it has been suggested that tracheal intubation should be accomplished during deep-inhalation anaesthesia without the use of neuromuscular blocking drugs. The loss of muscle tone associated with neuromuscular blocking agents may cause supraglottic tissues to prolapse over the airway, precluding effective bag-mask ventilation.

In children with Hurler syndrome the facemask positioning could be very difficult or even impossible. To solve this problem, it has been suggested that the regular facemask be used upside down with the narrower nasal bridge over the mouth (Baum & O'Flaherty, 2007).

Fiberoptic techniques have gained greater acceptance and should be used in children with known airway difficulties. Because of tissue infiltration of the nasopharynx and adenoidal hypertrophy, the nasal fiberoptic approach could be difficult in MPS children and may increase the risks of airway bleeding.

During induction of inhalation, upper airway obstruction may be controlled by changing the patient's position or with the use of an oral cannula or the placement of a stitch through the tongue to facilitate its anterior displacement.

Laryngeal mask airway (LMA) would be an easy and, in some cases, a life-saving choice in children with MPS. Furthermore, the use of LMA was advocated as a safe choice for fiberoptic-guided tracheal intubation (Walker et al., 2008). Children with MPS usually have augmented upper airway secretions and may present upper respiratory infections (URIs) more frequently than normal children do. The use of LMA in children with recent or actual URIs has been associated with a higher incidence of laryngospasm, cough, and oxygen desaturation compared with healthy children (von Ungern-Sternberg et al., 2007).

The use of various video laryngoscope models (Glidescope, AVIL, etc.) designed to give an improved glottic view on a video monitor with fiberoptic intubation has gained consensus among paediatric anaesthesiologists. The video laryngoscope blade is used to elevate the tongue or, if required, to lift up the epiglottis to provide a view of the larynx or eventually of the vocal cords. Once the vocal cords are visualized on the bedside video screen, the styletted endotracheal tube, bent to the form of a hockey stick, is guided under direct vision along the blade and then threaded through the vocal cords under monitor control. Conversely, if the video laryngoscope allows only a partial view of the laryngeal structures, fiberoptic intubation is performed using the video laryngoscope as a guide for the fiberoscope (Dullenkopf et al., 2002).

In patients with MPS, insertion of a supraglottic device as a conduit for fiberoptic-guided tracheal intubation can be very useful for difficult airway management. Varying techniques of either blind or fiberoptic-guided intubations through a supraglottic device (classic LMA, Pro-Seal LMA, I-gel) have been described for these patients. This aids maintenance of a relatively secured airway during intubation attempts, improves oxygenation by intermittent ventilation, and reduces the stress on the team dealing with difficult airway situations. It has been repeatedly described as a 'low skill technique', even for relatively inexperienced anaesthesiologists. (Michalek et al., 2008; Walker et al., 1997).

The atlanto-axial instability due to odontoid hypoplasia and ligamentous laxity renders endotracheal intubation in patients with MPS difficult. In the case of elective surgical procedures, the cervical spine instability should be addressed first by neurosurgical consultation. In the emergency situation, the approach to the airway and cervical spine should follow the same guidelines used for patients with traumatic injury and suspected cervical spine injury. Treatment may involve fixation with a rigid collar or placement of a halo traction device. Both of these devices, as in the trauma patient, can be expected to increase significantly the difficulty of airway management.

Cervical spine stability may not be preserved in the deeply anaesthetized patient with neuromuscular blockade. In smaller children, direct laryngeal visibility may be adequate in spite of cervical spine immobilization manœuvres. Direct laryngoscopy with manual in-line stabilization (MAIS) is an often successful and therefore suitable approach in these circumstances (Walker et al., 1997).

Birkinshaw (1975) described a specifically designed plaster bed that was used to fix the neck during intubation and operation in a patient with MPS IV and unstable neck. Nott and al Hajaj (1993) successfully performed awake intubation in a patient with unstable neck after spraying the pharynx with topical lidocaine, 4 per cent, and combined with intravenous fentanyl and ketamine. To avoid cervical cord damage in patients with cervical instability, Tzanova et al. (1993) suggested fiberoptic intubation of the spontaneously breathing child as the method of choice (Birkinshaw, 1975; Nott & al Hajaj, 1993; Tzanova et al., 1993) and they reported such successful anaesthesia in a 23-month-old girl with MPS IVA and unstable neck.

Anaesthesia

Anaesthetic options include both general anaesthesia as well as regional anaesthetic techniques. The latter may be chosen when underlying conditions such as airway abnormalities, cervical spine instability, or cardiorespiratory dysfunction increase the risks of general anaesthesia. In addition, the use of muscular relaxants is not advisable before the airway is completely secure.

Regional anaesthesia should constantly be considered for these patients, but always with a backup plan for airway management. For example, spinal (Tobias, 1999) or peripheral nerve blocks can be used for surgery of the extremities, which is very common for children with MPS. Nowadays peripheral nerve blocks under the vision of ultrasound (US) gained popularity as this provides greater safety and is easier to perform. Even with central blocks, US is suggested as an easy and safe method to improve efficacy. However, a case of failed epidural anaesthesia, despite good placement of the catheter, has been reported and ascribed to possible deposition of mucopolysaccharides in the epidural space or on the nerve sheath (Baum & O'Flaherty, 2007).

Positive end-expiratory pressure (PEEP) increases functional respiratory capacity (FRC) and dynamic lung compliance, decreases total airway resistance, and can be used to prevent alveolar collapse. An additional PEEP of 3 to 5 cm H_2O led to an increase of FRC by 10 per cent above baseline values in preschool children, whereas PEEP only restored FRC close to baseline in young infants.

Because extubation represents another major risk during anaesthesia in patients with MPS, after excluding any residual neuromuscular blockade, patients should be extubated while breathing spontaneously and when they are fully awake. However, it was suggested that extubation, when children are still under anaesthesia, reduces more than 10-fold the possibility of airway obstruction during awakening (Kamin, 2008).

Postoperative period

The postoperative period should be as short as possible. Day hospital surgery should be a primary objective for minor surgery or diagnostic procedures under anaesthesia. Postoperative measures include early extubation, trying to avoid the use of postoperative mechanical ventilation as much as possible, aggressive chest physiotherapy, and early investigation and treatment of respiratory infectious complications.

Overnight postoperative monitoring may be required in patients with a history of chronic airway obstruction, sleep apnoea, or respiratory dysfunction. Attention to maximizing respiratory function is crucial in the postoperative period. Its importance is highlighted by reports of postoperative respiratory arrests and deaths related to upper airway obstruction and respiratory failure in MPS patients, with a mortality rate as high as 20 per cent.

Patients undergoing major surgery, such as posterior spinal fusion, usually require postoperative observation in an intensive care unit. Recovery after general anaesthesia is often slow and accompanied by periods of apnoea, bronchospasm, and cyanosis. Therefore, postoperative ventilation is advisable, but weaning should be performed as soon as possible in order to minimize pulmonary complications and to assess neurologic function.

Conclusions

Children with MPS have special needs with respect to anaesthesia, and they need a highly dedicated and skilled team. Anaesthesia for children with MPS should be undertaken only by trained and skilled anaesthesiologists, nurses, and support staff in centres with appropriate facilities These patients need a detailed preoperative evaluation including a complete assessment of the airway, neck, and cardiopulmonary system. It is imperative to prepare an airway management plan before induction of anaesthesia. It is also necessary to be ready for the worst-case scenario for airway management, even when regional anaesthesia is used. Whenever possible regional anaesthesia alone or combined with light sedation should be the first option to avoid airway management problems and postoperative pulmonary complications. The postoperative period should be as short as possible. Day hospital surgery should be a primary objective for minor surgery or diagnostic procedures using anaesthesia.

References

Bartz, H.J., Wiesner, L. & Wappler, F. (1999): Anaesthetic management of patients with mucopolysaccharidosis IV presenting for major orthopaedic surgery. *Acta Anaesthesiol. Scand.* **43**, 679–683.

Baum, V.C. & O'Flaherty J.E. (2007): *Anesthesia for genetic metabolic, and dysmorphic syndromes of childhood*, 2nd ed., p. 256. Philadelphia, PA: Lippincott Williams & Wilkins.

Birkinshaw, K.J. (1975): Anaesthesia in a patient with an unstable neck: Morquio's syndrome. *Anaesthesia* **30**, 46–49.

Campling, E.A., Devlin, H.B. & Lunn, J.N. (1990): *The report of the national confidential enquiry into perioperative deaths 1989*. London: Disc to Print Ltd.

Diaz, J.H. & Belani, K.G. (1993): Perioperative management of children with mucopolysaccharidoses. *Anesth. Analg.* **77**, 1261–1270.

Dullenkopf, A., Holzmann, D., Feurer, R., Gerber, A. & Weiss, M. (2002): Tracheal intubation in children with Morquio syndrome using the angulated video-intubation laryngoscope. *Can. J. Anesth.* **49, 2**, 198–202.

Mauri, F. Ingelmo, P., Grimaldi, M., Parini, R., Melzi, M., Romagnoli, M., Tagliabue, G. & Fumagalli, R. (2009): *Multidetector computer tomography imagines for preoperative airway evaluation of children with mucopolisacaridosis*. [Free paper in SMART (Simposio Mostra Anestesia Rianimazione e Terapia Intensiva), Congress May 6–8, 2009, Milano].

Kamin, W. (2008): Diagnosis and management of respiratory involvement in Hunter syndrome. *Acta Paediat.* **97**, 57–60.

Lerman, J. (2009): A disquisition on sleep-disordered breathing in children. *Pediat. Anesth.* **19**, 100–108.

Michalek, P., Hodgkinson, P. & Donaldson, W. (2008): Fiberoptic intubation through an I-Gel supraglottic airway in two patients with predicted difficult airway and intellectual disability. *Anesth. Analg.* **106**, 1501–1504.

Nott, M.R. & al Hajaj, W.H. (1993): Anaesthesia for urinary diversion with ileal conduit in a patient with Morquio-Brailsford syndrome. *Anaesth. Intensive Care* **21**, 879–884.

Santamaria, F., Andreuci, M.V., Parenti, C., Polverino, M., Viggiano, D., Montella, S., Cesaro, A., Ciccarelli, R., Capaldo, B. & Andria, G. (2007): Upper airway obstructive disease in mucopolysaccharidoses: polysomnography, computed tomography and nasal endoscopy findings. *J. Inherit. Metab. Dis.* **30**, 743–749.

Tobias, J.D. (1999): Anesthetic care for the child with Morquio syndrome: general versus regional anesthesia. *J. Clin. Anesth.* **11**, 242–246.

Tzanova, I., Schwarz, M. & Jantsen, J.P. (1993): Securing the airway in children with the Morquio-Brailsford syndrome. *Anaesthetist.* **42,** 477–481.

von Ungern-Sternberg, B.S., Boda, K., Schwab, C., Sims, C., Johnson, C. & Habre, W. (2007): Laryngeal mask airway is associated with an increased incidence of adverse respiratory events in children with upper respiratory tract infections. *Anesthesiology* **107,** 714–719.

Walker, R.W., Darowski, M., Morris, P. & Wraith, J.E. (1994): Anaesthesia and mucopolysaccharidoses: a review of airway problems in children. *Anaesthesia* **49,** 1078–1084.

Walker, R.W.M., Allen, D.L. & Rothera, M.R. (1997): A fibreoptic intubation technique for children with mucopolysaccharidoses using the laryngeal mask airway. *Paediat. Anaesth.* **7,** 421–426.

Chapter 11

Neurosurgical complications and their management in mucopolysaccharidosis

Carlo Giussani, Sara Miori and Erik P. Sganzerla

Department of Neurosurgery, San Gerardo Hospital, via Pergolesi 33, 20052 Monza, Italy
carlo.giussani@libero.it

Summary

The major neurosurgical complications of mucopolysaccharidoses (MPSs) are associated with the development of communication hydrocephalus and craniovertebral junction instability. The management of both these complications is very challenging because of the diagnostic difficulties related to the association of an evolving cerebral atrophy with ventricular enlargement in hydrocephalus and to the technical complexity of craniovertebral junction surgery in paediatric patients with anatomic abnormalities in the case of instability of the craniovertebral junction. Communicating hydrocephalus is diagnosed by serial neurologic and neuroimaging techniques that look for signs and symptoms of increased intracranial pressure; the condition is managed by the implant of ventriculo-peritoneal shunts with programmable valves that can be regulated over time. Craniovertebral junction instability is associated with a number of anatomic abnormalities, each requiring highly demanding and precisely tailored surgical solutions.

Introduction

The MPSs are a heterogeneous group of lysosomal storage disorders caused by deficiency of an enzyme involved in the degradation of glycosaminoglycans. These enzyme deficiencies lead to the accumulation of glycosaminoglycans in the lysosomes, resulting in cell, tissue, and organ dysfunction. Recently, seven types of MPSs have been classified by Neufeld and coworkers in 2001 that can affect the central nervous system (CNS), with a wide range of intensity, determining different pathologic entities that can be faced by neurosurgeons in the milieu of multidisciplinary teamwork. Communicating hydrocephalus and craniovertebral junction (CVJ) instability in the context of diffuse spinal canal stenosis are the two major neurosurgical complications of the deposit of glycosaminoglycans in the lysosomes. In this chapter hydrocephalus and CVJ instability will be discussed separately in terms of pathophysiology, diagnosis, and treatment.

Communicating hydrocephalus

Pathophysiology

Hydrocephalus is characterized by an imbalance of cerebrospinal fluid (CSF) formation and absorption, with progressive dilatation of ventricles and cerebral parenchymal damage due to the increase of intracranial pressure (ICP). In fact, the Monro-Kellie theory defines the skull as a rigid container of constant volume that comprises three compartments: brain, cerebrospinal fluid, and blood; any increase in the volume of one of its contents causes IPC and the reduction of cerebral perfusion pressure and blood flow in the end stage. In infants and very young children this doctrine is not applicable because the sutures and fontanelles of these young children are not fused yet and the cranial volume can expand. Physiologically, 80 per cent of CFS is produced by the choroid plexuses, located in the lateral ventricles and 20 per cent in the parenchymal interstitial space and in the spine. CSF flows from the ventricular system into the ventral and dorsal subarachnoid space of the brain through three small foramina at the level of the fourth ventricle. At the level of the superior sagittal sinus, the CSF is reabsorbed *via* the arachnoid villi into the venous system. The arachnoid villi are protrusions of arachnoid inside the sagittal sinus, where they are gathered in macroscopically visible groups, defined as arachnoid granulation. The rate of absorption is pressure-dependent.

Physiopathologic criteria divide hydrocephalus into two categories: noncommunicating (or obstructive) and communicating (or nonobstructive):
• In noncommunicating or obstructive hydrocephalus, the blockage of CSF circulation is between the ventricular system and the subarachnoid spaces, with a dilatation that frequently involves the lateral and third ventricles. It can be caused by any process that obstructs the ventricular system (tumors, infections, hemorrhage, aqueductal stenosis). Different surgical options exist depending on the origin of the obstruction (endoscopic III ventriculostomy and ventriculoperitoneal shunt).
• In communicating or nonobstructive hydrocephalus, CSF flow between the ventricles and the extracerebral spaces is possible, but there is a block at the arachnoid granulation level or in the subarachnoid spaces.

In all cases there is a dilatation of the ventricular system that at the beginning does not cause any thinning of cerebral parenchyma and/or signs of transependymal CSF reabsorption as the direct sign of an increased ventricular pressure that forces the CSF into the periventricular brain parenchyma.

The pathogenesis of the ventricular enlargement in MPS patients is a combination of communicating hydrocephalus and cerebral atrophy. In fact, communicating hydrocephalus is not rare in MPS patients. The pathogenesis is the accumulation of storage material in the arachnoid villi, causing an impairment of CFS absorption. This view has been supported in the work of Glenn and Powell (1975), Sheridan and Johnson (1992), and Yatziv and Epstein (1977). In fact, in autopsies of children with MPS several instances of thickening of the leptomeninges, caused by an increase of collagen fibres and the presence of macrophages containing GAGs, have been found (Sheridan & Johnston, 1994). Less frequent is the obstructive hydrocephalus in children with MPS; its pathogenesis is the accumulation of GAGs in the periventricular spaces. Moreover, children with MPS frequently have severe central nervous system involvement, with progressing cerebral atrophy and a consequent *ex vacuo* hydrocephalus that makes a clear-cut diagnosis difficult in these patients. For these reasons, MPS hydrocephalus seems to be similar to normal-pressure hydrocephalus (NPH) in adults, with chronic overnight mild increases of the ICP instead of a rapidly evolving onset with high ICP. The typical signs and symptoms of hydrocephalus according to age are listed in Table 1. The development of hydrocephalus in children with MPS is generally slow and gradual, and therefore at the beginning typical symptoms of hydrocephalus as headache, vomiting, or papilledema are lacking. Moreover, the mixed origin of the ventricular enlargement makes it hard to differentiate true hydrocephalic symptoms from symptoms of MPS-related cerebral atrophy. Lethargy, irritability, and difficulty in walking, typical of children with MPS, can be symptoms caused by hydrocephalus and by the involvement of central nervous system by MPS as well. Besides, hydrocephalus by itself, if long-lasting, can contribute to the development of cerebral atrophy through the decrease of cerebral blood flow and the increase of intracranial pressure. Children with MPS are not always able to verbally communicate their symptoms and problems, which poses a further problem for the neurosurgeon and paediatrician.

Table 1. Signs and symptoms of hydrocephalus in children

Premature neonate	**Neonate**	**Children and adolescents**
Apnoea	Irritability	Headache
Bradycardia	Vomiting	Vomiting
Bulging fontanelle	Macrocephaly	Lethargy
Distension of the head veins	Sleepiness	Diplopia
Rapid increase of the circumference of the head	Poor head/neck control	Papilloedema
Vomiting	Psychomotor delay	Psychomotor delay
Alteration of the head shape		Imbalance
		Poor sphincter control
		Hyperreflexia, clonus

Radiologic signs of hydrocephalus

Radiologic diagnosis is not easy because the radiologist has to distinguish between a true hydrocephalus mixed with an *ex vacuo* component as the result of cerebral atrophy and just a severe cerebral atrophy that can occur alone (Fig. 1).

Different radiologic signs of hydrocephalus on a TC scan have been described that can help the neurosurgeon to make the diagnosis (Fig. 2) (Losowska-Kaniewska & Oleś, 2007):

• the size of both temporal horns (THs) is > 2 mm in width (in the absence of hydrocephalus, the temporal horns should be barely visible), and the sylvian and interhemispheric fissures and cerebral sulci are not visible;

• both temporal horns are > 2 mm, and the ratio of FH/ID is > 0.5 (FH, frontal horns; ID, internal diameter from inner table to inner table at this level);

• there is ballooning of the frontal horns of lateral ventricles ('Mickey Mouse' ventricles) and the third ventricle;

• periventricular low density is seen on CT or periventricular high density is seen on T2WI on MRI, suggesting transependymal absorption or filtration of CSF in the brain parenchyma;

• Evans' ratio (ratio of FH to maximal biparietal diameter) is > 30 per cent;

• dilatation of TH proportional to the dilatation of the body of lateral ventricles helps to differentiate hydrocephalus from cerebral atrophy.

As stated before, radiologic diagnosis is not easy because the enlargement of the ventricular chambers may be caused by the hydrocephalus itself as well as by the primitive atrophy typical of MPS. For the slowly progressing pattern of hydrocephalus development in these patients,

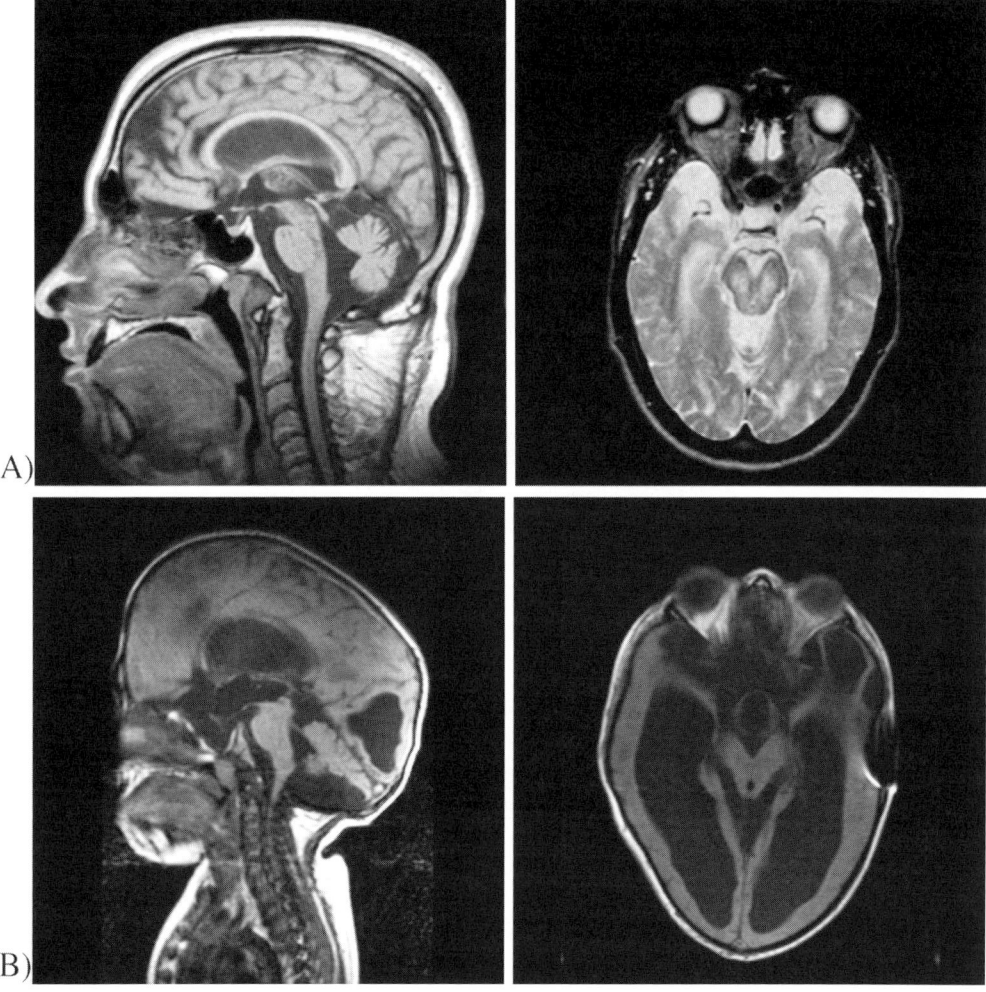

Fig. 1 (A) Cerebral atrophy in patient affected with MPS I-S. (B) Hydrocephalus in patient affected with MPS I-SH.

we think that it is essential to submit MPS patients with enlarged ventricles to neuroradiologic evaluation repeatedly over time to reach a correct diagnosis. The radiologic findings must be correlated to the clinical symptoms and, in rare cases, it is necessary to measure the intracranial pressure.

Treatment

Children affected by MPS with hydrocephalus should be treated by shunting the CSF (Drake, 2008). Various shunts have been described; the most commonly now used is the ventriculo-peritoneal shunt (VP shunt), whereas the ventriculo-atrial shunt is less often used. The goal of the shunt is to decrease intracranial pressure with the goal of alleviating the symptoms along with decreasing the size of the ventricles.

Chapter 11   Neurosurgical complications and their management in mucopolysaccharidosis

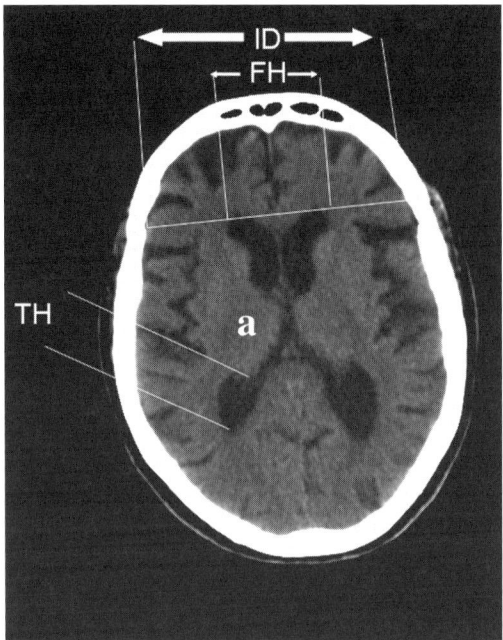

Fig. 2. Different measurable ventricular variables used to establish the presence of hydrocephalus.

The VP shunt device (Fig. 3) is composed of a proximal catheter placed into the frontal horn of the right lateral ventricle connected to a single one-way valve, which is connected to a distal catheter that is 'tunnelized' cranio-caudally under the skin up to the peritoneum, where it is inserted. In our experience it is preferable to implant a programmable valve. In fact, taking into account the mixed nature of the hydrocephalus and its consequent continuous slow progression (even after shunting), it is fundamental to be able to adjust over time the opening pressure of the valve according to changes seen on clinico-radiologic examination. The opening pressure of the valve is externally programmable, with an electromagnetic device allowing the neurosurgeon to choose between a wide range of pressures.

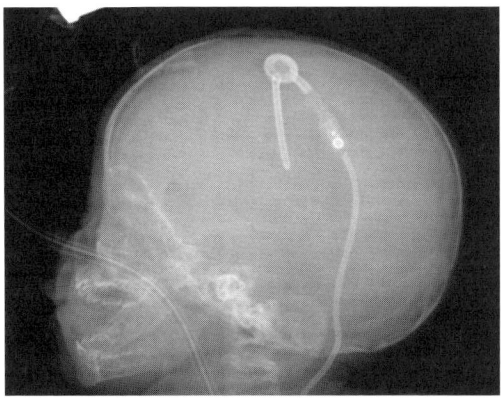

Fig. 3. Postsurgical shunt control in children.

Unfortunately, ventriculoperitoneal shunt complications are frequent; the most common are underdraining and overdraining (which can be easily corrected with a programmable valve), infections, and shunt device malfunctions (Table 2).

Table 2. Complications of shunts

Common complications	Rare complications		
	Cranial	Underskin	Distal catheter
Infection	Meningitis, ventriculitis, empyemas	Migration	Peritonitis from shunt infections
Underdraining	Subdural hygromas/ haematomas	Disconnection	Abdominal pseudo cyst
Overdraining	Hemiparesis, haematomas, etc.	Breaking	Hydrocele, inguinal hernia

Craniovertebral junction instability and spinal cord compression

The causes of spinal cord compression in children with MPS are the instability of the craniovertebral junction (CVJ) and the thickening of dura mater at the CVJ and cervical-dorsal spine. The CVJ is the most mobile joint of the upper cervical spine, particularly in children.

General anatomy and biomechanics (Menezes, 2008)

The CVJ has been identified as the most complex joint of the axial skeleton from an anatomic and kinetic point of view. CVJ instability of nontraumatic origin represents 27 per cent of all the CVJ instabilities in the paediatric age group and refers to the presence of different anatomic and motion abnormalities of the osteo-ligamentous elements; it carries an increased risk of developing severe cervico-medullary compression (Steinmetz et al., 2003). Consequently, the prompt recognition of even minor prodromal symptoms is mandatory in children at risk as MPS patients because surgical treatment can interrupt neurologic evolution The immature paediatric spine differs both biomechanically and physiologically from its adult counterpart. This is due to the presence at the occipito-atlanto-axial segments of several characteristics that predispose to injury: (1) an increased ligamentous laxity; (2) more horizontally oriented facets; (3) a less mature bone ossification (C1 ossification is not complete until 4–5 years of age and the subaxial cervical spine has not completed ossification until 2 to 4 years of age); (4) wedge-shaped vertebral bodies; (5) a higher fulcrum of cervical movement; and (6) higher inertia and torque forces associated with a larger head/body mass ratio (Eleraky & Theodore, 2000).

Pathogenesis of spinal cord compression in children with mucopolysaccaridosis

Menesez and Vogel (2008) have shown that, in addition to the normal anatomic developmental laxity and hypermobility in children with MPS, there are abnormalities of any component of the CVJ and thickening of dura mater and soft tissue.

Atlas arch abnormalities (Senoglu & Sonntag, 2007)

In the atlas arch there are three ossification centres: one anterior for the tubercle and two lateral for the lateral masses and the posterior arch. At birth, the posterior arch is almost completely fused, while the anterior centre joins together with lateral centres at the age of 5–9 years. Atlas posterior arch defects are variable (hypoplasia, aplasia, dysplasia) and more frequent than those of the anterior arch and are associated with mild clinical conditions. Lesions of the medulla oblongata are caused by the isolated posterior fragment that, in case of extension, moves forward and squeezes the medulla; the lesion is localized inferiorly with respect to the bone fragment level because the medulla moves downward during head extension. Generally, patients are asymptomatic, but can present symptoms after minor trauma like acute tetraparesis, with variable levels of sensibility loss and paresthesia that get worse with the head extended. Symptoms can develop slowly as a consequence of ligament hypertrophy, venous stasis, and edema of the medulla caused by micro-trauma.

Dens abnormalities

Dens aplasia with complete absence of its basilar portion or a hypoplasia with a rudimentary dens that does not reach the superior part of the atlas arch have been observed in children with a joint instability. An independent bone situated under C2, where the dens is generally present, is called *os odontoideum*: it should not be considered an isolated bone, but a separated part of a hypoplastic dens. Usually it is located at the top of the dens, or near the occipital base, in the foramen magnum area. The space between the free bone and the dens extends over the superior surfaces of C2, causing incompetence of the cruciate ligament and consequently an atlanto-axis instability. The biomechanics are very complex and different in each child: in some cases the major compression of CVJ occurs during flexion. The sliding of the cruciate ligament behind the *os odontoideum* and before the superior part of the dens can cause an irreducible dislocation; in this way the body axis and dens cause a spinal cord compression at the CVJ level. Patients with os odontoideum and cervical instability often present neurologic symptoms such as isolated occipital pain, myelopathy of variable severity, intracranial signs and symptoms, or vertebrobasilar compression (caused by the chronic instability). The alterations of dens are often associated with the finding of periodontal soft tissue that contributes to spinal cord compression. Some authors thought that these soft tissue masses were glycosaminoglycan deposits, but recent studies have demonstrated that they are a combination of nonossified fibrocartilagineous tissue and reactive granulation tissue, without any evidence of GAGs.

Dura mater thickening

As Taccone and Tortori-Donati (1993) state, dura mater thickening at the CVJ is a constant finding in radiologic investigation of patients with MPS; this thickening causes a decrease in subarachnoid space. However, the literature reports only few cases of spinal cord compression caused by thickening (Tamaki *et al.*, 1987). TC scans can show the dura thickening as a bulging soft tissue, but the gold standard examination is the MRI, which can show isointense or ipointense signal in T_1 and T_2 weighting, respectively, around the spinal cord. Only one case was reported of a cervical biopsy that identified this tissue as fibrotic, with poor capillary proliferation. Few studies are investigating the nature of this tissue by the administration of an intrathecal enzyme therapy in animal models and in human patients. Kakkis and Dickson (2004, 2007) demonstrated in dogs that this treatment decreases the accumulation of GAGs in the brain and at the meningeal level. In an animal model, with symptoms related to spinal cord compression, a remarkable reduction of symptoms was observed after intrathecal enzyme substitution, suggesting that the GAG accumulation can be one of the causes of dura thickening and spinal cord compression. Therefore, intrathecal enzyme therapy could be considered a promising treatment in asymptomatic patients who are not candidates, for other reasons, for surgery.

Summary of the findings of craniovertebral junction abnormalities related to the subtypes of mucopolysaccharidoses

Hunter syndrome (MPS I)

Spinal cord compression is not constant. The cervical vertebrae may have anomalies, with schisis of the posterior arch. Cervical disk herniations are frequent. The dens can present many anomalies too: hypoplasia, aplasia, or abnormal growth; however, severely symptomatic CVJ instability is less common than in the Morquio syndrome. Thickening of the ligaments and peridental mass may contribute to spinal cord compression. Thoracic and lumbar vertebral abnormalities are not typical of this form of MPS, but are described in literature.

Morquio syndrome (MPS IV)

The literature (Stevens & Ransford, 1991, 1996; Hughes & Jenkins, 1997) shows that bone anomalies are typical and distinctive of this MPS. All children affected by MPS IV have anomalies of the axis/dens: aplasia, hypoplasia, os odontoideum, or abnormal periodontoid tissue with a mass effect. Schisis of posterior and/or anterior arch of the atlas are common too and contribute to instability. Sudden flexion may cause spinal cord compression and acute respiratory failure and quadriplegia. The cervical myelopathy due to this instability is a common cause of disability and death in these children in the setting of even minor trauma. Many anomalies at all spine levels are also common.

Maroteaux-Lamy syndrome (MPS VI)

Spinal anomalies are less severe in Maroteaux-Lamy syndrome than in Morquio syndrome. Instability is not common. Nevertheless, spinal cord compression and myelopathy are common because of the thickening of the posterior-superior ligament and the dura as well as the presence of periodontoid hypertrophic mass (Thorne & Hughes, 2007; Vougiouskas & van Velthoven, 2001).

Sly syndrome (MPS VII)

Spinal anomalies are rare in the Sly syndrome, but when they exist, they often cause acute tetraparesis. For this reason children affected by the Sly syndrome need long-term radiologic screening (Dickerman & Schneider, 2004).

Signs and symptoms of spinal cord compression

Signs and symptoms of spinal cord compression are various (Table 3); children may be asymptomatic, but become symptomatic over the time. Neurologic symptoms are caused by spinal cord compression related to CVJ abnormalities, hypertrophy of the soft tissue, or spinal vascular involvement. Signs and symptoms begin insidiously, arising fairly late and progressing slowly. A very common symptom is cervical and occipital pain for compression of the greater occipital nerve, which originates from the second spinal nerve. Respiratory failure requiring intensive care occurs when the compression is acute.

Table 3. Signs and symptoms of spinal cord compression

Myelopathy	Brain stem dysfunction	Lower cranial nerve dysfunction	Vascular compromise	Spinal nerve dysfunction
Motor symptoms May be unobtrusive and nonspecific May be manifest only by lack of endurance Quadriparesis, triparesis, paraparesis, hemiparesis or monoparesis Sensory abnormalities Posterior column dysfunction Hypoalgesia-spino-thalamic tract dysfunction Bladder dysfunction	Nistagmus Apnoea Respiratory failure Ataxia Dysmetria Internuclear ophthalmoplegia	Hearing loss Dysphagia Soft palate paralysis Trapezius muscle weakness Tongue atrophy Hearing loss Dysphagia Soft palate paralysis	Syncope and vertigo	Cervical and occipital pain

Radiologic diagnosis

The common first radiologic imaging done is the X-ray examination of the cervical spine, with lateral, anterior-posterior, and open-mouth projection. TC scanning and MRI then provide more information about the peculiar anatomy of this region in each patient. MRI imaging is ideal for evaluating the presence of soft tissue, neural structures, and ligaments. TC with orthogonal reconstruction optimally defines the osseous anatomy and pathology of the CVJ. MRI and TC in flexion and extension are needed to evaluate spinal cord compression and instability. The presence of static spinal cord compression due to stenosis of the foramen magnum or dynamic spinal cord compression related to the decrease of spinal canal diameter during movement have to be evaluated as well. Stenosis is caused by bone anomalies and/or hypertrophic soft tissue; dynamic compression is caused by instability. To evaluate the instability the atlanto-odontoid interval (ADI; also called the predental space) is adopted. The ADI measures the distance between the posterior border of the anterior atlas arch and posterior border of the dens. In children, this space is 5–8 mm, whereas in adults it is less than 3 mm; this is because the child's ligaments are loose and the bone maturation is not complete. The predental space is more than 3 mm in MPS children with instability caused by the anomalies described (Smoker & Khanna, 2008).

Treatment

A child with MPS must be undergo both imaging and accurate, thorough clinical examination to facilitate the diagnosis of eventual CVJ anomalies before the appearance of acute neurologic symptoms. Cervical spine evaluation must be always done when acute neurologic symptoms occur, because minor trauma can also cause acute spinal cord compression in an abnormal spine. During the evaluation of a child with CVJ abnormalities and instability, other factors have to be considered:

- the possibility of physiologic realignment of the cervical spine, reducing the spinal cord compression;

- the causes of the pathologic process, including the study of bone abnormalities and eventual nervous system malformations;
- the child's age and the surgical possibilities related to individual anatomy and tissue maturity;
- the clinical condition of the patient.

Conservative treatment (wait and scan) can be used in asymptomatic patients with CVJ abnormalities without instability or spinal cord compression.

Goals of treatment for CVJ instability should be to provide neural decompression along with stabilization and fusion of the spine. As Menezes and Vogel (2008) and Chirossel and Palombi (2000) have shown, reducibility is one of the major criteria in choosing the correct therapeutic approach. Other important elements in the management of these children include the patient's dimensions, bone immaturity, ligament laxity, and specific anatomic abnormalities.

Reducible condition

Commonly the first step in the management of all patients is the external reduction of the dislocation, followed by immediate stabilization with a halo-orthosis. This device decreases the risk of worsening the neurologic conditions related to all the possible insults during the radiologic studies and during intubation and pronation. After external reduction and stabilization of the upper cervical spine, these patients should undergo a rehabilitation period in order to achieve the best neurologic and respiratory condition before surgery (Giussani & Sganzerla, 2009). The complex anatomy of the region and the young age of these patients has led to the development of many different surgical techniques employing both posterior and anterior approaches. The smaller physical size, the bone immaturity/ligamentous laxity, the abnormal anatomy, and growth potential are some of the important issues faced in the operative management of CVJ instability. In the past, some authors have noted a procedure-related morbidity in the management of CVJ instability, especially with the use of contoured loops and sublaminar wiring. Many researchers (Doyle *et al.*, 1996; Nader-Sepahi *et al.*, 2005; Taggard & Menezes, 2000; Nordt & Stauffer, 1981; Segal *et al.*, 1991; Inamasu *et al.*, 2005; Anderson & Brockmeyer, 2006) have shown that these devices can produce a posterior dural compression and have an intrinsic microinstability. Other authors (Rahimi & Stevens, 2003; Menezes & Ryken, 1992; Brockmeyer & Apfelbaum, 1999; Gluf & Brockmeyer, 2005) published reports of a series of CVJ instabilities in children treated by rigid internal fixation, reporting excellent fusion rates with minor complications. Many studies (Grob & Crisco, 1992; Hanley & Harvell, 1992; Oda, 1999; Bradford & Melcher, 2002) evaluated the efficacy of various techniques, without clearly answering which of them was preferable; the results were comparable concerning efficacy and biomechanical stability. Generally, every surgeon will choose the best technique in relation to his or her own personal confidence as well as the patient's anatomy and age. In all cases autologous bone grafts are placed. In children, the bone graft comes from parietal bone since it is more practical than iliac bone, which is commonly used in adults.

Irreducible conditions

Patients presenting anterior spinal cord compression with irreducible instability undergo transoral decompression before posterior instrumentation is performed. This condition is very rare in children with MPS. Patients with irreducible lesions and posterior compression undergo posterior decompression and fixation during the same surgical operation. To ensure long-lasting fusion after surgery, immobilization with a halo jacket for 40 to 80 days is recommended. Although the halo jacket is associated with frequent complications, this device is useful for stabilizing the fixed area and preventing dislocation and neurologic complications.

Case report

The patient was a 6-year-old girl with MPS type IVA. She had previously undergone cervical decompression at another institution, with partial removal of the posterior arch of C1 and of thickened atlanto-occipital membrane. After a backwards fall from a child's chair, she developed an acute quadriplegia with respiratory failure (Ranawat IIIB) and was admitted to our neurologic intensive care department. Neuroimaging studies showed an atlanto-axial instability with dens aplasia. MRI showed an altered spinal cord signal at C0–C1, with severe intramedullary malacia. The patient was initially treated with reduction and stabilization by halo-orthosis, and then received rehabilitative care for some weeks afterward. She then underwent a stabilization of the atlanto-axial segment by means of an occipital ring connected to C2 pedicle screws; the construct was augmented with split calvarian bone inserted between C0 and C2 (Fig. 4). After surgery, the restoration of a complete respiratory autonomy was assessed in our neurologic intensive care unit. At 3-year follow-up examination, she was able to walk with crutches (Ranawat IIIA). Radiologic follow-up examinations revealed a stable fixation with bone fusion and without signs of anomalous vertebral development.

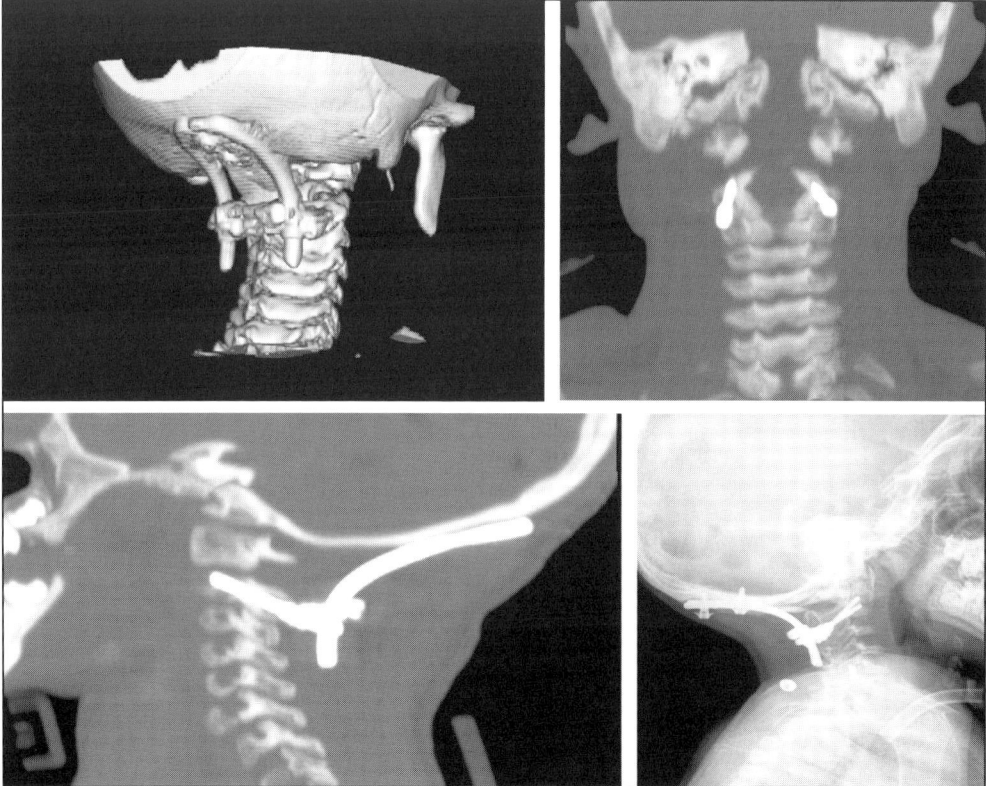

Fig. 4. Post-stabilization accomplished by the use of an occipital ring connected to C2 pedicle screws and split calvarian bone inserted between C0 and C2.

Conclusions

The major neurosurgical complications of MPS progression are (1) communicating hydrocephalus and (2) cervical spinal cord compression related to CVJ instability and/or thickening of the dura mater.

It is imperative that a multidisciplinary approach be used to address these complications. In particular, because of the slow progression of both these pathologic conditions, careful long-term clinical and radiologic follow-up is required. For hydrocephalus, surgical treatment with programmable valves should be done only in patients who show a clear correlation between radiologically determined progression and neurologic deterioration. On the other hand, surgical treatment of the cervical spine complications can be considered even in asymptomatic patients who present undoubtable radiologic signs of spinal cord compression or instability that make the patient prone to an increased risk of severe spinal cord damage even from minor trauma.

References

Anderson, R. & Brockmeyer, D. (2006): Long term maintenance of cervical alignment after occipitocervicale and atlantoaxial screw fixation in young children. *J. Neurosurg. Pediat.* **105**, 55–61.

Bradford, D.S. & Melcher, R.P. (2002): Biomechanical testing of posterior atlantoaxial fixation techniques. *Spine* **27**, 2435–2440.

Brockmeyer, D.L. & Apfelbaum, R.I. (1999): A new occipitocervical fusion construct in pediatric patients with occipitocervical instability. *J. Neurosurg.* **90**, 271–275.

Chirossel, J.P. & Palombi, O. (2000): Management of craniocervical junction dislocation. *Childs Nerv. Syst.* **16**, 697–701.

Condon, B.R. & Hadley, D.M. (1988): Quantification of cord deformation and dynamics during flexion and extension of the cervical spine using MR imaging. *J. Comput. Assist. Tomogr.* **12**, 947–955.

Dickerman, R. & Schneider J. (2004): Craniovertebral instability with spinal cord compression in a 17-month-old boy with Sly syndrome (MPS type VII). *Spine* **29**, E92–E94.

Doyle, J.S., Lauerman, W.C., Wood, K.B. & Krause, D.R. (1996): Complications and long-term outcome of upper cervical spine arthrodesis in patients with Down syndrome. *Spine* **21**, 1223–1231.

Drake, J.M. (2008): The surgical management of pediatric hydrocephalus. *Neurosurgery* **62** (Suppl. 2), 633–640.

Eleraky, M.A., Theodore, N., Adams, M., Rekate, H.L. & Sonntag, V.K. (2000): Pediatric cervical spine injuries: report of 102 cases and review of the literature. *J. Neurosurg.* **92** (Suppl.), 12–17.

Emans, J.B. & Rodgers, W.B. (1997): Increasing lordosis of the occipitocervical junction after arthrodesis in young children: the occipitocervical crankshaft phenomenon. *J. Pediat. Orthop.* **17**, 762–765.

Giussani, C. & Sganzerla, E. (2009): Severely symptomatic craniovertebral junction abnormalities in children. *Pediat. Neurosurg.* **45**, 29–36.

Glenn, W. & Powell, W. (1975): Communicating hydrocephalus in children with genetic inborn errors of metabolism. *Childs Brain* **1**, 251–254.

Gluf, W.M. & Brockmeyer, D.L. (2005): Atlantoaxial transarticular screw fixation: a review of surgical indications, fusion rate, complications, and lessons learned in 67 pediatric patients. *J. Neurosurg. Spine* **2**, 164–169.

Grob, D. & Crisco, J.J. (1992): Biomechanical evaluation of four different posterior atlantoaxial fixation techniques. *Spine* **17**, 480.

Hanley, E.N. & Harvell, J.C. (1992): Immediate postoperative stability of the atlantoaxial articulation: a biomechanical study comparing simple midline wiring, and the Gallie and Brooks procedures. *J. Spinal Dis.* **5**, 306.

Hughes, D. & Jenkins, J. (1997): MRI of the brain and craniocervical junction in Morquio's disease. *Neuroradiology* **39**, 381–385.

Inamasu, J., Kim, D. & Klugh, A. (2005): Posterior instrumentation surgery for craniocervical junction instabilities: an update. *Neurol. Med. Chir. (Tokyo)* **45**, 439–447.

Kakkis, E. & Dickson, P. (2004): Intrathecal enzyme replacement therapy reduces lysosomal storage in the brain and meninges of canine model of MPS I. *Mol. Genet. Metab.* **83**, 163.

Kakkis, E. & Dickson, P. (2007): Intrathecal enzyme replacement therapy: successful treatment of brain disease via the cerebrospinal fluid. *Mol. Genet. Metab.* **91**, 61–68.

Losowska-Kaniewska, D. & Oles, A. (2007): Imaging examinations in children with hydrocephalus *Adv. Med. Sci.* **52** (Suppl. 1), 176–179.

Mayer, B. & Schramm, J. (2001): Surgery for upper cervical spine instabilities in children. *Acta Neurochir.* **143,** 759–766.

Menezes, A.H. (1991–1992): Complications of surgery at the craniovertebral junction: avoidance and management. *Pediat. Neurosurg.* **17,** 254–266.

Menezes, A.H. (2008a): Decision making. *Childs Nerv. Syst.* (2008) **24,** 1147–1153.

Menezes, A.H. (2008b): Anatomy and biomechanics of normal craniovertebral junction and biomechanies of stabilization. *Childs Nerv. Syst.* **24,** 1091–1100.

Menezes, A.H. (2008c): Craniocervical developmental anatomy and its implications. *Childs Nerv. Syst.* **24,** 1109–1122.

Menezes, A.H. (2008): Craniovertebral junction database analysis: incidence, classification, presentation, and treatment algorithms. *Childs Nerv. Syst.* **24,** 1101–1108.

Menezes, A.H. & Ryken, T.C. (1992): Craniovertebral abnormalities in Down's syndrome. *Pediat. Neurosurg.* **18,** 24–33.

Menezes, A.H. & Traynelis, V. (2008): Fusion at the craniovertebral junction. *Childs Nerv. Syst.* **24,** 1209–1224.

Menezes, A.H. & Vogel, T.W. (2008): Specific entities affecting the craniocervical region: syndromes affecting the craniocervical junction. *Childs Nerv. Syst.* **24,** 1155–1163.

Nader-Sepahi, A., Casey, A.T., Hayward, R., Crockard, H.A. & Thompson, D. (2005): Symptomatic atlantoaxial instability in Down syndrome. *J. Neurosurg.* **103,** 231–237.

Nordt, J.C. & Stauffer, E.S. (1981): Sequelae of atlantoaxial stabilization in two patients with Down's syndrome. *Spine* **6,** 437–440.

Oda, I. (1999): Biomechanical evaluation of five different occipito-atlanto-axial fixation techniques. *Spine* **24,** 2377.

Rahimi, S.Y., Stevens, E.A., Yeh, D.J., Flannery, A.M., Choudhri, H.F. & Lee, M.R. (2003): Treatment of atlantoaxial instability in pediatric patients. *Neurosurg. Focus* **15,** ECP1.

Segal, L.S., Drummond, D.S., Zanotti, R.M., Ecker, M.L. & Mubarak, S.J. (1991): Complications of posterior arthrodesis of the cervical spine in patients who have Down syndrome. *J. Bone Joint Surg. Am.* **73,** 1547–1554.

Senoglu, M. & Sonntag, V. (2007): The frequency and clinical significance of congenital defects of the posterior and anterior arch of the atlas. *J. Neurosurg. Spine* **7,** 399–402.

Sheridan, M. & Johnston, H. (1992): Hydrocephalus, lumbar canal stenosis and Maroteaux-Lamy syndrome (MPS VI). *J. Neurosurg. Sci.* **36,** 215–217.

Sheridan, M. & Johnston, I. (1994): Hydrocephalus and pseudotumour cerebri in the mucopolysaccharidosis. *Childs Nerv. Syst.* **10,** 148–150.

Smoker, W. & Khanna, G. (2008): Imaging the craniocervical junction. *Childs Nerv. Syst.* **24,** 1123–1145.

Steinmetz, M.P., Lechner, R.M. & Anderson, J.S. (2003): Atlantooccipital dislocation in children: presentation, diagnosis, and management. *Neurosurg. Focus* **14,** ECP1.

Stevens, J. & Ransford, A. (1996): Occipito-atlanto-axial fusion in Morquio Brailsford syndrome. *J. Bone Joint Surg.* **78-B,** 307–313.

Stevens, J. & Ransford, A. (1991): The odontoid process in Morquio Brailsford's disease. *J. Bone Joint Surg.* **73-B,** 851–858.

Taccone, A. & Tortori-Donati, P. (1993): Mucopolysaccharidosis: thickening of dura mater at the craniovertebral junction and other CT/RMN finding. *Pediat. Radiol.* **23,** 349–352.

Taggard, D.A., Menezes, A.H. & Ryken, T.C. (2000): Treatment of Down syndrome-associated craniovertebral junction abnormalities. *J. Neurosurg.* **93,** 205–213.

Tamaki, N. *et al.* (1987): Myelopathy due to diffuse thickening of cervical dura mater in Maroteaux-Lamy syndrome: report of a case. *Neurosurgery* **21,** 416–419.

Thorne, J. & Hughes, D. (2007): Craniovertebral abnormalities in type VI mucopolysaccharidosis (Maroteaux-Lamy syndrome). *Neurosurgery* **48,** 852–853.

Visocchi, M. & Di Rocco, C. (2009): Pre-operative irreducible C1-C2 dislocation: intra-operative reduction and posterior fixation: the always posterior strategy. *Acta Neurochir.* **151,** 551–560.

Vougiouskas, V. & van Velthoven V. (2001): Neurosurgical interventions in children with Maroteaux-Lamy syndrome. *Pediat. Neurosurg.* **35,** 35–38.

Yatziv, S. & Epstein, C. (1977): Hunter syndrome presenting as macrocephaly and hydrocephalus. *J. Med. Genet.* **14,** 45–447.

Specific treatments
for lysosomal storage diseases

Chapter 12

Enzyme replacement therapy in lysosomal storage disorders: clinical effects and limitations

Michael Beck

Children's Hospital, University of Mainz, Langenbeckstrasse 1, 55101 Mainz, Germany
dr.m.beck@t-online.de

Summary

In 1991 it was demonstrated that the biweekly infusion of a modified β-glucocerebrosidase, extracted and purified from human placenta, had a significant therapeutic effect in patients affected by Gaucher disease. And in the last several years, enzyme preparations have been developed for several other lysosomal storage disorders. For patients with Fabry disease two different enzyme preparations have become available: agalsidase alfa (Replagal®), produced in a human cell line, and agalsidase beta (Fabrazyme®), produced in Chinese hamster ovary (CHO) cells. Both enzymes have been shown to be able to lessen pain, to reduce left ventricular mass, and to stabilize kidney function. However, they seem to do not have any effect on the cerebrovascular complications of Fabry disease. The formation of neutralizing antibodies reduces the clinical efficacy of the enzyme preparations. For three types of mucopolysaccharidoses, enzyme replacement therapy is available: laronidase (Aldurazyme®) for MPS I (Hurler and Scheie disease), idursulphase (Elaprase®) for MPS II (Hunter disease), and galsulphase (Naglazyme®) for MPS VI (Lamy-Maroteaux disease). Several studies have shown that treatment with these enzymes leads to increase of general endurance (as demonstrated by the 6-minute-walk test), improvement of lung function, reduction in liver size, and improvement of joint mobility. These enzymes do not have any effect on the manifestation of the central nervous system as they are not able to cross the blood–brain barrier. The clinical effects of long-term therapy are not known until now. The enzyme preparation alglucosidase alfa (Myozyme®) has been demonstrated to have positive clinical effects in patients with all forms of Pompe disease (the infantile, juvenile, and adult types). The presence of neutralizing antibodies diminishes the efficacy of Myozyme®.

In summary, all enzyme preparations are effective in alleviating some signs and symptoms and halting the progression of the disease, although they are not able to cure the patient of it.

Introduction

Lysosomes are membrane-delimited cell organelles containing a great number of acid hydrolases that are responsible for degradation of biological macromolecules. Newly synthesized lysosomal enzymes traverse the rough endoplasmic reticulum (RER) and Golgi apparatus, where they are modified by the formation of the mannose-6-phosphate recognition marker, which is essential for uptake into the lysosome *via* the mannose-6-phosphate receptor. A variable portion of newly synthesized lysosomal enzymes are not bound to the mannose-6-phosphate receptor and are secreted. These enzymes can be partially taken up and transported to the lysosomes through mannose-6-phosphate–mediated endocytosis. This mechanism is an essential prerequisite for the effectiveness of enzyme replacement therapy.

More than 40 years ago E. Neufeld and co-workers (Fratantoni et al., 1968) conducted pioneering experiments that revealed that the metabolic defect of cultured fibroblasts from mucopolysaccharidosis patients can be compensated by addition of corrective factors that are secreted by cells not having the same defect. Further studies have shown that the corrective factors represent enzymes that are taken up from outside the cell into the lysosomal compartment by receptor-mediated endocytosis via the mannose 6-phosphate receptor. On the basis of these experiments, clinical studies of enzyme replacement therapy were undertaken in the early 1970s in patients affected by Sandhoff, Pompe, and Fabry diseases. However, at that time it was not possible to obtain sufficient amounts of enzyme for life-long treatment of all patients, so it took many years before clinical trials with recombinant enzyme preparations could be performed.

Gaucher disease

In Gaucher disease (β-glucocerebrosidase deficiency), three phenotypes can be distinguished: About 90 per cent of all patients have the non-neuronopathic form, also called type I. Clinical manifestations include hepatosplenomegaly, anemia, thrombocytopenia, and skeletal complications. The acute neuronopathic form (type II) presents as acute severe illness, usually leading to death by the age of about 3 years. In type III, the so-called chronic neuronopathic form, first symptoms appear during infancy or childhood. Patients with type III Gaucher disease present most often with severe visceral, haematologic, and skeletal involvement, and neurologic symptoms such as supranuclear gaze palsy and seizures. Clinical evaluation in a large number of patients with a neuronopathic form of Gaucher disease has revealed that the chronic and acute neuronopathic form represents a phenotypic continuum rather than clearly distinguishable subtypes (Goker-Alpan et al., 2003).

Type I Gaucher disease has been the first lysosomal storage disorder for which enzyme replacement therapy became available. In 1991 Barton et al. reported the results of a clinical study in patients with Gaucher disease. In this trial, 12 patients with the non-neuronopathic form (type I) of the disease received β-glucocerebrosidase that was derived from human placenta and had to be de-glycosylated to expose mannose residues in the oligosaccharide chains because this enzyme has to be taken up by macrophages via the mannose receptor, and not by the mannose-6-phosphate receptor. The enzyme was administered at a dosage of 60 U/kg every two weeks. Within 9 to 12 months a significant increase in the haemoglobin and platelet count was observed in all patients, and liver and spleen volume decreased. On the basis of this trial, the enzyme preparation was approved for treatment of patients with Gaucher disease. Some years later the placenta-derived β-glucocerebrosidase (Ceredase®) was replaced by a recombinant form that is produced in CHO cells. Also, this enzyme preparation (Cerezyme®) needs to be modified for targeting mannose receptor sites on macrophages. Because the enzyme preparation isolated from placentas might theoretically be contaminated by pathogenic agents, it is no longer licensed.

In Gaucher disease enzyme replacement therapy leads to reduction of liver and spleen size and improvement in haematologic parameters within 1 year. In contrast, skeletal manifestations seem to respond more slowly (Grabowski et al., 1998). In 30 patients, the effect of enzyme replacement therapy (ERT) on skeletal disease was assessed by using coronal T_1- and

T_2-weighted spin echo MRI. Median MRI follow-up and duration of ERT were 36 months. During treatment an increased signal intensity consistent with partial reconversion of fatty marrow was seen in 19 of these patients. Not unexpectedly, focal bone lesions that correlated with the presence of bone infarcts did not respond to ERT (Poll et al., 2001).

The positive effect of ERT on skeletal manifestations of Gaucher disease was confirmed by an evaluation of data that were obtained from the International Gaucher Registry (Charrow et al., 2007). In this analysis only patients with bone crisis and/or bone pain data for 1 year prior to ERT, and for each of 3 years after the start of ERT, were included. After initiation of treatment, bone pain and frequencies of bone crises decreased significantly. This study has demonstrated that noteworthy improvements – not only in visceral signs, but also in decrease of symptoms of skeletal disease – can be achieved by enzyme replacement therapy.

The effect of enzyme replacement therapy on neurologic symptoms of type III Gaucher patients is still under discussion. Many studies were performed in order to evaluate the response of the central nervous system to various doses of enzyme (30 U/kg to 120 U/kg body weight every two weeks). Some authors reported a clear improvement not only of the visceral signs, but also of cerebral function, such as IQ and auditory evoked brain stem response, under therapy (Altarescu et al. 2001; Aoki et al. 2001).

In order to evaluate the effect of enzyme replacement therapy on the neurologic outcome of type III Gaucher disease in a greater number of persons, Davies et al. (2007) reviewed 55 patients from five European countries who had been on enzyme replacement therapy for different lengths of time. However, the analysis became very difficult because there was a significant variation in the study population regarding the dose of the enzyme, the age of the patients, and the presence or absence of risk factors such as splenectomy. Despite the difficulty of interpreting the study results, the authors could draw some conclusions from their data: The older patients appeared to remain relatively stable despite a low dose of enzyme and there was no clear effect of high-dose ERT in younger patients. Based on these data, a revision of guidelines for treatment of type III Gaucher patients has become necessary.

In an attempt to halt disease progression in the acute neuronopathic form of Gaucher disease, two patients received alglucerase at the age of 7 months and 4 days, respectively (Prows et al., 1997). However, the treatment could not alter the outcome, and both infants died before they reached 18 months of life. There is now a general agreement that enzyme replacement therapy is not indicated in the acute neuronopathic form of Gaucher disease.

Fabry disease

Kidney failure, cardiomyopathy, and cerebrovascular events are the complications that are mainly responsible for the morbidity and mortality of Fabry disease (α-galactosidase deficiency). Two different enzyme preparations have been developed to treat Fabry disease: algalsidase beta (Fabrazyme®; Genzyme Corp.), produced in Chinese hamster ovary cells, and agalsidase alfa (Replagal®; Shire Human Genetic Therapies, Inc.), produced in human cell lines. To prove the clinical efficacy of agalsidase alfa, Schiffmann and colleagues (2001) performed a randomized, placebo-controlled, double-blind trial in 26 males affected by Fabry disease. In this study, it was demonstrated that in patients treated with the enzyme the mean neuropathic pain severity score significantly declined from 6.2 to 4.3, whereas no significant change was seen in the placebo group ($p = 0.02$).

The analysis of the latest reports regarding the clinical efficacy and tolerability of agalsidase alfa in patients with Fabry disease have demonstrated that this enzyme preparation is effective in treating pain, reducing heart size and sweating, and improving hearing and quality of life (Beck, 2009). This drug is able to stabilize kidney function and slow progression of renal failure in patients with end-stage renal disease (West *et al.*, 2009).

As an alternative for a clinical parameter, a biomarker may also be used to demonstrate the efficacy of a drug. In a study by Eng *et al.* (2001), the clearance of microvascular endothelial deposits of storage material (globotriaosylceramide [Gb3]) from the kidney, heart, and skin was used as such a biomarker: Twenty of the twenty-nine patients in the treatment group (69 per cent) did not show any microvascular endothelial deposits of globotriaosylceramide in renal biopsy specimens after 20 weeks of treatment, as compared with none of the 29 patients in the placebo group ($p < 0.001$). Patients in the recombinant α-galactosidase A group also had decreased microvascular endothelial deposits of globotriaosylceramide in the skin and heart. Stabilization of kidney function by enzyme replacement therapy with agalsidase beta was reported by Wilcox *et al.* (2004), while Weidemann *et al.* (2009) observed an improvement of cardiac function by regular infusions of this enzyme preparation.

The clinical efficacy of agalsidase beta has been studied in a double-blind multicenter trial, in which 82 adult patients with Fabry disease with kidney dysfunction were randomly assigned to receiving infusions of enzyme replacement with agalsidase beta or placebo for up to 35 months (Banikazemi *et al.*, 2007). Data analysis at the end of the trial has shown that agalsidase beta was able to reduce the frequency of and to delay the time to clinical events (encompassing the composite outcome of renal, cardiac, and cerebrovascular events and death). Three patients withdrew from the study on account of positive or inconclusive serum IgE or skin results.

Mucopolysaccharidoses

Mucopolysaccharidosis type I (α-iduronidase deficiency)

Mucopolysaccharidoses are multisystemic disorders that affect several organ systems to individually variable degrees (Muenzer, 2004). They are characterized by a broad spectrum of clinical phenotypes, which makes it very difficult to evaluate the efficacy and safety of a recombinant enzyme preparation. In a randomized, double-blind, placebo-controlled multinational study, 45 patients with MPS I (Hurler-Scheie phenotype) received 100 U/kg (0.58 mg/kg) recombinant α-iduronidase (laronidase) or placebo intravenously weekly for 26 weeks. The laronidase and placebo groups had similar baseline values. After 26 weeks, patients receiving the enzyme showed an improvement in lung function and in the 6-minute-walk test (Wraith *et al.*, 2004). Furthermore, a significant reduction in liver volume and urinary glycosaminoglycan excretion was observed in the treated group. On the basis of the results of this study, the enzyme preparation Aldurazyme® (recombinant human α-L-iduronidase; laronidase; Genzyme Corporation; BioMarin Pharmaceuticals, Inc.) received approval in the United States, Europe, and many other countries.

In order to investigate long-term efficacy of recombinant α-iduronidase (laronidase), an extension study was initiated by Clarke *et al.* (2009): Forty-five patients with the attenuated form of the disease who had completed the 26-week, double-blind, placebo-controlled study were enrolled in this 3.5-year open-label trial. As shown in earlier trials, urinary glycosaminoglycan levels decreased within the first 12 weeks of treatment, and liver volume decreased within the first year. After 3.5 years of treatment liver volume normalized in 92 per cent of patients and lung function remained stable. The 6-minute-walk distance increased 31.7 ± 10.2 m in the first 2 years, with a final gain of 17.1 ± 16.8 m. In general, laronidase infusions were well tolerated, except in one patient, who experienced an anaphylactic reaction. One patient died from an upper respiratory infection unrelated to treatment.

The clinical efficacy in young, severely affected children with mucopolysaccharidosis type I has been investigated by Wraith *et al.* (2007). In this open-label trial, 20 patients (16 with Hurler syndrome and 4 with Hurler-Scheie syndrome) received laronidase for 52 weeks. A decline of urinary glycosaminoglycan excretion by ≈ 50 per cent was observed at week 13. In some patients, a decrease in left ventricular hypertrophy was found. All patients with Hurler-Scheie syndrome showed a normal course of development during the treatment period. An improvement of the general clinical status in 94 per cent of patients was reported by the investigators.

Laronidase does not cross the blood–brain barrier and will probably not have any positive effect on the central nervous system in severely affected patients with the Hurler phenotype; stem cell transplantation will therefore be the treatment of choice for this group of patients (Koc *et al.*, 2002). This procedure should be performed within the first years of life to prevent irreversible damage to the brain. However, enzyme replacement therapy could also be of importance for young patients with Hurler disease, as it may improve general lung and heart function, thereby making stem cell transplantation easier to tolerate (Wynn *et al.*, 2009).

Mucopolysaccharidosis type II (Hunter disease, iduronate sulphatase deficiency)

Major clinical manifestations of this X-linked disorder include joint contractures, obstructive and restrictive airway disease, cardiac disease, skeletal deformities, and mental retardation. Patients with the more attenuated (so-called adult) form are usually of normal intelligence, although they often have many complaints such as progressive loss of vision and severe hip disease.

After successful completion of a Phase I/II trial, a Phase III study was initiated to determine the efficacy of 0.5 mg/kg recombinant iduronate sulphatase [idursulphase (Elaprase®)], given weekly or biweekly *versus* placebo over 1 year. As the primary efficacy endpoint of this study a so-called two-component composite score was chosen, whereby the lung function and 6-minute-walk test were used (Muenzer *et al.*, 2006). A statistically significant improvement in this composite primary efficacy endpoint was seen in patients who received idursulphase compared to placebo ($P = 0.0049$). Urinary GAG levels were significantly lower in patients being treated with idursulphase in both the weekly or every-other-week dosing regimen compared to patients receiving placebo. A decrease of liver and spleen volume, a reduction of urinary glycosaminoglycan level, and improvement of joint range of motion were observed after one year in the treatment group.

Only patients older than 5 years have been enrolled in the clinical trials. Therefore, there is only limited experience in enzyme replacement therapy in patients younger than 5 years. In addition, it is unclear how to monitor the response to treatment, as these young patients may not be able to perform the tests used in the clinical trials (lung function and 6-minute-walk test). However, in spite of these challenges, treatment should be introduced in patients with Hunter disease under the age of 5 years after detailed discussion with the parents. In these patients careful clinical follow-up and annual developmental assessments will be necessary.

Enzyme replacement therapy probably does not have any positive effect on CNS manifestation in boys with severe Hunter disease, as idursulphase is not expected to cross the blood–brain barrier. However, the enzyme may be of benefit to these patients by improving respiratory function and joint mobility and by reducing liver and spleen size. Wraith *et al.* (2008) recommend offering the possibility of this treatment to patients with severe CNS involvement for a trial period of about one year. Thereafter a decision should be made together with the parents as to whether to continue or to stop the infusions.

Mucopolysaccharidosis type VI (Maroteaux-Lamy syndrome, arylsulphatase B deficiency)

Mucopolysaccharidosis type VI is characterized by severe skeletal deformities, enlargement of liver and spleen, obstructive lung disease, involvement of the eyes and the heart, and neurologic complications caused by nerve compression in the craniocervical region and the wrist. However, in contrast to children with the severe form of mucopolysaccharidosis type I (Hurler disease), patients with MPS VI always have normal intelligence.

The first preclinical studies with recombinant arylsulphatase B (rhASB) have been performed in a naturally occurring animal model of mucopolysaccharidosis type VI, a cat that shows many clinical features comparable to those observed in humans. The first studies in three MPS VI cats have shown that regular infusions of human recombinant enzyme, produced in Chinese hamster ovary cell, resulted in reduction of storage cells in liver Kupffer cells and connective tissues. One cat showed greater mobility under treatment.

After Crawley *et al.* (1996) showed in an animal model of MPS VI that regular infusions of recombinant human arylsulphatase B (rhASB) led to a reduction of storage vacuoles in Kupffer cells and connective tissue, clinical trials were initiated. In a Phase I/II trial it could be demonstrated that treatment with this recombinant enzyme was able to reduce urinary glycosaminoglycan excretion (Harmatz *et al.*, 2004). In all patients, general endurance and range of shoulder motion improved. After a Phase III study (double-blind, placebo-controlled) had demonstrated the clinical efficacy of weekly infusion of rhASB, this enzyme preparation (Naglazyme®) was approved by the FDA and EMEA for treatment of patients with mucopolysaccharidosis type VI.

In order to evaluate the long-term clinical benefits and safety of recombinant human arylsulphatase B (rhASB), 56 patients drawn from three clinical studies were followed in open-label extension studies for a total period of 97–260 weeks (Harmatz *et al.*, 2008). Efficacy was evaluated by the 12-minute-walk test and/or 6-minute-walk test, stair-climb test, and reduction in urinary glycosaminoglycans (GAG). Patients from all clinical trials showed an improvement in results of both the walk-tests as well of the stair-climb test. A significant reduction in urinary GAG was sustained. Only 560 of 4,121 reported adverse events (14 per cent) were related to treatment, whereas only 10 of 560 (2 per cent) were described as severe.

Pompe disease

In Pompe disease (glycogenosis type II, α-glucosidase deficiency) progressive cardiomyopathy, skeletal muscle weakness, and respiratory insufficiency are the leading clinical signs. Affected infants usually die within the first year of life. In contrast, patients with the later-onset form may survive longer, but may become bound to a wheelchair and may require artificial ventilation. Clinical trials of enzyme replacement therapy for patients with Pompe disease have been performed by several groups using enzymes produced either in the milk of transgenic rabbits or in CHO cells.

In a study performed by Amalfitano and co-workers (2001), three infants with Pompe disease received twice-weekly recombinant α-glucosidase (alglucosidase alfa) that was isolated from genetically modified CHO cells. The infusions were generally well tolerated. All infants survived the first year of life with well-preserved heart function. Muscle strength improved, too. Muscle biopsy showed a reduction of glycogen accumulation. The recombinant form α-glucosidase, produced in CHO cells [alglucosidase alfa (Myozyme®)], has been licensed for treatment of patients with Pompe disease based on the results of several clinical trials. In these trials, however, the study population was limited to young infants who were at a relatively early state of disease progression when enzyme replacement therapy was initiated. For evaluation of efficacy and safety of enzyme replacement therapy in a more heterogeneous population, Nicolino *et al.* (2009) performed a clinical trial in 21 infantile patients 3–43 months old (median 13 months), who were at variable stages of disease progression when treatment was initiated. Alglucosidase alfa was administered every 2 weeks for up to 168 weeks (median 120 weeks). At the end of the study, 71 per cent (15/21) of patients were alive and 44 per cent (7/16) of invasive-ventilator-free patients remained so. In addition, the treatment led to reduction of left ventricular mass, improvement of motor skills, and gain in functional independence.

Clinical studies have also been performed in patients with the late-onset form of Pompe disease. Merk *et al.* (2007) have investigated the clinical efficacy of enzyme replacement therapy in four adult Pompe patients aged between 39 and 68 years of age who received aglucosidase alfa over a period of 6 months. A significant improvement has been observed in three patients, whereby patients with pre-existing respiratory insufficiency seemed to benefit most. Further studies with adult patients are necessary in order to assess whether enzyme replacement therapy regularly leads to an improvement or at least to stabilization of clinical signs and symptoms.

Limitations of enzyme replacement therapy

In spite of the encouraging clinical results that have been observed in clinical trials of enzyme enzyme replacement therapy, it has become clear very soon that this therapeutic approach has some limitations and is not able to treat all aspects of the disorders equally. Several organs, such as cartilage, bone, and heart valve, are resistant to correction by intravenous ERT. Studies in an animal model (MPS VI cat) showed that very early treatment may possibly lead to a better skeletal response (Auclair *et al.*, 2003). In Pompe disease, the main limitation of enzyme replacement therapy is the significant variability of response by skeletal muscle. Major factors responsible for this variability include the lower number of mannose-6-phosphate receptors in skeletal muscle compared with the heart, the formation of antibodies, and the resistance to correction by type II myofibres (Raben *et al.*, 2005). Clinical trials in patients with Pompe disease have shown that in subjects who are negative for cross-reacting immunologic material (CRIM), the efficacy was markedly reduced in assocation with high-titre antibodies against human α-glucosidase (Kishnani *et al.*, 2007). In a mouse model of Pompe disease, it could be shown that the formation of antibodies can be prevented by AAV vector-mediated gene therapy that induced immune tolerance to the infused enzyme (Sun *et al.*, 2007).

The efficacy of enzyme replacement therapy is also limited by the fact that this therapeutic approach does not have any influence on the central nervous manifestations of the diseases as the enzymes cannot enter the brain because of the blood–brain barrier (Begley *et al.*, 2008). In order to learn how to overcome the blood–brain barrier, experiments were performed in sulphamidase-deficient (MPS IIIA) mice (Savas *et al.*, 2004). Recombinant human sulphamidase was injected directly into the brain of these animals at 6, 12, or 18 weeks of age. It could be shown that the enzyme reduced cytoplasmic vacuolation in neurons, glia, and perivascular cells. However, immunostaining for ubiquitin, a marker of neurodegeneration, was unaffected by enzyme replacement at any age, indicating the importance of early diagnosis and treatment.

Conclusions

In some lysosomal storage disorders, enzyme replacement therapy does not have an effect any more as specific organs are irreversibly damaged, as, for example, the kidney in the late stage of Fabry disease: Schiffmann et al. (2006) have reported that Fabry patients with stage III renal disease showed a decline of glomerular filtration rate despite long-term enzyme replacement therapy.

Some limitations of enzyme replacement therapy are possibly due to the timing of therapy, and early therapeutic intervention may be more efficient. Therefore newborn screening programmes for lysosomal storage disorders have been developed (Zhang et al., 2008). However, because a strict genotype–phenotype correlation does not exist for most of these conditions, screening programmes will probably not be generally introduced until the phenotype can be exactly predicted from a neonate.

References

Altarescu, G., Hill, S., Wiggs, E., Jeffries, N., Kreps, C., Parker, C.C., Brady, R.O., Barton, N.W. & Schiffmann, R. (2001): The efficacy of enzyme replacement therapy in patients with chronic neuronopathic Gaucher's disease. *J. Pediatr.* **138,** 539–547.

Amalfitano, A., Bengur, A.R., Morse, R.P., Majure, J.M., Case, L.E., Veerling, D.L., Mackey, J., Kishnani, P., Smith, W., Mcvie-Wylie, A., Sullivan, J.A., Hoganson, G.E., Phillips, J.A., 3rd, Schaefer, G.B., Charrow, J., Ware, R.E., Bossen, E.H. & Chen, Y.T. (2001): Recombinant human acid alpha-glucosidase enzyme therapy for infantile glycogen storage disease type II: results of a phase I/II clinical trial. *Genet. Med.* **3,** 132–138.

Aoki, M., Takahashi, Y., Miwa, Y., Iida, S., Sukegawa, K., Horai, T., Orii, T. & Kondo, N. (2001): Improvement of neurological symptoms by enzyme replacement therapy for Gaucher disease type IIIb. *Eur. J. Pediatr.* **160,** 63–64.

Auclair, D., Hopwood, J. J., Brooks, D.A., Lemontt, J.F. & Crawley, A.C. (2003): Replacement therapy in mucopolysaccharidosis type VI: advantages of early onset of therapy. *Mol. Genet. Metab.* **78,** 163–174.

Banikazemi, M., Bultas, J., Waldek, S., Wilcox, W.R., Whitley, C.B., Mcdonald, M., Finkel, R., Packman, S., Bichet, D.G., Warnock, D.G. & Desnick, R.J. (2007): Agalsidase-beta therapy for advanced Fabry disease: a randomized trial. *Ann. Intern. Med.* **146,** 77–86.

Barton, N.W., Brady, R.O., Dambrosia, J.M., Di Bisceglie, A.M., Doppelt,S. H., Hill, S.C., Mankin, H.J., Murray, G.J., Parker, R.I., Argoff, C.E., et al. (1991): Replacement therapy for inherited enzyme deficiency macrophage-targeted glucocerebrosidase for Gaucher's disease. *N. Engl. J. Med.* **324,** 1464–1470.

Beck, M. (2009): Agalsidase alfa for the treatment of Fabry disease: new data on clinical efficacy and safety. *Expt. Opin. Biol. Ther.* **9,** 255–261.

Begley, D.J., Pontikis, C.C. & Scarpa, M. (2008): Lysosomal storage diseases and the blood-brain barrier. *Curr. Pharm. Des.* **14,** 1566–1580.

Charrow, J., Dulisse, B., Grabowski, G.A. & Weinreb, N.J. (2007): The effect of enzyme replacement therapy on bone crisis and bone pain in patients with type 1 Gaucher disease. *Clin. Genet.* **71,** 205–211.

Clarke, L.A., Wraith, J.E., Beck, M., Kolodny, E.H., Pastores, G.M., Muenzer, J., Rapoport, D.M., Berger, K.I., Sidman, M., Kakkis, E.D. & Cox, G.F. (2009): Long-term efficacy and safety of laronidase in the treatment of mucopolysaccharidosis I. *Pediatrics* **123,** 229–240.

Crawley, A.C., Brooks, D.A., Muller, V.J., Petersen, B.A., Isaac, E.L., Bielicki, J., King, B.M., Boulter, C.D., Moore, A.J., Fazzalari, N.L., Anson, D., Byers, S. & Hopwood, J.J. (1996): Enzyme replacement therapy in a feline model of Maroteaux-Lamy syndrome. *J. Clin. Invest.* **97,** 1864–1873.

Davies, E.H., Erikson, A., Collin-Histed, T., Mengel, E., Tylki-Szymanska, A. & Vellodi, A. (2007): Outcome of type III Gaucher disease on enzyme replacement therapy: review of 55 cases. *J. Inherit. Metab. Dis.* **30,** 935–942.

Eng, C.M., Guffon, N., Wilcox, W.R., Germain, D.P., Lee, P., Waldek, S., Caplan, L., Linthorst, G.E. & Desnick, R.J. (2001): Safety and efficacy of recombinant human alpha-galactosidase A replacement therapy in Fabry's disease. *N. Engl. J. Med.* **345,** 9–16.

Fratantoni, J.C., Hall, C.W. & Neufeld, E.F. (1968): Hurler and Hunter syndromes: mutual correction of the defect in cultured fibroblasts. *Science* **162,** 570–572.

Goker-Alpan, O., Schiffmann, R., Park, J.K., Stubblefield, B.K., Tayebi, N. & Sidransky, E. (2003): Phenotypic continuum in neuronopathic Gaucher disease: an intermediate phenotype between type 2 and type 3. *J. Pediatr.* **143**, 273–276.

Grabowski, G.A., Leslie, N. & Wenstrup, R. (1998): Enzyme therapy for Gaucher disease: the first 5 years. *Blood Rev.* **12**, 115–133.

Harmatz, P., Whitley, C.B., Waber, L., Pais, R., Steiner, R., Plecko, B., Kaplan, P., Simon, J., Butensky, E. & Hopwood, J.J. (2004): Enzyme replacement therapy in mucopolysaccharidosis VI (Maroteaux-Lamy syndrome). *J. Pediatr.* **144**, 574–580.

Harmatz, P., Giugliani, R., D. Schwartz, I.V., Guffon, N., Teles, E.L., Miranda, M.C.S., Wraith, J.E., Beck, M., Arash, L., Scarpa, M., Ketteridge, D., Hopwood, J.J., Plecko, B., Steiner, R., Whitley, C.B., Kaplan, P., Yu, Z.-F., Swiedler, S.J. & Decker, C. (2008): Long-term follow-up of endurance and safety outcomes during enzyme replacement therapy for mucopolysaccharidosis VI: final results of three clinical studies of recombinant human N-acetylgalactosamine 4-sulphatase. *Mol. Genet. Metab.* **94**, 469–475.

Kishnani, P.S., Corzo, D., Nicolino, M., Byrne, B., Mandel, H., Hwu, W.L., Leslie, N., Levine, J., Spencer, C., Mcdonald, M., Li, J., Dumontier, J., Halberthal, M., Chien, Y.H., Hopkin, R., Vijayaraghavan, S., Gruskin, D., Bartholomew, D., Van Der Ploeg, A., Clancy, J.P., Parini, R., Morin, G., Beck, M., De La Gastine, G.S., Jokic, M., Thurberg, B., Richards, S., Bali, D., Davison, M., Worden, M.A., Chen, Y.T. & Wraith, J.E. (2007): Recombinant human acid α-glucosidase: Major clinical benefits in infantile-onset Pompe disease. *Neurology* **68**, 99–109.

Koc, O.N., Day, J., Nieder, M., Gerson, S.L., Lazarus, H.M. & Krivit, W. (2002): Allogeneic mesenchymal stem cell infusion for treatment of metachromatic leukodystrophy (MLD) and Hurler syndrome (MPS-IH). *Bone Marrow Transplant.* **30**, 215–222.

Merk, T., Wibmer, T., Schumann, C. & Kruger, S. (2007): [Enzyme replacement therapy in Pompe's disease]. *Med. Klin. (Munich)* **102**, 570–573.

Muenzer, J. (2004): The mucopolysaccharidoses: a heterogeneous group of disorders with variable pediatric presentations. *J. Pediatr.* **144**, S27–34.

Muenzer, J., Wraith, J.E., Beck, M., Giugliani, R., Harmatz, P., Eng, C.M., Vellodi, A., Martin, R., Ramaswami, U., Gucsavas-Calikoglu, M., Vijayaraghavan, S., Wendt, S., Puga, A., Ulbrich, B., Shinawi, M., Cleary, M., Piper, D., Conway, A.M. & Kimura, A. (2006): A phase II/III clinical study of enzyme replacement therapy with idursulphase in mucopolysaccharidosis II (Hunter syndrome). *Genet. Med.* **8**, 465–473.

Nicolino, M., Byrne, B., Wraith, J.E., Leslie, N., Mandel, H., Freyer, D.R., Arnold, G.L., Pivnick, E.K., Ottinger, C.J., Robinson, P.H., Loo, J.C., Smitka, M., Jardine, P., Tato, L., Chabrol, B., Mccandless, S., Kimura, S., Mehta, L., Bali, D., Skrinar, A., Morgan, C., Rangachari, L., Corzo, D. & Kishnani, P.S. (2009): Clinical outcomes after long-term treatment with alglucosidase alfa in infants and children with advanced Pompe disease. *Genet. Med.* **11**, 210–219.

Poll, L.W., Koch, J.A., Vom Dahl, S., Willers, R., Scherer, A., Boerner, D., Niederau, C., Haussinger, D. & Modder, U. (2001): Magnetic resonance imaging of bone marrow changes in Gaucher disease during enzyme replacement therapy: first German long-term results. *Skel. Radiol.* **30**, 496–503.

Prows, C.A., Sanchez, N., Daugherty, C. & Grabowski, G.A. (1997): Gaucher disease: enzyme therapy in the acute neuronopathic variant. *Am. J. Med. Genet.* **71**, 16–21.

Raben, N., Fukuda, T., Gilbert, A.L., De Jong, D., Thurberg, B.L., Mattaliano, R.J., Meikle, P., Hopwood, J.J., Nagashima, K., Nagaraju, K. & Plotz, P.H. (2005): Replacing acid alpha-glucosidase in Pompe disease: recombinant and transgenic enzymes are equipotent, but neither completely clears glycogen from type II muscle fibers. *Mol. Ther.* **11**, 48–56.

Savas, P.S., Hemsley, K.M. & Hopwood, J.J. (2004): Intracerebral injection of sulphamidase delays neuropathology in murine MPS-IIIA. *Mol. Genet. Metab.* **82**, 273–285.

Schiffmann, R., Kopp, J.B., Austin, H.A., 3rd, Sabnis, S., Moore, D.F., Weibel, T., Balow, J.E. & Brady, R.O. (2001): Enzyme replacement therapy in Fabry disease: a randomized controlled trial. *JAMA* **285**, 2743–2749.

Schiffmann, R., Ries, M., Timmons, M., Flaherty, J.T. & Brady, R.O. (2006): Long-term therapy with agalsidase alfa for Fabry disease: safety and effects on renal function in a home infusion setting. *Nephrol. Dial. Transplant* **21**, 345–354.

Sun, B., Bird, A., Young, S.P., Kishnani, P.S., Chen, Y.T. & Koeberl, D.D. (2007): Enhanced response to enzyme replacement therapy in Pompe disease after the induction of immune tolerance. *Am. J. Hum. Genet.* **81**, 1042–1049.

Weidemann, F., Niemann, M., Breunig, F., Herrmann, S., Beer, M., Stork, S., Voelker, W., Ertl, G., Wanner, C. & Strotmann, J. (2009): Long-term effects of enzyme replacement therapy on Fabry cardiomyopathy: evidence for a better outcome with early treatment. *Circulation* **119**, 524–529.

West, M., Nicholls, K., Mehta, A., Clarke, J.T.R., Steiner, R., Beck, M., Barshop, B A., Rhead, W., Mensah, R., Ries, M. & Schiffmann, R. (2009): Agalsidase alfa and kidney dysfunction in Fabry disease. *J. Am. Soc. Nephrol.* **20**, 1132–1139.

Wilcox, W.R., Banikazemi, M., Guffon, N., Waldek, S., Lee, P., Linthorst, G.E., Desnick, R.J. & Germain, D.P. (2004): Long-term safety and efficacy of enzyme replacement therapy for Fabry disease. *Am. J. Hum. Genet.* **75,** 65–74.

Wraith, J.E., Clarke, L.A., Beck, M., Kolodny, E.H., Pastores, G.M., Muenzer, J., Rapoport, D.M., Berger, K.I., Swiedler, S.J., Kakkis, E.D., Braakman, T., Chadbourne, E., Walton-Bowen, K. & Cox, G.F. (2004): Enzyme replacement therapy for mucopolysaccharidosis I: a randomized, double-blinded, placebo-controlled, multinational study of recombinant human alpha-L-iduronidase (laronidase). *J. Pediatr.* **144,** 581–588.

Wraith, J.E., Beck, M., Lane, R., Van Der Ploeg, A., Shapiro, E., Xue, Y., Kakkis, E.D. & Guffon, N. (2007): Enzyme replacement therapy in patients who have mucopolysaccharidosis I and are younger than 5 years: results of a multinational study of recombinant human alpha-L-iduronidase (laronidase). *Pediatrics* **120,** e37–46.

Wraith, J.E., Scarpa, M., Beck, M., Bodamer, O.A., De Meirleir, L., Guffon, N., Meldgaard Lund, A., Malm, G., Van Der Ploeg, A.T. & Zeman, J. (2008): Mucopolysaccharidosis type II (Hunter syndrome): a clinical review and recommendations for treatment in the era of enzyme replacement therapy. *Eur. J. Pediatr.* **167,** 267–277.

Wynn, R.F., Mercer, J., Page, J., Carr, T.F., Jones, S. & Wraith, J.E. (2009): Use of enzyme replacement therapy (Laronidase) before hematopoietic stem cell transplantation for mucopolysaccharidosis I: experience in 18 patients. *J. Pediatr.* **154,** 135–139.

Zhang, X.K., Elbin, C.S., Chuang, W.L., Cooper, S.K., Marashio, C.A., Beauregard, C. & Keutzer, J.M. (2008): Multiplex enzyme assay screening of dried blood spots for lysosomal storage disorders by using tandem mass spectrometry. *Clin. Chem.* **54,** 1725–1728.

Chapter 13

Gaucher disease: clinical follow-up and management with individualized treatment

Elena Cassinerio, Irene Motta and Maria Domenica Cappellini

Centro Anemie Congenite, Dipartimento di Medicina Interna 1 A, Fondazione IRCCS Ospedale Maggiore Policlinico Ca' Granda, Università di Milano, via F. Sforza 35, 20122 Milan, Italy
maria.cappellini@unimi.it

Summary

Gaucher disease (GD), the most common inherited lysosomal storage disorder, is a multisystem disease resulting from an autosomal recessive defect of the gene encoding the glucocerebrosidase enzyme, which is responsible for accumulation of glucosylceramide into reticuloendothelial cells, particularly in liver, spleen, and bone marrow. Gaucher disease is a clinically heterogeneous disorder and it is traditionally classified as type 1 (non-neuronopathic disease) and types 2 and 3 (acute and chronic neuronopathic disease, respectively). The manifestations and the clinical progression of GD are highly variable between affected patients as is age, features of clinical presentation, and organ involvement. Each patient needs an accurate initial multisystem assessment and staging of damage to varying organs and the burden of the disease, followed by periodic evaluation. Over the years, authors have proposed several index scores to stage the severity of the disease. The presence of complications, such as anaemia, thrombocytopenia, and bleeding tendencies, organomegaly, liver or pulmonary dysfunction, or bone disease, is an indication for starting therapy. The heterogeneity of GD requires an individualized therapeutic approach. The aim of treatment should be directed to eliminate the symptoms, improving the patient's well-being, and preventing irreversible organ damage. The current standard treatment of GD is enzyme replacement therapy (ERT) with imiglucerase, a recombinant form of glucocerebrosidase. An alternative oral treatment has become available (substrate reduction therapy) and the development of new therapies (such as those using small molecules or chaperones) look to become possible in the future. Therapeutic goals are identified for each manifestation of the disease and their achievement and maintenance should be continually monitored.

Introduction

Gaucher disease is a progressive lysosomal storage disease due to an autosomal recessive deficiency of glucocerebrosidase, associated with the pathologic accumulation of glucosylceramide in the reticuloendothelial cells (monocytes/macrophages), particularly in liver, spleen, bone marrow, and lung, and thus rendering GD a multiorgan chronic disorder (Neufeld *et al.*, 1991). The accumulation of glucosylceramide in reticuloendothelial cells is the main pathologic mechanism leading to GD that was first described in 1934 by Aghion. Only in 1965 the glucocerebrosidase deficiency was demonstrated to be the cause of this storage disease (Brady et al., 1965). The defective gene (the *GBA* gene) is located on chromosome 1, and to date more than 300 different mutations have been described and a striking difference in their distribution has been observed in different populations. Also, recombination events between the *GBA* gene and its highly homologous pseudogene downstream have been identified, resulting from gene conversion, fusion, or duplication. The most common genotypes are N370S, L444P, IVS2^{+1}, and 84GG (Grace et al., 1994). Large macrophages, loaded with glucosylceramide, are called 'Gaucher cells' (Fig. 1). The macrophage origin of Gaucher cells has been demonstrated by the presence of surface macrophage markers, intense phagocytic activity, and characteristic cytoplasmic inclusions (Trajkovic-Bodennec et al., 2004; Jmoudiak & Futerman, 2005; Bitton et al., 2004; Boven et al., 2004). Thus, all the organs containing cells derived from the mononuclear phagocyte system (liver, bones, central nervous system, lung, spleen, lymph nodes, bone marrow, gastrointestinal and genitourinary tracts, pleura, and peritoneum) may be affected by Gaucher disease. Recent studies have shown that macrophagic activation, resulting in elevated serum levels of IL-1β, IL-6, IL-10, IL 8, TNF-α, and soluble IL-2 receptor, is one of the drivers of the GD pathogenesis (Parkin & Brunning, 1982). Moreover, the presence of systemic inflammation has been shown, demonstrated by elevated levels of inflammatory indicators (immunoglobulins and ferritin), and there is an increased risk of developing lymphoproliferative disorders and myeloma (Rosenbloom et al., 2005; Boven et al., 2004). The macrophage activation could potentially explain some clinical features of adult type 1 GD such as osteopenia and skeletal abnormalities, anaemia, activation of the coagulation cascade, or platelet activation (Moran et al., 2000; Hollak et al., 1997; Altarescu et al., 2005). Moreover, chitotriosidase, a human chitinase produced from activated macrophages, is markedly elevated in GD, and the chitotriosidase plasma level is used to determine the severity of the disease and to monitor the response to therapy (Aerts et al., 2005; Deegan & Cox, 2005; Vellodi et al., 2005). The clinical progression of the disease is highly variable, with different effects on the involved organs among affected patients (Maaswinkel-Mooij et al., 2000; Beutler & Grabowsky, 2006). Three major forms of GD have been clinically described (Table 1). About 90 per cent of all patients have the non-neuronopathic form, also called type 1. Type 1 GD patients are usually young adults, but manifestation of GD type 1 may become evident at any age; however, early clinical presentation predicts a more severe course of disease (Zimran et al., 1992). For this reason it is imperative to identify GD as early as possible so that monitoring and treatment begin at once. The incidence of type 1 GD in the overall population ranges from 1:40,000 to 1:60,000, but the incidence is higher in the Ashkenazi Jewish population (from 1:450 to 1:1,500). Clinical manifestations include anaemia, thrombocytopenia, enlargement of the spleen, skeletal abnormalities (osteopenia, lytic

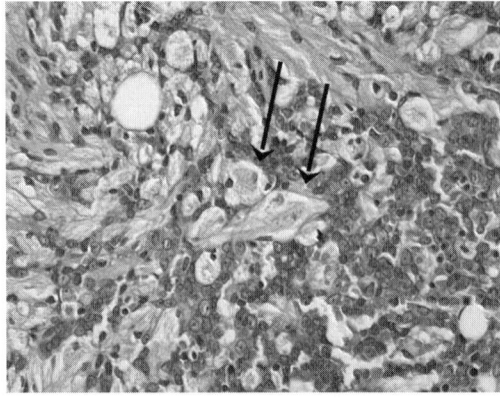

Fig. 1. Gaucher cells in a bone marrow biopsy.

Table 1. Different types of Gaucher disease

Characteristics and form of the disease	Type 1 Non-neuronopathic (adult form)	Type 2 Acute neuronopathic (< 1 year-old)	Type 3 Chronic neuronopathic (childhood-young)
Incidence	1:40,000 to 1:60,000 (1:450 to 1:1,500 in Ashkenazi Jews)	< 1:100,000	< 1:50,000 to < 1:100,000
Ethnic group	Pan-ethnic (Ashkenazi Jews)	Pan-ethnic	Pan-ethnic (northern Sweden)
Age of onset	Every age	< 1 year	Childhood
Life expectancy	6 to 80 years	< 2 years	2 to 60 years
Neurologic involvement	–	+++	+/+++ (progressive)
Hepatosplenomegaly	+/+++	++	+/+++
Haematologic involvement	+/+++	+++	+/+++
Skeletal involvement	+/+++	–	–/+++

lesions, pathologic fractures, chronic bone pain, bone crisis, bone infarcts, osteonecrosis, and skeletal deformities) and, in a small number of patients, lung involvement with interstitial lung disease and pulmonary hypertension (Vellodi *et al.*, 2005). The neuronopathic forms (type 2 and type 3) are pan-ethnic, although a particularly high prevalence of neurologic involvement has been documented among patients with GD in northern Sweden, Poland, and in the Jenin Arab population (Vellodi *et al.*, 2009). Type 2 is an acute neuronopathic form with a severe prognosis, leading to death by the age of 2 years. This disease variant may be characterized by neurologic symptoms due to pyramidal involvement (opisthotonus, head retroflexion, spasticity, trismus) and cognitive impairment (Vellodi *et al.*, 2001). Type 3 GD is characterized by a chronic neurologic involvement that usually appears later in life as compared to type 2. An intermediate form of neurologic GD has been described: this is characterized by a relatively late age at onset, but eventually rapidly progressive neurologic disease (Goker-Alpan *et al.*, 2003). A relationship between genotype and phenotype has been established, although a great heterogeneity of phenotype expression is observed: homozygosity for N370S is mainly associated with 'mild' type 1 GD, whereas homozygous L444P and D409H genotypes are related to neurologic forms of the disease (Vellodi *et al.*, 2009). The diagnosis of GD is based on the presence of reduced or absent glucocerebrosidase activity in peripheral blood leukocytes or in line cells obtained from blood or skin biopsy (Neufeld *et al.*, 1991). Molecular analysis confirms the diagnosis. The current standard therapy for treatment of GD is ERT with imiglucerase (Cerezyme®, Genzyme Corporation), a recombinant form of glucocerebrosidase. Alglucerase, introduced in 1991, was a first-generation placental glucocerebrosidase. The drug was extracted from a large pool of human placental tissue, and it remained the standard therapy for symptomatic GD patients for many years (Barton *et al.*, 1991). Recently, an oral alternative therapeutic approach (miglustat; Zavesca®, Actelion Pharmaceuticals) has become available for GD type 1, based on the principle of reducing substrate load: miglustat is actually an inhibitor of glucosylceramide synthase (the first committed step in the biosynthesis of glycosphingolipids). Miglustat is licensed in Europe, United States, and Israel for oral treatment of mild to moderate type 1 GD or where ERT is not suitable due to allergy, hypersensitivity, or poor venous access (Cox *et al.*, 2000; Weinreb *et al.*, 2008; Cox *et al.*, 2003).

Gaucher disease: review of monitoring and treatment

Clinical monitoring of the disease

The assessment of the development and progression of GD is essential in disease management and plays a major role in deciding to start treatment (Jmoudiak & Futerman, 2005). The initial assessment of a patient with GD is based on physical examination, blood tests, and visceral, skeletal, heart, and pulmonary evaluation to stage the disease and the organ burden (Fig. 2). In particular, white blood cell and platelet counts, haemoglobin levels, kidney and liver function, bleeding tendencies, and iron balance must be evaluated at diagnosis and regularly thereafter to follow disease progression and response to treatment. Organomegaly (spleen and liver enlargement) has to be evaluated by ultrasound (US) or better by computerized tomography (TC) or magnetic resonance imaging (MRI) to define liver and spleen volume and their eventual structural abnormalities. Electrocardiographic (ECG) and Doppler echocardiographic examination, and chest X-ray are used to define myocardial or valvular abnormalities and to show the presence of signs of pulmonary hypertension. Different imaging techniques are available to estimate the skeletal involvement in GD (vom Dahl et al., 2006): they can be categorized as qualitative, semi-quantitative, and quantitative imaging methods (Table 2). X-ray examination is a qualitative technique and it can detect Erlenmeyer-flask deformity (a typical sign consisting of distal femur enlargement), remodeling changes, osteosclerosis, osteolytic lesions (in advanced GD), osteonecrotic lesions, and fractures. The gold standard for assessing bone marrow infiltration of Gaucher cells is magnetic resonance imaging (MRI), with T_1- and T_2-weighted spin echo sequences. Spin echo sequence MRI is sensitive to changes in the fat content of adult yellow bone marrow, it shows irreversible lesions of GD (bone infarctions or fibrosis areas), and it is the most sensitive method for detecting femoral head necrosis. MRI is a qualitative method, but many scoring systems are available to render this technique also semi-quantitative (Rosenthal et al., 1986; Poll et al., 2001; Terk et al., 2000). Moreover, dual-energy X-ray absorptiometry (DEXA) is a technique validated for the assessment of bone mineral density (BMD) in patients with osteoporosis. In Gaucher disease DEXA is used to stage osteopenia/osteoporosis, monitoring the results during treatment. The severity of osteopenia assessed by DEXA in GD patients seems to be related to genotype, splenomegaly and hepatomegaly (Pastores et al., 1996). However, DEXA may lead to false normal or high values in patients with GD and severe skeletal disease, with sclerotic areas, avascular necrosis, or collapsed vertebrae (Kinoshita et al., 1998; Liu et al., 1997; Pye et al., 2007). Furthermore, the use of specific biomarkers can indirectly reflect the burden of the disease, its activity or complications, and the response to treatment. In GD, angiotensin-converting enzyme (ACE), tartrate-resistant acid phosphate (TRAP), and chitotriosidase are useful indicators of the disease progression and the response to therapy (Weinreb et al., 2004; Cabrera-Salazar et al., 2004). Chitotriosidase, a protein secreted from activated macrophages, is the most used biomarker in GD. It is markedly increased in treatment-naïve patients with GD and will decrease in response to ERT, in conjunction with improvements in haematologic and visceral parameters (Kovolenko et al., 2000). Moreover, a dose–response relationship has been described for plasma chitotriosidase activity and abnormal bone marrow infiltration in GD (de Fost et al., 2006). It is important to note that up to 6 per cent of the population does not have any chitotriosidase activity because of a common deletion in the chitotriosidase gene (Aerts & Hollak, 1997). A newly described surrogate biomarker is CCL18/PARC, which is particularly useful in patients with chitotriosidase deficiency to monitor the response to treatment (Cox et al., 2008). Actually, the

Chapter 13 Gaucher disease: clinical follow-up and management with individualized treatment

Blood tests	
Primary tests	**Additional tests as indicated** [5]
Haemoglobin	White blood cell count
Platelet count	AST and/or ALT (SGOT and/or SGPT)
Biochemical markers [3] - chitotriosidase	Alkaline phosphatase
Glucocerebrosidase activity	Total and direct bilirubin
Mutation analysis	Hepatitis profile
Antibody sample [4]	Albumin
	Total protein
	Serum immunoelectrophoresis
	Calcium
	Phosphorus
	Iron
	Iron-binding capacity
	Ferritin
	Vitamin B12
	PT
	PTT

Visceral [6]
Spleen and liver volume (volumetric MRI or CT)

Skeletal
X-ray: AP view of entire femora and lateral view of spine [7]
MRI (coronal: T1 & T2 weighted) of entire femora, and if possible of hips and lumbar vertebrae (QCSI) [b]
DEXA: lumbar spine and femoral neck [8]

Pulmonary
ECG, chest X-ray, and Doppler echocardiogram (right ventricular systolic pressure) for patients > 18 years

	Patients not on ERT		Patients on ERT			
			Therapeutic goals not achieved or maintained		Therapeutic goals achieved	At dosage change or significant clinical complication
	Every 12 months	Every 12-24 months	Every 3 months	Every 12 months	Every 12-24 months	
Blood tests [5]						
Haemoglobin	X		X		X	X
Platelet count	X		X		X	X
Biochemical markers [3] - chitotriosidase	X		X		X	X
Visceral [6]						
Spleen volume		X		X	X	X
Liver volume		X		X	X	X
Skeletal [9]						
MRI [b]		X		X	X	X
DEXA [8]		X		X	X	X
X-ray [7,10]		X		X	X	X
Pulmonary [11]						

1. A complete patient and family history, preferably including a pedigree, should be conducted.
2. A comprehensive physical examination and patient-reported functional health and well being survey should be performed at least annually.
3. One or more biochemical markers should be initially measured and consistently monitored at least every 12 months. Of the recommended markers (chitotriosidase or ACE or TRAP), chitotriosidase - when available as a validated procedure from an experienced laboratory - may be the most sensitive indicator of changing disease activity, and is therefore preferred.
4. A baseline sample should be drawn and may be stored at Genzyme. A subsequent sample is suggested to be drawn at 6 months after starting Cerezyme. The baseline and additional samples may be tested only if clinically indicated, such as for a suspected immune-mediated adverse event, prior to a switch to home therapy, or for suspected loss of efficacy of Cerezyme.
5. Additional blood tests, initially evaluated selectively based on each patient's age and clinical status, should be followed appropriately if initially abnormal.
6. Obtain contiguous transaxial 10 mm-thick sections for sums of regions of interest.
7. Plain X-ray can be used to detect deformity or fractures, and assess cortical thickness and skeletal age, but is of limited value to detect early signs of marrow involvement or osteopenia.
8. Dual-energy X-ray absorptiometry: for measuring bone mineral density, to detect and monitor osteopenia.
9. Additional anatomical skeletal sites should be evaluated if symptoms develop in such locations.
10. Optional in absence of new symptoms or evidence of disease progression; should not play major role in monitoring skeletal response to therapy.
11. Repeated pulmonary assessments are recommended every 12-14 months for patients with borderline or above normal pulmonary pressure at baseline.
a Weinreb NJ, Aggio MC, Andersson HC, et al. Gaucher disease type 1: revised recommendations on evaluations and monitoring for adult patients. Semin Hematol 2004;41(4 Suppl 5):15-22.
b Maas M, Poll LW, Terk MR. Imaging and quantifying skeletal involvement in Gaucher disease. Br J Radiol 2002; 75 (Suppl 1):A13-A24.

Abbreviations: ALT: alanine aminotransferase; AP: anteroposterior; AST: aspartate aminotransferase; CT: computed tomography; DEXA: dual-energy X-ray absorptiometry; ECG: electrocardiogram; MRI: magnetic resonance imaging; PT: prothrombin time; PTT: partial thromboplastin time

Fig. 2. Schematic assessment of complications and organ burden in Gaucher disease [from International Collaborative Gaucher Group (ICGG), Gaucher Registry Annual Report 2009].

Table 2. Some methods for the assessment of skeletal pathology in Gaucher disease

Method	Advantages	Disadvantages
X-ray	• Available worldwide • Standardized • Inexpensive and easy to perform • Indicated in fractures, exposure; local skeletal complaints or arthroplasty	• Lack of sensitivity for pathologic pattern and for follow-up of GD • Cumulative radiation
MRI (magnetic resonance imaging)	• Gold standard for assessment of bone marrow changes • No radiation exposure • Available in developed countries • Semi-quantitative assessment is possible • Easy to perform • Standardized MRI-investigations protocols • Sensitivity to skeletal changes in response to therapy	• High investigational costs • Not available in all countries • Use in paediatric patients requires further research
Scintigraphic imaging with ^{99m}Tc-sestamibi	• Widely available • Semi-quantitative score possible • Localized evaluation with correlation with systemic burden of GD and with other imaging methods	• Low specificity
QCSI (quantitative chemical shift imaging)	• More-sensitive MRI method measuring fat fraction • Early changes in fat fraction can be measured during therapy • Correlates with clinical bone complications	• Limited experience worldwide • Not widely available
DEXA (dual-energy X-ray-absorptiometry)	• Relatively inexpensive • Low radiation exposure • Widely available • Severity of osteopenia correlates with visceromegaly	• False positive and confounding findings in areas of avascular necrosis, infarction, vertebral collapse, lytic and sclerotic lesions

[Modified from vom Dahl (2006)]

use of biomarkers is intended to establish the activity of the disease during follow-up, but they have to be considered as an adjunct to clinical and other laboratory measurements to predict the evolution of GD. Particular attention must be paid in clinical assessment and follow-up in splenectomized patients with GD as they have a higher risk of severe bone disease, malignancies, and portal and pulmonary hypertension (Cox et al., 2008). In the past years, before the availability of ERT, splenectomy was carried out quite frequently because of spleen size and severe pancytopenia. At present, splenectomy is only used to control life-threatening thrombocytopenia, pressure effects (hydronephrosis), spleen rupture, and, in rare cases, autoimmune haemolytic anaemia or idiopathic thrombocytopenic purpura associated with GD; rarely splenectomy is indicated if tumour or lymphoma are present (Hughes et al, 2007). Splenectomy may have a severe impact on the course of GD: It has been shown to be associated with aggressive bone disease (Fleshner et al., 1991; Ida et al., 1999; Schiffmann et al., 2002), such as lytic lesions (Ashkenazi et al., 1996), osteonecrosis (Rodrigue et al., 1999), and reduction of body mass density (Pastores et al., 1996). An increased risk of malignancies in splenectomized patients affected by GD has also been suggested by Fleshner et al. (1991). Mistry et al. (2002) also reported that pulmonary hypertension is a more frequent complication in splenectomized patients with GD. Finally, an accurate bone and pulmonary follow-up is mandatory in this group of patients. For clinical follow-up, different indexes have been proposed for assessing the severity of the disease at baseline and then after each round of scheduled follow-up examinations. The aims of having a scoring index are to stage and to quantify the burden of GD. The first score index was devised by Zimran *et al.* in 1992 for the objective determination of the phenotypic expression of the disease, with criteria based on the extent of organ involvement. Recently, a new scoring system, the Gaucher Disease Severity Score Index–Type I (GAUSSI–I), has been proposed by Di Rocco *et al.* (2008) as a reliable method for staging the severity of adult type 1 GD and for evaluating responses to treatment. It consists in evaluation of different domains, represented by complications of the disease. Each domain has a score that can be evaluated at baseline and then followed thereafter. The follow-up for the assessment of the burden of the disease has to be repeated every 12 to 24 months, depending on the evolution of the disease and on the achievement and maintenance of therapeutic goals (Fig. 2).

Treatment and tailored therapeutic goals

GD is a clinically heterogeneous disorder and it needs an individualized approach and treatment to achieve a good response for all organs involved by the disease in each patient. This process requires a comprehensive initial assessment of all organs involved and the establishment of therapeutic goal. A definition of therapeutic goals for each component affected is important to establish the correct treatment (dose and timing of therapy), to assess expectations of both the physicians and patients, and to adjust therapy when goals are not met (Pastores *et al.*, 2004). For each patient a starting dosage has to be established and then adjusted with resepect to the achievement of therapeutic goals. The response to therapy is influenced by different factors such as concomitant pathologic conditions and age at presentation (Fig. 3). The standard therapy for GD is ERT with imiglucerase, and its dosage and frequency of administration has to be individualized to achieve and maintain the therapeutic aims. The initial treatment dose has to be based on the severity of the disease and on the likelihood for progressive or new-onset complications (Andersson *et al.*, 2005). The initial dosage of ERT can be established by dividing patients into low-risk and high-risk groups, as shown in 2005 by Andersson *et al.* (Tables 3 and 4). The recommended initial ERT dosage in adults and children at high risk is 60 U/kg body weight every 2 weeks; lower-risk adults start ERT at 30–45 U/kg every 2 weeks. In 2003, a panel of experts reviewed all the literature, their clinical experience and data from the International Gaucher Registry, and they proposed therapeutic goals for GD patients with reference to each organ system (Pastores *et al.*, 2004). The goals included improvement of the following conditions: anaemia, thrombocytopenia, visceral involvement (hepatomegaly and splenomegaly), skeletal pathology, growth, pulmonary involvement, functional health and well-being, physical examination, and biomarkers (Fig. 4). After the achievement of therapeutic goals, the decision to change the dose should take into account the history and course of the disease. Reduction of ERT is not appropriate in the presence of stable or minimally improved severe skeletal disease (Andersson *et al.*, 2005). Imiglucerase doses should not be decreased only on the basis of haematologic or organ volume improvement, but considering potentially reversible skeletal or pulmonary persistent disease. In some cases, increasing the dose leads to the achievement of therapeutic goals or it can help patients who relapse after dose reduction (Pastores *et al.*, 2004). Adult patients at high risk at baseline and who have achieved all therapeutic goals can have a decreased dose (by 15 to 25 per cent) until their next evaluation and if the therapeutic goals are maintained. The minimum recommended long-term dose in this group of patients is 30 U/kg every 2 weeks. In adult patients with less-severe GD (low-risk patients), a higher dose reduction may be tolerated (25 to 50 per cent): however, the minimum recommended

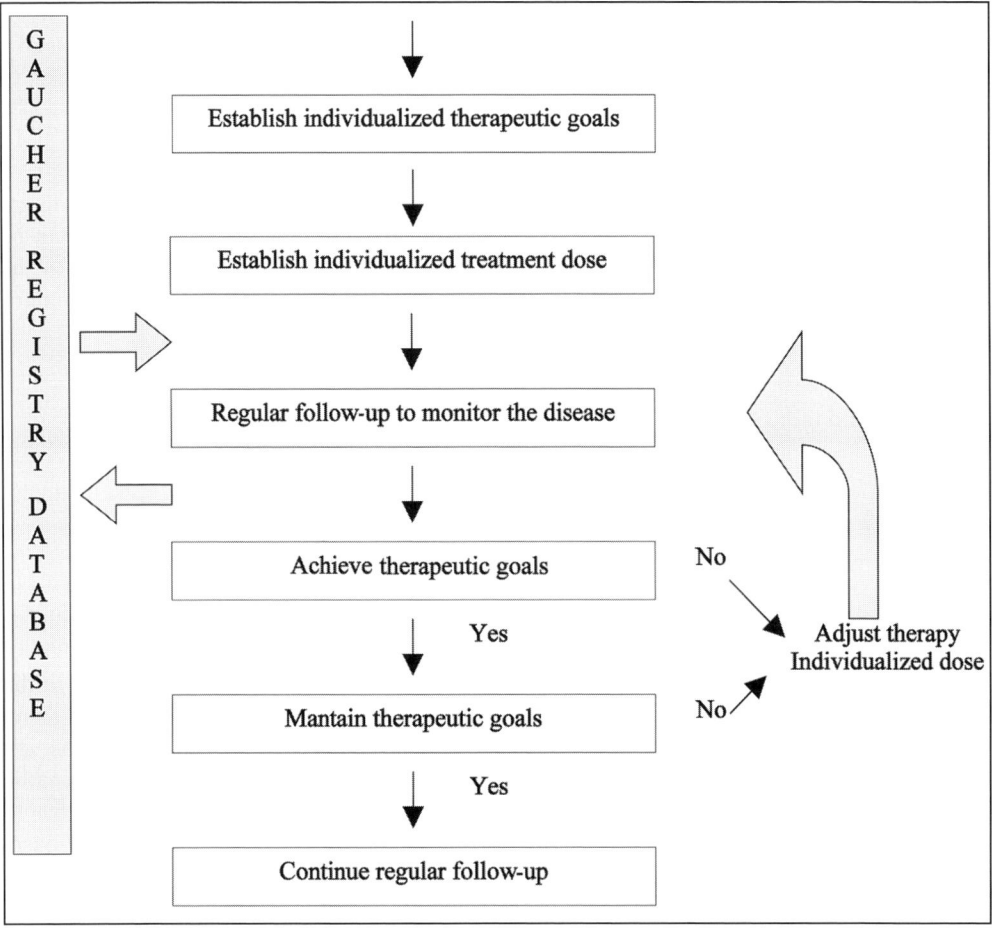

Fig. 3. Process for individualized treatment in Gaucher disease (modified from Pastores et al., 2004).

maintenance dose should not be lower than 20 U/kg every 2 weeks (Andersson et al., 2005). After dose changes, if therapeutic goals are not maintained, an increase or return to previous dosage must be considered.

Other treatment options for individual complications

Skeletal complications

Skeletal involvement in GD may lead to avascular necrosis and osteoporosis with fractures. Biphosphonates, acting directly on osteoclasts, are used to reduce bone resorption, increase calcium absorption, improve calcium balance, and maintain or improve bone density indices, preventing complications (Ostlere & Gold, 1991). In GD oral biphosphonate associated with ERT rapidly increases bone density (Wenstrup et al., 2004), but its effect on bone strength or on fracture risk is unknown. Although there is evidence that biphosphonates may alleviate bone pain in children (Bembi et al., 1994), it is not sufficient to recommend their standard use in adult patients with GD. Some patients can benefit from biphosphonate therapy, but a clear end-point has to be determined before starting treatment, and administration ceased once the

Table 3. Risk assessment in adults with Gaucher disease

High-risk adult GD patients – one or more of the following:	Low-risk adult GD patients
Symptomatic skeletal disease	Normal liver, cardiac, lung and renal function
• moderate to severe osteopenia	Minimal impairment of quality of life
• avascular necrosis	No obvious or recent rapid progression of disease manifestations
• chronic bone pain	Skeletal disease limited to mild osteopenia and Erlenmeyer-flask deformity
• pathologic fractures	Haemoglobin > 10.5 g/dl for females and > 11.5 g/dl for males (or not more than 2.0 g/dl below lower limit of normal for age and sex)
• bone crises	Platelet count > 60,000 mm^3 on three determinations
• joint replacement(s)	Liver volume < 2.5 × normal
Impaired QOL due to Gaucher disease	Spleen volume < 15 × normal
Cardiopulmonary disease, including pulmonary hypertension	
Platelet count ≤ 60,000 mm^3 or documented abnormal bleeding episodes	
Symptomatic anaemia or haemoglobin ≤ 8.0 g/dl	
Transfusion dependency	
Significant liver disease	
• severe hepatomegaly (> 2.5 × normal)	
• infarcts	
• portal hypertension	
• hepatitis	
Significant splenic disease	
• severe splenomegaly (≤ 15 × normal)	
• infarcts	
Significant renal disease	
Any concomitant disease that can complicate or exacerbate GD	

From Andersson et al. (2005)

Table 4. Risk assessment in children with Gaucher disease

High-risk children with Gaucher disease – one or more of the following:
• Sympomatic disease, including abdominal or bone pain, fatigue, exertion limitations, weakness or cachexia • Growth failure • Any evidence of skeletal involvement, including Erlenmeyer-flask deformity • Haemoglobin ≤ 2.0 g/dl below lower limit of normal for age and sex • Platelet count ≤ 60,000 mm^3 and/or documented abnormal bleeding episode(s) • Impaired quality of life

From Andersson et al. (2005)

desired bone mineralization density and reduction of fracture risk are achieved. In the presence of avascular necrosis or fractures, orthopaedic intervention may be necessary. Lebel et al. (2001) reported enhancement of quality of life, improvement of function, and restoration of normal activities in 23 patients with GD undergoing total hip arthroplasty.

Thrombocytopenia and bleeding tendencies

Surgical procedures may be complicated by the presence of thrombocytopenia as well as abnormalities in platelet function, increased prothrombin time (PT), or activated partial thromboplastin time (aPTT). Surgeons should pay attention to bleeding complications in GD patients, particularly those with platelet count of $100 \times 10^3/mm^3$ or below (Hughes et al., 2007). A complete coagulation assessment in GD patients is recommended before any surgical procedure. The use of desmopressin acetate (DDAVP) is recommended before major surgery with the aim of increasing factor VIII activity and improving platelet function. Deficiencies in specific coagulation factors can be countered by using recombinant factors or factor concentrates. When PT or aPTT are prolonged and no specific factor deficiency is detected, infusion of fresh frozen plasma is recommended. Platelet infusion should be done before surgery and when the platelet count is reduced to less than $50 \times 10^3/mm^3$ (Hughes et al., 2007).

Malignant haematologic disease

An increased risk of developing multiple myeloma is present in GD patients (Rosenbloom et al., 2005). A regular check for monoclonal abnormalities is recommended in patients with GD. There are no data on the effects of high-dose ERT on MGUS and potential B-cell malignancies, but when there is evidence of multiple myeloma in patients with GD, treatment options should be considered. Chemotherapy to treat myeloma may worsen the cytopenia of GD. Patients with a concomitant diagnosis of myeloma should not to be excluded from receiving ERT, which may be useful to improve the patient's overall condition and in particular alleviate cytopenia. Few cases have been reported in the literature of the co-occurrence of multiple myeloma with GD nor do guidelines exist for their treatment (Hughes et al., 2007).

Neuronopathic Gaucher disease

In neuronopathic GD, ERT has an excellent safety profile and it ameliorates systemic involvement; however, there is no evidence that it has reversed, stabilized, or slowed the progression of neurologic involvement (Vellodi et al., 2009). Children with chronic neuronopathic GD should start ERT at a dosage of 60 U/kg every 2 weeks, whereas in adults a dose of 30–60 U/kg every 2 weeks should be sufficient. In patients with the acute neurologic form of the disease, ERT has little effect on the progressively downhill course (Bove et al., 1995).

Chapter 13 Gaucher disease: clinical follow-up and management with individualized treatment

Haematology	Time frame
- increase haemoglobin ≥12.0 g/dL (7.4 mmol/l) for males and ≥11.0 g/dL (6.8 mmol/l) for females and children	1-2 years
Intact spleen:	
- in severe thrombocytopenia increase platelet count to level sufficient to prevent bleeding, usually ≥ 30 x 10⁹/L	year 1
- upon moderate baseline thrombocytopenia increase count 1.5 - 2 fold	year 1
Splenectomised patients:	
- normalization of platelet count	year 1

Visceral	
- reduce liver volume	
- by 20% - 30%	1-2 years
- by 30% - 40%	3-5 years
- reduce spleen volume	
- by 30% - 50%	year 1
- by 50% - 60%	2-5 years

Skeletal	
- reduce or eliminate bone pain	1-2 years
- prevent bone crises	1-2 years
- prevent osteonecrosis and subchondral joint collapse	1-2 years
- increase cortical and trabecular bone mineral density (adults)	3-5 years
- decrease bone marrow infiltration by ≥2 out of 8 BMB points [d,e]	2-5 years

Paediatric patients	
- attain normal or ideal peak skeletal mass (children)	year 2
- normalize growth	year 3
- achieve normal onset of puberty	

Other	
- prevent pulmonary disease by timely initiation of Cerezyme and avoidance of splenectomy	
- prevent rapid deterioration of pulmonary disease and sudden death	
- reverse hepatopulmonary syndrome and dependency on oxygen	
- ameliorate pulmonary hypertension	
- improve functional health and well being	
- reduce plasma chitotriosidase activity > 15%	year 1

[*] Pastores GM, Weinreb NJ, Aerts H, et al. Therapeutic goals in the treatment of Gaucher disease. Semin Hematol 2004;41(4 Suppl 5):4-14.

[d] Vom Dahl S, Poll L, Di Rocco M, et al. Evidence-based recommendations for monitoring bone disease and the response to enzyme replacement therapy in Gaucher patients. Curr Med Res Opin 2006; 22 (6): 1045-1064.

[e] de Fost M, Hollak CEM, Groener JEM, et al. Superior effects of high dose enzyme replacement therapy in type 1 Gaucher disease on bone marrow involvement and chitotriosidase levels : a 2-center retrospective analysis. Blood 2006; 108 (3): 830-835.

Fig. 4. Therapeutic goals in treatment Gaucher disease [from International Collaborative Gaucher Group (ICGG), Gaucher Registry Annual Report 2009].

Conclusions

Gaucher disease is an inherited lysosomal storage disease resulting from an autosomal recessive defect of the gene encoding the glucocerebrosidase enzyme (GlcCerase) responsible for accumulation of glucosylceramide into reticuloendothelial cells, particularly in liver, spleen, bone marrow, and lung, and thus rendering GD a multiorgan chronic disorder. This multiorgan, chronic, heterogeneous disorder requires an individualized treatment approach. Many variables, such as severity and rate of disease progression, concomitant pathologic conditions, the impact of disease manifestations on quality of life, and the phenotype/genotype relationship, should be considered prior to initiation of treatment in a patient with GD. The current standard therapy for treatment of GD is ERT with imiglucerase (Cerezyme®), a recombinant form of glucocerebrosidase. Recently, an oral alternative therapeutic approach (miglustat [Zavesca®], Actelion Pharmaceuticals) has become available for GD type 1, based on the principle of reducing substrate load. The correct assessment of the burden of the disease and proper follow-up helps to determine an individualized therapy. Guidelines for the evaluation and monitoring of the disease and therapeutic goals were published in 2004, but they require periodic update to reflect emerging knowledge about the many aspects of GD. This knowledge may be tapped by consulting the data and information found at the International Gaucher Registry, the largest database, which contains the data of the 5,323 patients enrolled up to December 2008-2009 (International Collaborative Gaucher Group [ICGG], Gaucher Registry Annual Report 2009).

References

Aerts, J.M. & Hollak, C.E. (1997): Plasma and metabolic abnormalities in Gaucher's disease. *Baillieres Clin. Haematol.* **10**, 691–709.

Aerts, J.M., Hollak, C.E., van Breemen, M., Groener, J.E. & Boot, R.G. (2005): Identification and use of biomarkers in Gaucher disease and other lysosomal storage disease. *Acta Paediatr.* **94** (Suppl.), 43–46.

Altarescu, G., Zimran, A., Michelakakis, H. & Elstein, D. (2005): TNF alpha levels and TNF alpha gene polymorphism in type I Gaucher disease. *Cytokine* **31**, 149–152.

Andersson, H.C., Charrow, J., Kaplan, P., Mistry, P., Pastores, G.M., Prakesh-Cheng, A., Rosenbloom, B.E., Scott, R.C., Wappner, R.S. & Weinreb, N.J. for the International Collaborative Group U.S. Regional Coordinators (2005): Individualization of long-term enzyme replacement therapy for Gaucher disease. *Genet. Med.* **7**, 105–110.

Ashkenazi, A., Zaizov, R. & Matoth, Y. (1986): Effect of splenectomy on destructive bone changes in children with chronic (Type I) Gaucher disease. *Eur. J. Pediatr.* **145**, 138–141.

Barton, N.W., Brady, R.O., Dambrosia, J.M., Di Bisceglie, A.M., Doppelt, S.H., Hill, S.C., Mankin, H.J., Murray, G.J., Parker, R.I. & Argoff, C.E. (1991): Replacement therapy for inherited enzyme deficiency: Macrophage-targeted glucocerebrosidase for Gaucher disease. *N. Engl. J. Med.* **324**, 1464–1470.

Bembi, B., Zanatta, M., Carrozzi, M., Baralle, F., Gornati, R., Berra, B. & Agosti, E. (1994): Enzyme replacement treatment in type 1 and type 3 Gaucher's disease. *Lancet* **344**, 1679–1682.

Beutler, E. & Grabowsky, G.A. (2006): Gaucher disease. In: *Metabolic and molecular bases of inherited disease*, eds. C. Scriver *et al.*, pp. 3635–3668. New York: McGraw-Hill.

Bitton, A., Etzell, J., Grenert, J.P. & Wang, E. (2004): Erythrophagocytosis in Gaucher cells. *Arch. Pathol. Lab. Med.* **128**, 1191–1192.

Bove, K.E., Daugherty, C. & Grabowski, G.A. (1995): Pathological findings in Gaucher disease type 2 patients following enzyme therapy. *Hum. Pathol.* **26**, 1040–1045.

Boven, L.A., van Meurs, M., Boot, R.G., Mehta, A., Boon, L., Aerts, J.M. & Laman, J.D. (2004): Gaucher cells demonstrate a distinct macrophage phenotype and resemble alternatively activated macrophages. *Am. J. Clin. Pathol.* **122**, 359–369.

Brady, R.O., Gal, A.E., Canfer, J.N. & Bradley, R.M. (1965): The metabolism of glucocerebroside purification and properties of a glucosyl- and galactosylceramide-cleaving enzyme from rat intestinal tissue. *J. Biol. Chem.* **240**, 3766–3770.

Cabrera-Salazar, M.A., O'Rourke, E., Henderson, N., Wessel, H. & Barranger, J.A. (2004): Correlation of surrogate markers of Gaucher disease: implications for long-term follow-up of enzyme replacement therapy. *Clin. Chim. Acta* **344**, 101–107.

Cox, T.M., Lachmann, R., Hollak, C., Aerts, J., van Weely, S., Hrebicek, M., Platt, F., Butter, T., Dwek, R., Moyses, C., Gow, I., Elstein, D. & Zimran, A. (2000): Novel oral treatment of Gaucher's disease with N-butyldeoxynojirimycin (OGT 918) to decrease substrate biosynthesis. *Lancet* **355**, 1481–1485.

Cox, T.M., Aerts, J.M., Andria, G., Beck, M., Belmatoug, N., Bembi, B., Chertkoff, R., Vom Dahl, S., Elstein, D., erikson, A., Giralt, M., Heitner, R., Hollak, C., Hrebicek, M., Lewis, S., Mehta, A., Pastores, G.M., Rolfs, A., Miranda M.C. & Zimran, A. (2003): The role of iminosugar N-butyldeoxynojirimycin (miglustat) in the management of type I (non neuronopathic) Gaucher disease: a position statement. *J. Inherit. Metab. Dis.* **26**, 513–526.

Cox, T.M., Aerts, J.M., Belmatoug N., Cappellini, M.D., vom Dahl, S., Goldblatt, J., Grabowsky, G.A., Hollak, C., Hwu, P., Maas, M., Martins, A.M., Mistry, P., Pastores, G.M., Tylki-Szymanska, A., Yee, J. & Weinreb, N. (2008): Management of non-neuronopathic Gaucher disease with special reference to pregnancy, splenectomy, bisphosphonate therapy, use of biomarkers and bone disease monitoring. *J. Inherit. Metab. Dis.* **31**, 319–336.

Deegan, P.B. & Cox, T.M. (2005): Clinical evaluation of biomarkers in Gaucher disease. *Acta Paediatr. Suppl.* **94** (447), 47–50.

de Fost, M., Hollak, C.E., Groener, J.E., Aerts, J.M., Maas, M., Poll, L.W., Wiersma, M.G., Haussinger, D., Brett, S., Brill, N. & vom Dahl, S. (2006): Superior effect of high-dose enzyme replacement therapy in type 1 Gaucher disease on bone marrow involvement and chitotriosidase levels: a 2-center retrospective analysis. *Blood* **108**, 830–835.

Di Rocco, M., Giona, F., Carubbi, F., Linari, S., Minichilli, F., Brady, R.O., Mariani, G. & Cappellini, M.D. (2008): A new severity score index for phenotypic classification and evaluation of responses to treatment in type I Gaucher disease. *Haematologica* **93**, 1211–1218.

Fleshner, P.R., Aufses, A.H. Jr., Grabowsky, G.A & Elias, R. (1991): A 27-year experience with splenectomy for Gaucher's disease. *Am. J. Surg.* **161**, 69–75.

Goker-Alpan, O., Schiffmann, R., Park, J.K., Stubblefield, B.K., Tayebi, N. & Sidransky, E. (2003): Phenotypic continuum in neuronopathic Gaucher disease: an intermediate phenotype between type 2 and type 3. *J. Pediatr.* **143**, 273–276.

Grace, M.E., Newman, K.M., Scheinker, V., Berg-Fussman, A. & Grabowsky, G.A. (1994): Analysis of human acid β-glucosidase by site-directed mutagenesis and heterogeneous expression. *J. Biol. Chem.* **269**, 2283–2291.

Hollak, C.E., Evers, L., Aerts, J.M. & van Oers, M.H. (1997): Elevated levels of M-CSF, sCD14, and IL8 in type 1 Gaucher disease. *Blood Cells Mol. Dis.* **23**, 201–212.

Hughes, D., Cappellini, M.D., Berger, M., Droogenbroeck, J.V., de Fost, M., Janic, D., Marinakis, T., Rosenbaum, H., Villarubia, J., Zhukovskaya, E. & Hollak, C. (2007): Recommendations for the management of the haematological and onco-haematological aspects of Gaucher disease. *Br. J. Haematol.* **138**, 676–686.

Ida, H., Rennert, O.M., Kato, S., Ueda, T., Oishi, K., Maekawa, K. & Eto, Y. (1999): Severe skeletal complications in Japanese patients with type 1 Gaucher disease. *J. Inherit. Metab. Dis.* **22**, 63–73.

International Collaborative Gaucher Group (ICGG), Gaucher Registry Annual Report 2009. <www.gaucherregistry.com>

Jmoudiak, M. & Futerman, A. (2005): Gaucher disease: pathological mechanisms and modern management. *Br. J. Haematol.* **129**, 178–188.

Kinoshita, H., Tamaki, T., Hashimoto, T. & Kasaqui, F. (1998): Factors influencing lumbar spine bone mineral density assessment by dual-energy X-ray absorptiometry: comparison with lumbar spinal radiogram. *J. Orthop. Sci.* **3**, 3–9.

Kovolenko, T.A., Zhanaeva, S.Y., Falameeva, O.V., Kaledin, V.I., Filyushina, E.E., Buzueva, I.I. & Paul, G.A. (2000): Chitotriosidase as a marker of macrophage stimulation. *Bull. Exp. Biol. Med.* **130**, 948–950.

Lebel, E., Itzchaki, M., Hadas-Halpern, I., Zimran, A. & Elstein, D. (2001): Outcome of total hip arthroplasty in patients with Gaucher disease. *J. Arthroplasty* **16**, 7–12.

Liu, G., Peacock, M., Eilam, O., Dorulla, G., Braunstein, E. & Johnston, C.C. (1997): Effect of osteoarthritis in the lumbar spine and hip on bone mineral density and diagnosis of osteoporosis in elderly men and women. *Osteoporos. Int.* **7**, 564–569.

Maaswinkel-Mooij, P., Hollack, C., van Eysden-Plaisier, M., Prins, M., Aerts, H. & Poll, R. (2000): The natural course of Gaucher disease in the Netherlands: implications for monitoring of disease manifestation. *J. Inherit. Metab. Dis.* **23**, 77–82.

Mistry, P.K., Sirrs, S. & Chan, A. (2002): Pulmonary hypertension in type 1 Gaucher's disease: genetic and epigenetic determinants of phenotype and response to therapy. *Metabolism* **77**, 91–98.

Moran, M.T., Schofield, J.P., Hayman, A.R., Shi, G.P., Young, E. & Cox, T.M. (2000): Pathologic gene expression in Gaucher disease: up-regulation of cysteine proteinases including osteoclastic cathepsin K. *Blood* **96**, 1969–1978.

Neufeld, E.F. (1991): Lysosomal storage disease. *Annu. Rev. Biochem.* **60**, 257–280.

Ostlere, S.J. & Gold, R.H. (1991): Osteoporosis and bone density measurements methods. *Clin. Orthop. Relat. Res.* **271**, 149–163.

Parkin, J. & Brunning, R. (1982): Pathology of the Gaucher cell. In: *Gaucher disease: a century of delineation and research*, eds. R. Desnick, S. Gatt & G. Grabowski, pp. 151. New York: Alan R. Liss.

Pastores, G.M., Wallenstein, S., Desnick, R.J. & Luckey M.M. (1996): Bone density in type 1 Gaucher disease. *J. Bone Miner. Res.* **11**, 1801–1807.

Pastores, G.M., Weinreb, N.J., Aerts, H., Andria, G., Cox, T.M., Giralt, M., Grabowski, G.A., Mistry P.K. & Tylki-Szymanska, A. (2004): Therapeutic goals in the treatment of Gaucher disease. *Semin. Hematol.* **41**, 4–14.

Poll, L.W., Koch, J.A., vom Dahl, S., Willers, R., Scherer, A., Boerner, D., Niederau, C., Haussinger, D. & Modder U. (2001): Magnetic resonance imaging of bone marrow changes in Gaucher disease during enzyme replacement therapy: first German long-term results. *Skeletal Radiol.* **9**, 496–503.

Pye, S.R., Reid, D.M., Lunt, M., Adams, J.E., Silman, A.J. & O'Neill T.W. (2007): Lumbar disc degeneration: association between osteophytes, and-plate sclerosis and disc space narrowing. *Ann. Rheum. Dis.* **66**, 330–333.

Rodrigue, S.W., Rosenthal, D.I. & Barton, N.W. (1999): Risk factors for osteonecrosis in patients with type I Gaucher's disease. *Clin. Orthop. Relat. Res.* **362**, 201–207.

Rosenbloom, B.E., Weinreb, N.J., Zimran, A., Kacena, K.A., Charrow, J., & Ward, E. (2005): Gaucher disease and cancer incidence: a study from the Gaucher Registry. *Blood* **105**, 4569–4572.

Rosenthal, D.I., Scott, J.A., Barranger, J., Mankin, H.J., Saini, S., Brady, T.J., Osier, L.K. & Doppelt, S. (1986): Evaluation of Gaucher disease using magnetic resonance imaging. *J. Bone Joint Surg. Am.* **68**, 802–808.

Schiffmann, R., Mankin, H., Dambrosia, J.M., Xavier, R.J., Kreps, C., Hill, S.C., Barton, N.W. & Rosenthal, D.I. (2002): Decreased bone density in splenectomized Gaucher patients receiving enzyme replacement therapy. *Blood Cells Mol. Dis.* **28**, 288–296.

Terk, M.R., Dardashti, S. & Liebman H.A. (2000): Bone marrow response in treated patients with Gaucher disease: evaluation by T1-weighted magnetic resonance images and correlation with reduction in liver and spleen volume. *Skeletal Radiol.* **29**, 563–571.

Trajkovic-Bodennec, S., Bodonnec, J. & Futerman, A.H. (2004): Phosphatidylcholine metabolism is altered in a monocyte-derived macrophage model of Gaucher disease but not in lymphocytes. *Blood Cells Mol. Dis.* **33**, 77–82.

Vellodi, A., Bembi, B., de Villemeur T.B., Collin-Histed, T., Erikson, A., Mengel, E., Rolfs, A. & Tylki-Szymanska, A. Neuropathic Gaucher Disease Task Force. (2001): Management of neuronopathic Gaucher disease: a European consensus. *J. Inherit. Metab. Dis.* **24**, 319–327.

Vellodi, A., Foo, Y. & Cole, T.J. (2005): Evaluation of three markers in the monitoring of Gaucher disease. *J. Inherit. Metab.* Dis. **28**, 585–592.

Vellodi, A., Tylki-Szymanska, A., Davies, E.H., Kolodny, E., Bembi, B., Collin-Histed, T., Mengel, E., Erikson, A. & Schiffmann, R. (2009): Management of neuronopathic Gaucher disease: revised recommendations. *J. Inherit. Metab. Dis*. DOI 10.1007/s10545-009-1164-2.

vom Dahl, S., Poll, L., Di Rocco, M., Ciana, G., Denes, C., Mariani G. & Maas, M. (2006): Evidence-based recommendations for monitoring bone disease and the response to enzyme replacement therapy in Gaucher patients. *Curr. Res. Med. Opin.* **22**, 1045–1064.

Weinreb, N.J., Aggio, M.C., Andersson, H.C., Andria, G., Charrow, J., Clarke, J.T.R., Erikson, A., Giraldo, P., Goldblatt, J., Hollak, C., Ida, H., Kaplan, P., Kolodny, E.H., Mistry, P., Pastores, G.M., Pires, R., Prakesh-Cheng, A., Rosenbloom, B.E., Scott, C.R., Sobreira, E., Tylki-Szymanska, A., Velodi, A., vom Dahl, S., Wappner, R.S. & Zimran, A (2004): Gaucher disease type I: revised recommendations on evaluations and monitoring for adult patients. *Semin. Hematol.* **41**, 15–22.

Weinreb, N., Tayor, J., Cox, T., Yee, J. & vom Dahl, S. (2008): A benchmark analysis of the achievement of therapeutic goals for type 1 Gaucher disease patients treated with imiglucerase. *Am. J. Hematol.* **83**, 890–895.

Wenstrup, R.J., Bailey, L., Grabowsky, G.A., Moskovitz, J., Oestreich, A.E., Wu, W. & Sun, S. (2004): Gaucher disease: alendronate disodium improves bone mineral density in adults receiving enzyme therapy. *Blood* **104**, 1253–1257.

Zimran, A., Kay, A., Gelbart, T., Garver, P., Thurston, D., Saven, A. & Beutler, E. (1992): Gaucher disease: clinical, laboratory, radiologic and genetic features of 53 patients. *Medicine (Baltimore)* **71**, 337–353.

Chapter 14

Enzyme replacement therapy in glycogenosis type II

Giovanni Ciana and Bruno Bembi

Centro Coordinamento Regionale Malattie Rare, Azienda Ospedaliero Universitaria 'S. Maria della Misericordia', piazzale S. Maria della Misericordia 15, 33100 Udine, Italy
ciana.giovanni@aoud.sanita.fvg.it

Summary

Glycogenosis type II or Pompe disease is an inherited autosomal recessive metabolic myopathy caused by deficiency of the enzyme acid α-glucosidase, which hydrolyzes lysosomal glycogen. It has a wide spectrum of clinical presentations: the classic infantile form is seen soon after birth, with muscle weakness, cardiomyopathy, respiratory insufficiency, and a rapidly fatal course. The late-infantile phenotype shows less acute cardiac involvement, with the fatal course during early childhood. On the contrary, the late-onset forms generally do not manifest cardiac involvement, but present with progressive skeletal muscle impairment and a variable degree of respiratory insufficiency. With disease progression, many patients are confined to wheelchairs or need walking aids and ventilatory support. Age of death varies from early childhood to late adulthood. Enzyme replacement therapy (ERT) with recombinant human alpha glucosidase (rhGAA) has been available since 1999 and received marketing approval in 2006 (alglucosidase alpha; Myozyme, Genzyme Corporation). The availability of ERT has changed clinical expectation for affected patients. In the classic infantile phenotype ERT has significantly improved cardiac function, with marked reduction of storage material, improved motor skills, reduced the need for ventilation, and improved the survival rate. A patient's clinical conditions at baseline and the age at initiation of therapy are the most important factors in predicting clinical outcome. Only few data about ERT in the late-onset phenotype are available at present. However, published studies have shown that ERT improved motor and pulmonary function, even if it is not yet clear whether all patients may benefit from ERT. It has been suggested that ERT be started as soon as possible when the patients' clinical conditions are still reasonably good and muscle architecture has not yet been much compromised.

Introduction

Glycogenosis type II (known also as Pompe disease or acid maltase deficiency) is an inherited autosomal recessive metabolic myopathy, characterized by lysosomal glycogen storage due to the deficiency of the lysosomal enzyme acid α-glucosidase. Its incidence is estimated to be about 1:40,000 neonates/year (Hirschhorn & Reuser, 2001).

Three clinical forms of the disease have been described: (1) 'classic infantile' glycogenosis type II, which is manifested during the first few months of life and includes hypertrophic cardiomyopathy. The disease rapidly progresses and it is almost invariably fatal within the first

2 years (van den Hout *et al.*, 2003). (2) The 'nonclassic infantile' phenotype is seen between the first and second year of life and is characterized by a more attenuated course of the disease. (3) The 'late-onset' phenotype, which is characterized by the absence of cardiomyopathy and the progressive involvement of skeletal and respiratory muscles presents at any time after the age of 2 years.

Although this classification is still used, glycogenosis type II should be considered as a disease that encompasses a continuous spectrum of phenotypes with different age at onset, organ involvement, and degree of myopathy (Table 1).

Table 1. Glycogenosis type II: phenotypic continuum

Infantile onset	Late onset
Rapidly progressive muscle weakness	Progressive muscle weakness
Feeding difficulties	No cardiac involvement
Cardiomegaly	Swallowing difficulty
Moderate hepatomegaly	Respiratory infections
Macroglossia	Respiratory distress
Respiratory infections	Exercise intolerance
Respiratory diseases	Elevated muscular enzymes
Delayed motor milestones	Moderate hepatomegaly
Elevated muscular enzymes	Residual GAA activity
Rapidly progressive fatal course	
No/residual GAA activity	

For a long time glycogenosis type II has been considered to be untreatable. Nutrition and exercise therapy, being the only supportive treatment, have been shown to slow disease progression, even if not uniformly, in late-onset form (Slonim *et al.*, 1983, 2007). In 1999, ERT became available as the human recombinant enzyme (hrGAA) was first purified from rabbit milk and then from Chinese hamster ovary (CHO) cells.

Currently, a number of reports have been published on the efficacy and safety of ERT in infantile phenotypes, whereas data concerning late-onset phenotypes are still limited. This review summarizes the results reported in the literature so far.

Enzyme replacement therapy in infantile phenotypes

The feasibility of ERT in Pompe disease was first demonstrated during the 1980s by Reuser *et al.* (1984) and van der Ploeg *et al.* (1988), who, by using α-glucosidase purified from bovine testis and human urine, corrected the defect in cultured skeletal muscle cells. They also demonstrated that the enzyme targeting was mediated by the mannose 6-phosphate receptor. These first experiments gave evidence of the difficulty of reaching the muscle tissue: a large amount of the protein was sequestered in the liver and the spleen, and only a small fraction reached heart and skeletal muscles. On the basis of these results, these authors predicted that high doses of enzyme would be necessary to efficiently reach the muscle tissues. During the 1990s, the cloning of the GAA gene and advances in recombinant technology led to the industrial production of rhGAA both in the milk of transgenic rabbits and in CHO cells (Bijovet *et al.*, 1999; van Hove *et al.*, 1996), opening the era of enzyme replacement therapy.

Different studies in the animal model of glycogenosis II have shown that a dosage of enzyme $\geq$ 10 mg/kg i.v. was necessary to reduce the lysosomal storage of glycogen in muscle cells (Kikuchi *et al.*, 1998; Bijovet *et al.*, 1999; van Hove *et al.*, 1996; Raben *et al.*, 2003).

The first therapeutic human clinical trial was performed in 1999, when four patients with classic infantile Pompe disease were infused with the rabbit-derived enzyme (van den Hout et al., 2000). Almost concomitantly, Amalfitano et al. (2001) conducted a pilot study with the CHO-derived recombinant enzyme in three infants. Subsequently, Klinge et al. (2005) reported the results in two infants receiving enzyme replacement therapy over a 48-week period, while Kishnani et al. (2006) reported the results of a 1-year follow-up of eight patients with the infantile form of the disease who also received CHO-derived enzyme. ERT was started during the first 6 months of life in all the 17 patients involved in these four studies. Data analysis showed a prominent effect of ERT in reducing cardiomegaly and improving heart function. Ten patients also showed a marked improvement in their motor skills and reached important milestones such as sitting, rolling, standing, and walking. Five of them learned to walk without needing supportive ventilation. Not all children responded equally well. Ten remained ventilator-dependent, of whom five died. A further patient died while not receiving any respiratory support. However, in comparison with the natural history of untreated children, in which the mean age of survival is less than 1 year, the overall rate of survival was significant improved: the longest survivors in this population were 8-year-old children.

All these studies underline the severity of initial clinical conditions as major prognostic factor.

During the last 2 years, three different studies, involving larger groups of patients with a prolonged follow-up, have been published (Kishani et al., 2007, 2009; Nicolino et al., 2009).

The first study of Kishnani et al. (2007) evaluated the ERT effect of CHO-derived rhGAA up to 106 weeks of follow-up in 18 classic infantile patients diagnosed before the first 6 months of age. Patients were divided in two groups: those receiving 20 mg/kg and those receiving 40 mg/kg every other week, respectively.

All patients were alive at the end of the study: six became ventilation-dependent, seven were able to walk, three could stand up, and three learned to sit or roll over, whereas three did not manifest any significant improvement. No differences in the clinical outcome were reported between the two groups.

The same cohort was then enrolled in an extended study (Kishnani et al., 2009) and continued to receive ERT for up to a total of 3 years. Survival rate and ventilatory use were analysed at 24 and 36 months. Cardiomyopathy continued to lessen in ERT-responding patients, and an improvement in motor skills was detected in 11 children, seven of whom were walking by the time of their final assessment, while the other four were sitting independently at that time.

The survival rate was 94.4 per cent and 72 per cent at 24 and 36 months, respectively. At the end of the study or at the age of death, an overall number of 9 children required invasive ventilator support.

The authors concluded that in this patient population ERT reduced (*a*) the risk of death by 95 per cent; (*b*) the risk of invasive ventilation or death by 91 per cent; and (*c*) the risk of any type of ventilation or death by 87 per cent, in comparison with untreated historical groups.

In the study performed by Nicolino et al. (2009), 21 infants aged 3 to 43 months (median 13 months) received ERT for up to 168 weeks (median 120 weeks, range 0.6–168 weeks). Survival rate was 71 per cent (16/21) at the end of the study. Left ventricular mass index improved in all patients and 13 patients (62 per cent) achieved new motor milestones: 86 per cent (18/21) gained functional independence skills and five walked without support. Sixteen patients were free of invasive ventilation (*via* tracheostomy) at the beginning of the study. By the end of the study, seven of them were alive and free of invasive ventilation, four needed continued ventilatory support, and five died.

These authors concluded that ERT reduced the risk of death by 79 per cent and the risk of invasive ventilation by 58 per cent, when compared to untreated reference cohorts.

Both these long-term follow-up studies showed a positive effect of ERT on cardiac and skeletal muscles, respiratory function and survival. If the study of Kishnani et al. underlines the importance of beginning ERT in the first 6 months of life, the one of Nicolino et al. shows that treatment may be efficacious even if started beyond this age. It suggests that baseline clinical status is a better indicator of the progression of Pompe disease and of the potential response to treatment than age alone.

These data seem very encouraging in view of the upcoming use of ERT in late-onset phenotypes. However, studies in larger series of patients as well as longer periods of follow-up are needed in order to understand the still persisting 'gray areas' of the disease in early life.

Enzyme replacement therapy in late-onset phenotypes

Three main studies on the natural history of late-onset glycogenosis have been published in the last 4 years, the first in 2005 by Winkel et al. and the other two by Hagemans et al. in 2005 and 2006. The analysis of these data showed a median age at onset of 24 years and a median age at diagnosis of 33 years. The first symptoms were mainly related to muscle weakness. Muscle enzymes were frequently, but not always, elevated and respiratory failure was the main cause of death.

Regarding the respiratory and mobility impairment, the studies demonstrated a direct correlation between the duration of disease and the percentage of patients needing ventilatory support and mobility devices, particularly the wheelchair. At present, only few studies have been published reporting the first results of ERT effectiveness in late-onset glycogenosis II patients.

Positive effects on muscular strength and mobility have been reported by different authors. Winkel et al. (2004) followed three patients who had been receiving rabbit milk–derived rhGAA since 1999, when they were 11, 16, and 32 years old, respectively. They were all wheelchair-bound. After 3 years of treatment, the youngest and least-affected patient showed a drastic gain of muscle strength and function, while the other two showed some increase of muscle strength. These patients were followed for another 5 years (van Capelle et al., 2008). During that period a stabilization of muscle function was observed in the two more severely affected, while the youngest one achieved normal muscle strength for all muscle groups: he could rise from a squatting position and did not present any limitation in sport and social activities.

Case et al. (2008) showed the regained ability to walk without any assistive device and to climb stairs with railings in a 63-year-old female. Merk et al. (2009) described a positive effect on muscle strength of the thighs and the pelvic girdle in four patients aged 39 to 68 years after 6 months of ERT.

A quantitative magnetic resonance imaging study was performed by Ravaglia et al. in 2008. These authors described an increase in muscle mass of the lower limbs in a severely affected 49-year-old male treated with ERT, with a concomitant increase in body mass index.

The first results of a phase III multicentre, double-blind, randomized placebo-controlled trial, involving a series of 90 ambulatory patients (free of invasive ventilation prior to ERT and older than 8 years of age) followed for 78 weeks, was presented at the 2008 Annual Symposium of the SSIEM (Society for the Study of Inborn Errors of Metabolism) in Lisbon by van der Ploeg et al., who reported a significant improvement in patients' walking capacity, measured by the 6-minute walk test.

Finally, a very recent study by Strothotte et al. (2009) has shown a significant improvement in the modified Gowers' test and the 6-minute-walk test in a group of 44 patients with late-onset disease.

In all these studies a significant decrease in the plasma levels of muscle enzymes was observed during ERT.

Despite the positive clinical results of ERT in patients affected by glycogenosis type II, studies performed by Fukuda et al. (2006) and Raben et al. (2007) raise some doubt about the real effect of ERT in correcting the mechanism of muscle cellular damage. These authors demonstrated a dramatic expansion of vesicles of the endocytic/autophagic pathways caused by the storage process, both in alpha-glucosidase (GAA) knock-out mice and in patients' myoblasts. The autophagic build-up seems to alter the trafficking and processing of the therapeutic enzyme along the endocytic pathway, particularly in type II myoblasts. This abnormality seems to be responsible for the increased ERT resistance of these cells in comparison with type I fibres. Further studies are needed to better understand the mechanisms involved in the cellular damage and to improve the enzymatic uptake and targeting to the lysosome.

Less conclusive are the data concerning respiratory involvement. Winkel et al. (2004) and van Capelle et al. (2008) have described a stabilization of respiratory function in their patients, even in those more severely affected and ventilator-dependent. Merk at al. (2009) reported an improvement of pulmonary function in two of four patients over a 6-month treatment period. In the same study, the maximal inspiration pressure improved in all four patients, even if two of them did not suffer from respiratory insufficiency. Also, the study of van der Ploeg et al. (2008) showed an improvement of pulmonary function in treated patients compared to the placebo group, whereas Strothotte et al. (2009) did not observe any significant result on respiratory parameters.

Our personal experience in a multicentre Italian study of 29 late-onset patients (13 females, 16 males; 7 juveniles, 22 adults) treated for at least 36 months has shown significant results in terms of muscular improvement (improving results of the 6-minute-walk test in all of them and decreasing the Walton scale severity index in five patients), reduction in mean daily ventilation time (from 15.5 to 9.6 hours), reduction of plasma muscular enzyme values (CK, LDH, AST, and ALT), and improvement in subjective symptoms such as headache and muscular pain (Bembi et al., 2009; and unpublished results)

No severe secondary effects have been reported in any of the aforementioned studies.

Conclusions

ERT in glycogenosis type II has been shown to change patients' prospects in terms of quality of life and life expectancy.

Many factors may influence the therapeutic response: the age of the patient at the beginning of ERT, the severity of muscle involvement at baseline, the mechanisms of tissue diffusion and cellular uptake of the therapeutic enzyme, and finally the influence of the autophagic build-up. Although these are still open issues, the first clinical trials have clearly demonstrated that:

a) In classic infantile phenotypes, ERT markedly improves survival and reduces the risk of any type of ventilation; it also dramatically reduces cardiac storage, improving both cardiac and skeletal muscle function. However, new issues related to the longer survival period, such as long-term muscular response, hearing loss, possible arrhythmic complications, and the secondary involvement of bone metabolism need to be discussed.

b) In late-onset phenotypes, ERT improves or stabilizes motor and pulmonary function, independently of patients' age and disease severity. The positive results also appear to be directly related to the early start of therapy.

Acknowledgments: The authors would like to thank Sarah Tripepi Winteringham, BA, MCIL, and Andrea Dardis, PhD, for their support in proofreading and editing this manuscript.

References

Amalfitano, A., Bengur, A.R, Morse, R.P., Majure, J.M., Case, L.E., Veerling, D.L., Mackey, J, Kishnani, P., Smith, W., McVie-Wylie, A., Sullivan, J.A., Hoganson, G.E., Phillips, J.A., 3rd, Schaefer, G.B., Charrow, J., Ware, R.E, Bossen, E.H. & Chen, Y.Y. (2001): Recombinant human acid alpha-glucosidase enzyme therapy for infantile glycogen storage disease type II: results of a phase I/II clinical trial. *Genet. Med.* **3,** 132–138.

Bembi, B., Ravaglia, S., Pisa, F.E., Ciana, G., Fiumara, A., Confalonieri, M., Parini, R., Rigoldi, M., Moglia, A., Costa, A., Danesino, C., Pittis, M.G. & Dardis, A. (2009): Enzyme replacement therapy in late-onset phenotypes of glycogenosis 2: a 24 months follow-up. Submitted for publication.

Bijovet, A.G., van Huirtum, H., Kroos, M.A., van de Kamp, E.H., Schoneveld, O., Visser, P., Brakenhoff, J.P., Weggeman, M, van Corven, E.J., van der Ploeg, A.T. & Reuser, A.J. (1999): Human acid alpha-glucosidase from rabbit milk has therapeutic effect in mice with glycogen storage disease type II. *Hum. Mol. Genet.* **8,** 2145–2153.

Case, L.E., Koeberl, D.D., Young, S.P., Bali, D., DeArmey, S.M., Mackey, J. & Kishnani, P.S. (2008): Improvement with ongoing enzyme replacement therapy in advanced late-onset Pompe disease: a case study. *Mol. Genet. Metab.* **95,** 233–235.

Fukuda, T., Roberts, A., Ahearn, M., Zaal, K., Ralston, E., Plotz, P.H. & Raben, N. (2006): Autophagy and lysosomes in Pompe disease. *Autophagy* **2,** 318–320.

Hagemans, M.L., Winkel, L.P., Hop, W.C., Reuser, A.J., van Doorn, P.A. & van der Ploeg, A.T. (2005): Disease severity in children and adults with Pompe disease related to age and disease duration. *Neurology* **64,** 2139–2141.

Hagemans, M.L., Hop, W.J., van Doorn, P.A., Reuser, A.J. & van der Ploeg, A.T. (2006): Course of disability and respiratory function in untreated late-onset Pompe disease. *Neurology* **66,** 581–583.

Hirschhorn, R. & Reuser, A. (2001): Glycogen storage disease type II: acid alpha-glucosidase (acid maltase) deficiency. In: *The metabolic and molecular bases of inherited disease,* vol. 3, eds. C. Scriver, A. Beaudet, W. Sly & D. Valle, pp. 3389–3420. New York: McGraw-Hill.

Kikuchi, T., Yang, H.W., Pennybacker, M. Ichicara, N., Mizutani, M., van Hove, J.L. & Chen, Y.T. (1998): Clinical and metabolic correction of Pompe disease by enzyme therapy in acid-maltase-deficient quail. *J. Clin. Invest.* **15,** 827–833.

Kishnani, P.S., Nicolino, M., Voit, T., Rogers, R.C., Tsai, A.C., Waterson, J., Herman, G.E., Amalfitano, A., Thurberg, B.L., Richards, S., Davison, M., Corzo, D. & Chen, Y.T. (2006): Chinese hamster ovary cell-derived recombinant human acid alpha-glucosidase in infantile-onset Pompe disease. *J. Pediatr.* **149,** 89–97.

Kishnani, P.S, Corzo, D., Nicolino, M., Byrne, B., Mandel, H., Hwu, W.L., Leslie, N., Levine, J., Spencer, C., McDonald, M, Li, J., Dumontier, J., Halberthal, M., Chien, Y.H., Hopkin, R., Vijayaraghavan, S., Gruskin, D., Bartholomew,D., van der Ploeg, A. Clancy, J.P, Parini, R., Morin, G., Beck, M., De la Gastine, G.S, Jokic, M., Thurberg, B., Richards, S., Bali, D., Davison, M., Worden, M.A., Chen, Y.T. & Wraith, J.E. (2007): Recombinant human acid alpha glucosidase: major clinical benefits in infantile-onset Pompe disease. *Neurology* **68,** 99–109.

Kishnani, P.S., Corzo, D., Leslie, N.D., Gruskin, D., van der Ploeg, A., Clancy, J.P., Parini, R., Morin, G., Beck, M., Bauer, M.S., Jokic, M., Tsai, C.E,., Tsai, B.W., Morgan, C., O'Meara, T., Richards, S., Tsao, E.C. & Mandel, H. (2009): Early treatment with alglucosidase alpha prolongs long term survival of infants with Pompe disease. *Pediatr. Res.* **66,** 329–335.

Klinge, L., Straub, V., Neudorf, U., Schaper, J., Bosbach, T., Görlinger, K., Wallot, M., Richards, S. & Voit, T. (2005): Safety and efficacy of recombinant acid alpha-glucosidase (rhGAA) in patients with classical infantile Pompe disease: results of a phase II clinical trial. *Neuromusc. Disord.* **15,** 24–31.

Merk, T., Wibmer, T., Schumann, C. & Krüger, S. (2009): Glycogen storage disease type II (Pompe disease): influence of enzyme replacement therapy in adults. *Eur. J. Neurol.* **16,** 274–277.

Nicolino, M., Byrne, B., Wraith, J.E., Leslie, N., Mandel, H., Freyer, D.R., Arnold, G.L., Pivnick, E.K., Ottinger, C.J., Robinson, P.H., Loo, J.C., Smitka, M., Jardine, P., Tatò, L., Chabrol, B., McCandless, S., Kimura, S., Mehta, L., Bali, D., Skrinar, A., Morgan, C., Rangachari, L., Corzo, D. & Kishnani, P.S. (2009): Clinical outcomes after long-term treatment with alglucosidase alpha in infants and children with advanced Pompe disease. *Genet. Med.* **11,** 210–219.

Raben, N., Danon, M., Gilbert A.L., Dwivedi, S., Collins, B., Thurberg, B.L., Mattaliano, R.J., Nagaraju, K. & Plotz, P.H. (2003): Enzyme replacement therapy in the mouse model of Pompe disease. *Mol. Genet. Metab.* **80,** 159–169.

Raben, N., Takikita, S., Pittis, M.G., Bembi, B., Marie, S.K., Roberts, A., Page, L., Kishnani, P.S., Schoser, B.G., Chien, Y.H., Ralston, E., Nagaraju, K. & Plotz, P.H. (2007): Deconstructing Pompe disease by analyzing single muscle fibers: to see a world in a grain of sand. *Autophagy* **3,** 546–552.

Ravaglia, S., Danesino, C., Pichiecchio, A., Repetto, A., Poloni, G.U., Rossi, M., Fratino, P., Moglia, A. & Costa, A. (2008): Enzyme replacement therapy in severe adult-onset glycogen storage disease type II. *Adv. Ther.* **25,** 820–829.

Reuser, A.J, Kroos, M.A., Ponne, N.J., Wolterman, R.A., Loonen, M.C, Busch, H.F., Visser, W.J. & Bolhuis, P.A. (1984): Uptake and stability of human bovine acid alpha-glucosidase in cultured fibroblasts and skeletal muscle cells from glycogenosis type patients. *Exp. Cell Res.* **155,** 178–189.

Slonim, A.E., Coleman, R.A., McElligot, M.A., Nassar, J., Hirshorn, K. & Labadie, G.U. (1983): Improvement of muscle function in acid maltase deficiency by high-protein therapy. *Neurology* **33,** 24–38.

Slonim, A.E., Bulone, L., Goldberg, T., Minikes, J., Slonim, E., Galanko, J. & Martinuik, F. (2007): Modification of the natural history of adult-onset acid maltase deficiency by nutrition and exercise therapy. *Muscle Nerve* **35,** 70–77.

Strothotte S, Strigl-Pill, N., Grunert, B., Kornblum, C., Eger, K., Wessig, C., Deschauer, M., Breunig, F., Glocker, F.X., Vielhaber, S., Brejova, A., Hilz, M., Reiners, K., Müller-Felber, W., Mengel, E., Spranger, M. & Schoser, B. (2010): Enzyme replacement therapy with alglucosidase alpha in 44 patients with late-onset glycogen storage disease type 2: 12-month results of an observational clinical trial. *J. Neurol.* **257,** 91–97.

Van Capelle, C.I., Winkel, L.P., Hagemans, M.L., Shapira, S.K., Arts W.F., van Doorn, P.A., Hop, W.C., Reuser, A.J. & van der Ploeg, A.T. (2008): Eight years experience in two children and one adult with Pompe disease. *Neuromusc. Disord.* **18,** 447–452.

Van den Hout, H., Reuser, A.J., Vulto, A.G., Loonen, M.C.B., Cromme-Dijkhuis, A. & van der Ploeg, A.T. (2000): Recombinant human alpha-glucosidase from rabbit milk in Pompe patients. *Lancet* **356,** 397–398.

Van den Hout, H.M., Hop, W., van Diggelen, O.P., Smeitinnk, J.A., Smit, G.P., Poll-The, B.T., Bakker, H.D., Loonen, M.C., de Klerk, J.B., Reuser, A.J. & van der Ploeg, A.T. (2003): The natural course of infantile Pompe's disease: 20 original cases compared with 133 cases from the literature. *Pediatrics* **112,** 332–340.

Van der Ploeg, A.T., Loonen, M.C., Bolhuis, P.A., Busch, H.F., Reuser, A.J & Galjard, H. (1988): Receptor-mediated uptake of acid alpha-glucosidase corrects lysosomal glycogen storage in cultured skeletal muscle. *Pediatr. Res.* **24,** 90–94.

Van der Ploeg, A.T., Clemens, P.R., Corzo, D., Escolar, D., Florence, J., Laforet, P., Lake, S., Mayhew, J., Morgan, C., Pestronk, A., Rosenbloom, B., Skrinar, A. & Wasserstein, M. (2008): *Placebo controlled study of alglucosidase alpha in adults with Pompe disease* [abstract]. In: Annual Symposium of the Society for the Study of Inborn Errors of Metabolism, Lisbon, Portugal, 2–5 September, 2008.

Van Hove, J.L., Yang, H.W., Wu, J.Y., Brady, R.O. & Chen, Y.T. (1996): High level production of recombinant human lysosome acid alpha-glucosidase in Chinese hamster ovary cells which targets to heart muscle and corrects glycogen accumulation in fibroblasts from patients with Pompe disease. *Proc. Natl. Acad. Sci. USA* **93,** 65–70.

Winkel, L.P., van den Hout, J.M., Kamphoven, J.H., Disseldorp, J.A., Remmerswaal, M., Arts, W.F., Loonen, M.C., Vulto, A.G., van Doorn, P.A., De Jong, G., Hop, W., Smit, G.P., Shapira, S.K., Boer, M.A., van Diggelen, O.P., Reuser, A.J. & van der Ploeg, A.T. (2004): Enzyme replacement therapy in late-onset Pompe's disease: a three-year follow-up. *Ann. Neurol.* **55,** 495–502.

Winkel, L.P., Hagemans, M.L., van Doorn, P.A., Loonen, M.C., Hop, W.J., Reuser, A.J. & van der Ploeg, A.T. (2005): The natural course of non-classic Pompe's disease: a review of 225 published cases. *J. Neurol.* **252,** 875–884.

Chapter 15

Haematopoietic stem cell transplantation for lysosomal storage diseases

Giovanna Lucchini, Paola Corti and Attilio Rovelli

*BMT Unit, Paediatric Department, Milano – Bicocca University, San Gerardo Hospital,
via Pergolesi 33, 20052 Monza, Italy*
a.rovelli@hsgerardo.org

Summary

Haematopoietic stem cell transplantation (HSCT) can benefit some selected subsets of patients with lysosomal storage diseases. Results have been impressive in children with MPS I-H, but poor in other disorders. Careful, multidisciplinary decision-making regarding whether to recommend HSCT and how to provide optimal pre- and post-HSCT care has proven essential to increase the likelihood of a good outcome. This is a review of the state of the art in this field and current indications for the procedure.

Introduction

Lysosomal storage diseases (LSDs) are more than 40 different disorders having an aggregate estimated incidence of 1 in 7,000–10,000 live births. For most of these disorders medical management is extremely difficult and disease-specific, requiring an experienced base in many specialties in order to provide appropriate care. Until recently, management of most LSDs consisted only of supportive care, but during the last decade, much progress has been made in this field towards treatment.

At present, LSDs are at the convergence of many basic science discoveries and clinical trials of experimental treatments, which makes them appropriately recognized as a paradigm for overcoming many of the problems of orphan diseases. Since enzyme replacement therapy (ERT) was successfully introduced in 1991 for patients with Gaucher disease, this principle of treatment has been considered for other disorders as well. Currently available treatment options for many LSDs include enzyme replacement therapy, substrate reduction with imino sugar, chaperones, and haematopoietic stem cell transplantation (HSCT). Further drugs might soon become available for individual diseases, an enormous effort has been directed at developing new strategies for crossing the blood–brain barrier, and clinical trials of gene therapy are in an advanced preclinical phase.

Haematopoietic stem cell transplant for LSDs was pioneered nearly 30 years ago by Hobbs, who performed HSCT in a patient with mucopolysaccharidosis type I-H (MPS I-H). Since then, HSCT has been carried out for at least 20 of the known lysosomal storage diseases so far. The results have provided proof of principle that donor bone marrow generates a permanent endogenous supply of enzyme-producing cells. However, in view of the advent of new therapies and technologies and increased understanding of the factors for successful transplantation, with constantly improving HSCT results, the correct place of HSCT needs constant redefinition, and current practice might be expected to change in the coming years (Beck, 2007; Boelens, 2006; Prasad & Kurtzberg, 2008; Vellodi, 2005).

Haematopoietic stem cell transplantation

Over the past 30 years, nearly 1,000 HCSTs have been performed worldwide for patients with a wide range of different LSDs. With the exception of a few diseases, such as MPS I-H and globoid cell leukodystrophy (GLD), most published data in this field are single case reports or small series with short follow-up. The most relevant reasons for this are that, until recently, data collection for these diseases has never become as routine as for patients undergoing transplantation for malignancies, follow-up has not been performed in a systematic fashion, and cooperative trials for such rare diseases are often impossible to set up. The issue of the length of follow-up is particularly important when evaluating the outcome of 'indolent' forms of LSDs. A careful collection of information about the genotype, the specific organ damage, and the neuropsychological status at the time of HSCT is essential to correctly evaluate the long-term results (Martin *et al.*, 2006; Pastores *et al.*, 2007; Peters *et al.*, 1996, 1998; Rovelli & Steward, 2005; Staba *et al.*, 2004).

The rationale of HSCT in LSDs is based on the repopulation of the recipient with metabolically normal donor-derived cells. HSCT repopulates mononuclear phagocytic cells (macrophages, Kupffer cells, pulmonary alveolar macrophages) and provides replacement of non-neuronal cells in the central nervous system (CNS). After HSCT, donor-derived cells are identified throughout the CNS (including perivascular and parenchymal regions) and over time they completely repopulate the microglial compartment. Macrophages and microglia represent major effectors of the catabolism of the storage material, and their replacement by normal cells has also the potential to restore a critical scavenger function. The exact mechanisms involved in infiltration of brain parenchyma by blood-circulating precursors and in their differentiation into microglia are yet poorly characterized (Proia & Wu, 2004). Following transplantation, the normal enzyme is released by donor-derived cells and taken up by defective cells by receptor-mediated endocytosis (intercellular transport). Also other mechanisms, such as the direct intercellular transfer occurring from adjacent cells (cell-to-cell contact), could play a role. The enzyme is targeted to the lysosome by the mannose or mannose-6-phosphate (M6P) tag on that enzyme, which binds to the appropriate receptor on the cell surface. The heterogeneity of receptor-mediated endocytosic systems influences the extent to which uptake of hydrolase occurs in various cells and tissues after transplantation (Vellodi, 2005).

HSCT is a complex medical procedure that involves the administration of high-dose chemotherapy (conditioning regimen) to the recipient, aiming at ablating the haematopoietic cells in the marrow (creation of space) and immune system (immunosuppression), and replacing them with donor stem cells (engraftment), which are capable of producing normal amounts of the deficient enzyme. Conditioning is central to HCST: host stem cells must be eradicated to allow donor stem cells to access the defined niches within the marrow stroma for engraftment, and immunosuppression is required to prevent rejection of the incoming donor cells by host immune cells (host-versus-graft disease). Metabolic transplant procedures have relied mostly on a backbone of busulphan and cyclophosphamide conditioning and, until a few years ago, a relevant number of patients (at least one-third of those undergoing transplantation in Europe) had a T-cell-depleted graft because of concerns about the potential for graft-versus-host disease (GvHD) to aggravate the inflammatory components of leukodystrophy. In the last decade there has been experimentation with increased immunosuppression, alternative agents such as melphalan, fludarabine, and thiotepa, reduced-intensity conditioning regimens, and the use of high stem cell doses, but controlled data are lacking. However, it has been clearly shown in a recent retrospective study that both T-cell depletion and reduced-intensity conditioning regimens were found to be risk factors for rejection, whereas a busulphan-based conditioning regimen with busulphan pharmacokinetic targeting and an unmanipulated graft protected against graft failure (Boelens *et al.*, 2007). Furthermore, at least in childen with MPS I-H, a remarkably low incidence of GvHD, in comparison with other transplant settings, has been reported by different studies without *ex vivo* T-cell depletion (Souillet *et al.*, 2003).

HSCT creates a short-term risk to the life of the patient and presents him or her with some long-term complications. However, the quality of life of most long-term survivors is highly improved, and in almost all cases, immunosuppressive therapy can be discontinued as the new immune system becomes tolerated by the recipient, in contrast to solid organ transplantation, for which life-long immune suppression is required.

During the 1980s and '90s, the success of HSCT was hindered by limited donor availability, the high rate of transplant-related morbidity and mortality (GvHD, idiopathic pneumonia, lung haemorrhage, *etc.*) and graft loss (15–75 per cent). However, in the past five years, almost all highly experienced transplant centres have been reporting engrafted survival rates of more than 90 per cent, with most donations being unrelated or mismatched cord blood units. The highest rate of survival and success is achieved in patients with MPS I-H when they receive a transplant at a younger age, soon after the diagnosis, with a fully matched cord blood unit, following a fully myeloablative conditioning and achieving a long-lasting full donor chimerism. These results arise as a consequence of improved transplant practice mainly due to *(a)* advances in HLA typing with better matching of unrelated donors, *(b)* larger unrelated donor pools and improved supportive care, *(c)* an increased understanding of the factors associated with failure of the transplant in the LSD setting and increased availability and use of alternative stem cell sources (cord blood), and *(d)* standardization of protocols. HSCT is currently without any doubt a much safer procedure with an estimated greater survival. These results might foster a reconsideration of the role of HSCT in children with more attenuated disease, where previously the procedure would have been considered too risky, and in children with significant co-morbidities, where outcome was previously unacceptably poor (Prasad & Kurtzberg, 2008).

HSCT creates a dynamic chimera involving the transplanted donor cells and the recipient–host. For this reason, an accurate assessment of chimerism in the patient's blood or bone marrow provides critical information on the progress of engraftment, and serves as a key element in predicting rejection. Quantitative methodologies enable estimating the magnitude of chimerism in the patient based on the ratio between the donor and recipient blood cells, which is usually expressed as per cent donor chimerism. The greatest challenge in the area of transplantation for LSDs is the high frequency of primary and secondary graft rejection and incomplete donor chimerism. Initial engraftment has been reported to occur in 63 to 85 per cent of MPS I-H patients according to donor type and other transplant factors. Second graft procedures are needed in many patients, even where sibling donors have been used, increasing the risk of transplant-related morbidity and mortality. At least 15–30 per cent of patients with MPS I-H need a second graft, although the second procedure is usually well tolerated by children with that disorder and the rate of success is unexpectedly high (approximately 80 per cent).

Insufficiency of the myeloablative regimen and immunosuppression have been considered the possible cause of the high rate of rejection. It has been suggested that earlier achievement of more complete donor chimerism by increasing cyclophosphamide doses may enhance long-term outcome. However, increasing regimen potency could enhance toxicity to fragile organ systems with pathologic accumulation.

Recently it has become clear from registry data that the use of cord blood as a donor cell source is associated with improved rates of engraftment and complete donor chimerism (Boelens et al., 2009). Furthermore, the use of umbilical cord blood increases the unrelated donor pool for children requiring HSCT, as less precise matching is required. More than 90 per cent of children with MPS I-H receiving a cord blood graft achieve a full donor chimerism and nearly 100 per cent of them show a fully normal enzyme activity level. Therefore cord blood is currently the recommended cell source for transplantation in MPS I-H patients (Martin et al., 2006). A concomitant search for unrelated cord blood should be started as soon as eligibility has been defined for a patient with an LSD. Since the cell dose seems to influence the outcome, it is recommended to select a cord blood unit with a high number of nucleated cells per kilogram (possibly from 5 to 10, but no less than 3.5×10^7/kg).

It has been generally believed for a long time that incomplete donor chimerism might not affect outcome since it is likely that as little as 10 per cent of normal enzyme levels are required for full therapeutic effect. This supposition should be considered with care, particularly because of the lag phase to clinical stability. Many sibling donors will be carriers, with approximately half of normal enzyme levels. When added to slow ingress of microglial cells and protracted washout of toxic metabolites, it seems likely that partial chimerism can only compromise the long-term benefit to the CNS of the transplant procedure. Recently, a markedly different transplant outcome, expressed in terms of deficient enzyme level and residual substrate, has been shown in allografted MPS I-H patients. When a normal donor was used, there was significantly higher enzyme than when a heterozygous donor was used or when there was mixed chimerism after transplant. The higher enzyme level was associated with significantly reduced substrate. Since HSCT outcome improved, particularly with the higher levels of donor chimerism following cord blood grafts, this information might influence donor selection when a heterozygote-matched family member is available.

ERT is now available for some LSDs (Fabry, Gaucher, and Pompe diseases, and MPS I, II, and VI) or is under development for others, which has raised interest in evaluating the potential role of pre-transplant ERT in reducing treatment-related mortality and enhancing engraftment. Higher alpha-L-iduronidase levels are likely to result in more rapid and more complete clearance of substrates from visceral organs, which would be expected to translate into clinical benefit to the MPS I-H patients eligible for HSCT. Initial reports seemed to show no effect on treatment-related morbidity and mortality or engraftment. However, improved survival expectancy after HSCT has been recently reported in high-risk patients. Therefore, pre-transplant ERT could be useful in those patients lacking the prompt availability of a banked umbilical cord blood unit, while waiting for the identification of a potential unrelated donor or in those at high risk (due to cardiomyopathy or previous lung complications, for example) for transplantation. Our current practice is to treat all MPS I-H patients with ERT until engraftment (based on chimerism and alpha-L-iduronidase activity) (Cox-Brinkman et al., 2006; Grewal et al., 2005).

At present, HSCT is the only available treatment that can prevent CNS disease progression (e.g., in MPS I-H patients) and is effective in improving or normalizing functions in many organs. However, musculoskeletal abnormalities can become worse despite continued engraftment, and orthopaedic and neurosurgical interventions are still necessary in several patients. This is currently one of the major limitations of HSCT in patients with LSDs characterized by skeletal involvement. Details about results of HSCT and specific organ and neuropsychological outcome in MPS I-H patients have been recently reviewed (Aldenhoven et al., 2008; Pitt et al., 2009) and are also reported by Jaap Boelens in another chapter in this volume.

Current indications for haematopoietic stem cell transplantation

From the impressive results in MPS I-H, it was expected that most storage disorders could be alleviated by HSCT. However, it was found that benefit from HSCT appeared limited only to selected subsets of patients with a few types of LSDs. HSCT is not effective in patients with overt neurologic symptoms or in those with aggressive infantile forms (Peters & Steward, 2003).

The primary goals of HCT have been to promote long-term survival with donor-derived engraftment and to optimize the quality of life by switching the patient's phenotype to a less severe one.

The main reason for HSCT failure is the slow pace of replacement of fixed tissue macrophages/histiocytes and microglial populations by the transplanted haematopoietic cell progeny compared to the quick progression of the primary disease. This lag period (12–24 months) before disease stabilization after HCT makes it necessary to extrapolate the likely condition of the patient at that future stage before deciding eligibility for transplantation: the more severe the phenotype and the longer the interval from onset of first obvious symptoms to HCT, the poorer the outcome.

Indications, practice suggestions, and guidelines have been published, and open issues in this field have been frequently reviewed. Detailed guidelines for HSCT in MPS I-H are also available at the European Blood and Marrow Transplantation Group website (www.ebmt.org). However, indications and guidelines should be cautiously used and interpreted in the context of emerging information and progress. Eligibility for HSCT in patients with LSDs has to be defined by a multidisciplinary team of expert investigators to reach the best therapeutic decision for the individual patient. As well, HSCT should be performed in centres whose physicians possess all the comprehensive skills needed to treat these disorders since optimal pre- and post-HSCT care is essential in increasing the likelihood of a good outcome.

HSCT is reported to arrest neurologic deterioration in severe forms of MPS I-H, but it is thought to have relatively little impact on the neurologic disease of other forms of MPS (MPS II and MPS III). Studies showing the potential advantages of cord blood transplantation in LSDs unfortunately confirmed that very early transplantation is necessary to alter the natural history of storage leukodystrophies. HSCT seems effective in patients with globoid cell leukodystrophy only if performed when the patient is asymptomatic and at a very early age (neonates) (Escolar et al., 2005). Late infantile metachromatic leukodystrophy (MLD) is apparently not effectively treated by HSCTs of any type, cord blood or bone marrow, while the reported course following HSCT in juvenile/adult MLD seems, more or less, comparable to the expected natural course, which is usually characterized by a slow progression of the disease. The assertion that MLD patients undergoing transplantation when asymptomatic (at birth or at least 1 year before the age of onset in the affected sibling) remain asymptomatic has never been proven (Martin, 2007). At least in Europe, the practice of prenatal diagnosis makes it unlikely that a sufficient cohort of affected newborn siblings can be found for a cord blood transplantation research protocol.

The current indications for HSCT in LSDs are summarized in Table 1.

Table 1. Indications for haematopoietic stem cell transplantation (HSCT) for lysosomal diseases

Standard[a]	Mucopolysaccharidosis type I-H (< 2 years of age)
Clinical option[b]	Alpha-mannosidosis Aspartylglucosaminuria Globoid cell leukodystrophy (asymptomatic neonates and selected late-onset cases) Metachromatic leukodystrophy (asymptomatic neonates only) Mucolipidosis type II (I-cell disease) Mucopolysaccharidosis type VI (where antibody attenuates efficacy of ERT; severe phenotype) Mucopolysaccharidosis type VII Wolman disease
Developmental[c]	Fucosidosis (early diagnosis) Gaucher disease type III Juvenile Sandhoff disease Juvenile Tay-Sachs disease Mucopolysaccharidosis type II (early diagnosis, very young age) Pompe disease
Not recommended or contraindicated	Globoid cell leukodystrophy (symptomatic early onset) GM1 gangliosidosis Infantile Sandhoff disease Infantile Tay-Sachs disease Metachromatic leukodystrophy (early-onset disease or symptomatic patients) Mucopolysaccharidosis type II, III, IV Niemann-Pick disease types B and C

[a] Standard-of-care transplants may be performed in any specialized centre experienced with HSCT procedures for lysosomal diseases provided the centre has an appropriate infrastructure as defined by national and international guidelines and can provide the multidisciplinary care needed by these patients. In the Standard indication there is clear evidence supporting the use of HSCT. The results are reasonably well defined and are superior to results obtained through other approaches.
[b] Although HSCT is thought to be of potential benefit, there are insufficient data to be certain; HSCT might be a valuable option for individual patients after careful discussion of risks and benefit with the family.
[c] The decision to offer HSCT is not supported by data, but is thought reasonable for individual patients as part of such evidence gathering; these HSCTs should be done within the framework of an approved clinical study protocol.

Perspectives

Innovative approaches are needed to improve the efficiency of HSCT, to overcome refractory disease manifestations and, particularly, to find other means of treating disorders that do not benefit from HSCT. Many projects are under development including those evaluating potential novel sources of adult stem cells and the effects of co-transplantation of specialized cells.

The role of transplantation of mesenchymal stem cells (MSCs) at or after HSCT, particularly in patients with those LSDs that include skeletal manifestations or peripheral nervous involvement, is a further area of interest. The potential of MSCs in differentiating into osteoblasts and chondrocytes and the data available from children with osteogenesis imperfecta should also stimulate investigation in the field of mucopolysaccharidoses (Horwitz et al., 2002; Koc et al., 2002).

Gene therapy is the insertion of a functional gene to produce a working enzyme and replace the defective one and it promises a potential cure for inherited disorders. Currently, several different LSD animal models are being studied in which either direct gene transfer is done using viral vectors, or defective haematopoietic stem cells are genetically altered and then returned to the donor. One possible advantage of gene therapy is the potential for overexpression of enzyme, which may achieve better results than conventional HSCT, which is only likely to result in enzyme expression at donor levels. A clinical trial using transplantation of autologous $CD34^+$ cells, transfected with lentiviral vector containing the human arylsulphatase A cDNA, for treatment of MLD (Telethon Institute for Gene Therapy, Milan) is under the final process of review and approval (Biffi, 2004).

Conclusions

The results of HSCT proved that donor-derived macrophages and microglia become a stable source of endogenous enzyme cross-correcting defective cells in the central nervous system. Clinical experience, however, showed that HSCT can significantly benefit only selected subsets of patients. Results were impressive in children with MPS I-H, otherwise fated to premature death, but were often poor in other disorders. The correct role for transplant procedures in LSDs needs to be constantly re-thought as new therapies and technologies emerge and, with the exception of MPS I-H, the use of transplantation is still not yet well defined and remains problematic and challenging. Over the next decade, combining improved transplant procedures with new drugs and novel cell sources along with advances in gene therapy might significantly change the prospects for success in this field (Beck, 2007).

References

Aldenhoven M., Boelens J.J. & de Koning T.J. (2008): The clinical outcome of Hurler syndrome after stem cell transplantation. *Biol. Blood Marrow Transplant.* **14,** 485–498.

Beck, M. (2007): New therapeutic options for lysosomal storage disorders: enzyme replacement, small molecules and gene therapy. *Hum. Genet.* **121,** 1–22.

Biffi, A., De Palma, M., Quattrini, A., Del Carro, U., Amadio, S., Visigalli, I., Sessa, M., Fasano, S., Brambilla, R., Marchesini, S., Bordignon, C. & Naldini, L. (2004): Correction of metachromatic leukodystrophy in the mouse model by transplantation of genetically modified hematopoietic stem cells. *J. Clin. Invest.* **113,** 1118–1129.

Boelens, J.J. (2006): Trends in hematopoietic stem cell transplantation for inborn errors of metabolism. *J. Inherit. Metab. Dis.* **29,** 413–420.

Boelens, J.J., Wynn, R.F., O'Meara, A., Veys, P., Bertrand, Y., Souillet, G., Wraith, J.E., Fischer, A., Cavazzana-Calvo, M., Sykora, K.W., Sedlacek, P., Rovelli, A., Uiterwaal, C.S. & Wulffraat, N. (2007): Outcomes of haematopietic cell transplantation for MPS-I in Europe: a risk factor analysis for graft-failure. *Bone Marrow Transplant.* **40,** 225–233.

Boelens J.J., Rocha V., Aldenhoven M., Wynn R., O'Meara A., Michel G., Ionescu I., Parikh S., Prasad V.K., Szabolcs P., Escolar M., Gluckman E., Cavazzana-Calvo M., Kurtzberg J., EUROCORD, Inborn error Working Party of EBMT and Duke University (2009): Risk factor analysis of outcomes after unrelated cord blood transplantation in patients with Hurler syndrome. *Biol. Blood Marrow Transplant.* **15,** 618–625.

Cox-Brinkman, J., Boelens, J.J., Wraith, J.E., O'Meara, A., Veys, P., Wijburg, F.A., Wulffraat, N. & Wynn, R.F. (2006): Haematopoietic cell transplantation (HCT) in combination with enzyme replacement therapy (ERT) in patients with Hurler syndrome. *Bone Marrow Transplant.* **38,** 17–21.

Escolar, M.L., Poe, M., Provenzale, J.M., Richards, K.C., Allison, J., Wood, S., Wenger, D.A., Pietryga, D., Wall, D., Champagne, M., Morse, R., Krivit, W. & Kurtzberg, J. (2005): Transplantation of umbilical cord-blood in babies with infantile Krabbe's disease. *N. Engl. J. Med.* **352,** 2069–2081.

Grewal, S.S., Wynn, R., Abdenur, J.E., Burton, B.K., Gharib, M., Haase, C., Hayashi, R.J., Shenoy, S., Sillence, D., Tiller, G.E., Dudek, M.E., van Royen-Kerkhof, A., Wraith, J.E., Woodard, P., Young, G.A., Wulffraat, N., Whitley, C.B. & Peters, C. (2005): Safety and efficacy of enzyme replacement therapy in combination with hematopoietic stem cell transplantation in Hurler syndrome. *Genet. Med.* **7,** 143–146.

Horwitz, E.M., Gordon, P.L., Koo, W.K., Marx, J.C., Neel, M.D., McNall, R.Y., Muul, L. & Hofmann, T. (2002): Isolated allogeneic bone marrow-derived mesenchymal cells engraft and stimulate growth in children with osteogenesis imperfecta: implications for cell therapy of bone. *Proc. Natl. Acad. Sci. USA* **99,** 8932–8937.

Koc, O.N., Day, J., Nieder, M., Gerson, S.L., Lazarus, H.M. & Krivit, W. (2002): Allogeneic mesenchymal stem cell infusion for treatment of metachromatic leukodystrophy (MLD) and Hurler syndrome (MPS-IH). *Bone Marrow Transplant.* **30,** 215–222.

Martin, P.L., Carter, S.L., Kernan, N.A., Sabdev, I., Wall, D., Pyetriga, D., Wagner, J.E. & Kurtzberg, J. (2006): Results of the cord blood transplantation study (COBLT): outcomes of unrelated donor umbilical cord blood transplantation in pediatric patients with lysosomal and peroxisomal storage diseases. *Biol. Blood Marrow Transplant.* **12,** 184–194.

Pastores, G.M., Arn, P., Beck, M., Clarke, J.T.R., Guffon, N., Kaplan, P., Muenzer, J., Norato, D.Y., Shapiro, E., Thomas, J., Viskochil, D. & Wraith, J.E. (2007): The MPS I registry: design, methodology, and early findings of a global disease registry for monitoring patients with mucopolysaccharidosis type I. *Mol. Genet. Metabol.* **91,** 37–47.

Peters, C., Balthazor, M., Shapiro, E.G., King, R.J., Kollman, C., Hegland, J.D., Henslee-Downey, J., Trigg, M.E., Cowan, M.J., Sanders, J., Bunin, N., Weinstein, H., Lenarsky, C., Falk, P., Harris, R., Bowen, T., Williams, T.E., Grayson, G.H., Warkentin, P., Sender, L., Cool, V.A., Crittenden, M., Packman, S., Kaplan, P., Lockman, L.A., Anderson, J., Krivit, W., Dusenbery, K. & Wagner, J. (1996): Outcome of unrelated donor bone marrow transplantation in 40 children with Hurler syndrome. *Blood* **87,** 4894–4902.

Peters, C., Shapiro, E.G., Anderson, J., Henslee-Downey, P.J., Klemperer, M.R., Cowan, M.J., Saunders, E.F., de Alarcon, P.A., Twist, C., Nachman, J.B., Hale, G.A., Harris, R.E., Rozans, M.K., Kurtzberg, J., Grayson, G.H., Williams, T.E., Lenarsky, C., Wagner, J.E. & Krivit, W. (1998): Hurler syndrome: II. Outcome of HLA-genotypically identical sibling and HLA-haploidentical related donor bone marrow transplantation in fifty-four children. *Blood* **91,** 2601–2608.

Peters, C. & Steward, C.G. (2003): Hematopoietic cell transplantation for inherited metabolic diseases: an overview of outcomes and practice guidelines. *Bone Marrow Transplant.* **31,** 229–239.

Pitt, C., Lavery, C. & Wager, N. (2009): Psychosocial outcomes of bone marrow transplant for individuals affected by mucopolysaccharidosis I Hurler disease: patient social competency. *Child Care Health Dev.* **35,** 271–280.

Prasad, V.K. & Kurtzberg, J. (2008): Emerging trends in transplantation of inherited metabolic diseases. *Bone Marrow Transplant.* **41,** 99–108.

Proia, R.L. & Wu, Y.P. (2004): Blood to brain to the rescue. *J. Clin. Invest.* **113,** 1108–1110.

Rovelli, A.M. & Steward, C.G. (2005): Hematopoietic stem cell transplantation activity in Europe for inherited metabolic diseases: open issues and future directions. *Bone Marrow Transplant.* **35,** S23–S26.

Souillet, G., Guffon, N., Maire, I., Pujol, M., Taylor, P., Sevin, F. Bleyzac, N., Mulier, C., Durin, A., Kebaili, K., Galambrun, C., Bertrand, Y., Froissart, R., Dorche, C., Gebuhrer, L., Garin, C., Berard, J. & Guibaud P. (2003): Outcome of 27 patients with Hurler's syndrome transplanted from either related or unrelated haematopoietic stem cell sources. *Bone Marrow Transplant.* **31,** 1105–1117.

Staba, S.L., Escolar, M.L., Poe, M., Kim, Y., Martin, P.L., Szabolcs, P., Allison-Thacker, J., Wood, S., Wenger, D.A., Rubinstein, P., Hopwood, J.J., Krivit, W. & Kurtzberg, J. (2004): Cord-blood transplants from unrelated donors in patients with Hurler's syndrome. *N. Engl. J. Med.* **350,** 1960–1969.

Vellodi, A. (2005): Lysosomal storage disorders. *Br. J. Haematol.* **128,** 413–431.

Chapter 16

Allogeneic stem cell transplantation for Hurler syndrome: graft outcome and long-term clinical outcomes

Jaap Jan Boelens and Mieke Aldenhoven

Department of Immunology/Hematology and Stem Cell Transplantation, University Medical Centre Utrecht, KC.03.063.0, Lundlaan 6, 3584 EA Utrecht, the Netherlands
j.j.boelens@umcutrecht.nl

Summary

Hurler syndrome (HS) is a severe inborn error of metabolism causing progressive multisystem morbidity, including developmental deterioration, and death in early childhood. Stem cell transplantation (SCT) is the only treatment able to prevent disease progression in these patients, especially when the SCT is performed early in life and before cerebral involvement has occurred.

Published data regarding SCT in HS patients appear to be promising. There were, however, some major limitations, including a high rate of graft failure and transplantation-related mortality and morbidity. Over the last 5 years, various collaborative studies on graft outcomes have been done. These studies have prompted new international guidelines, subsequently resulting in lower transplantation-related morbidity and mortality rates. SCT for inborn errors of metabolism (IEM) has consequently become a safer procedure.

Successful SCT in HS patients has clearly been shown to be effective, with an improvement of various important clinical outcome parameters (e.g., neuropsychological outcome) and a significantly prolonged survival. However, certain clinical manifestations appear to be irreversible or continue to progress despite successful SCT, causing residual disease burden which varies considerably between patients. Since long-term follow-up data are sparse, knowledge is lacking about the long-term effects and the factors that influence them in HS patients undergoing successful transplantation. This chapter provides an overview on what is so far known regarding the long-term follow-up. In order to evaluate the natural course and the influence of various patient, donor, and transplantation variables on the long-term outcome of HS patients after successful SCT, an international long-term follow-up study has recently been initiated. This multicentre study, a collaborative effort of EBMT, Eurocord, CIBMTR, Duke University, and the University of Minnesota, will further optimize the selection criteria and the transplantation techniques used. Furthermore, analysis of the needs and processes of care in patients, parents, and families will help to plan for innovation in their care. It is hoped that the results of this study will help to significantly improve the outcome and quality of life of HS patients and their families.

Introduction

Hurler syndrome (HS) is the most severe phenotype in the spectrum of mucopolysaccharidosis type I, an autosomal recessive lysosomal storage disorder. Patients suffering from HS develop progressive and ultimately fatal multisystem deterioration including psychomotor retardation, severe skeletal deformities, and life-threatening cardiac and pulmonary complications due to lack of the lysosomal enzyme alpha-L-iduronidase (Neufeld & Muenzer, 2001).

Intravenous enzymes, administered during enzyme replacement therapy, which has been available for MPS I patients since 2003, are incapable of crossing the blood–brain barrier and so this therapy is not able to prevent central nervous system deterioration (Kakkis et al., 2001; Wraith, 2005). Enzyme replacement therapy is consequently only indicated in patients without central nervous system involvement, such as the milder phenotype MPS I – Scheie disease.

The donor-derived stem cells engrafted after successful stem cell transplantation (SCT) are, however, able to provide a continuous endogenous source of the missing enzyme throughout the body, including the peripheral tissues as well as the central nervous system. Therefore allogeneic SCT is still considered the treatment of choice in several lysosomal storage disorders characterized by central nervous system involvement, including HS (Aldenhoven et al., 2009; Aldenhoven et al., 2008). At present, more than 500 SCTs have been performed in HS patients worldwide, making HS the inborn error of metabolism for which transplantation has been most frequently used (EBMT Registry, 2007; IBMTR Registry, 2007). This chapter will focus on the progress that has been made in recent years regarding the graft outcome as well as what is known regarding the clinical long-term outcome of HS patients after successful SCT.

Graft outcome: transplantation procedure and the use of cord blood

Although significant successful clinical results have been reported in HS patients after SCT, provided that the transplantation was performed early in life (Aldenhoven et al., 2008), the success of SCT has been limited by various factors including donor availability, high rates of graft failure, mixed chimerism (presence of both autologous and allogeneic hematopoietic cells) and transplantation-related morbidity and mortality (Boelens et al., 2007). In order to reduce these limitations, a risk-factor analysis was performed in HS patients registered in the European Blood and Marrow Transplantation (EBMT) database (Boelens et al., 2007). In this European retrospective study ($n = 146$ HS patients undergoing transplantation between 1994 and 2004) the probability of being 'alive and engrafted' (A&E) was only 53 per cent (Fig. 1). Predictors for graft failure in this study were T-cell depletion (OR, 0.18; $P = 0.02$) and reduced-intensity conditioning regimen (OR, 0.08; $P = 0.002$). Higher rates of A&E could be predicted when pharmacokinetic targeting with busulphan was used, which appeared to protect against graft failure (OR, 8.05; $p = 0.028$). These data have resulted in new EBMT guidelines for SCT in HS (<www.ebmt.org>).

During this retrospective European study, it was also found that significantly more patients receiving cord blood achieved full-donor chimerism (93 per cent) in comparison with patients receiving bone–marrow or peripheral–blood stem cells (67 per cent; OR, 9.31; $p = 0.044$). Furthermore, all patients receiving a cord blood transplant attained normal enzyme levels, compared with 60 per cent in the other group (Boelens et al., 2007). Other studies using cord blood as a stem cell source also showed high incidences of full-donor chimerism and normal enzyme levels in HS patients (Church et al., 2007; Martin et al., 2006; Prasad et al., 2008; Staba et al.,

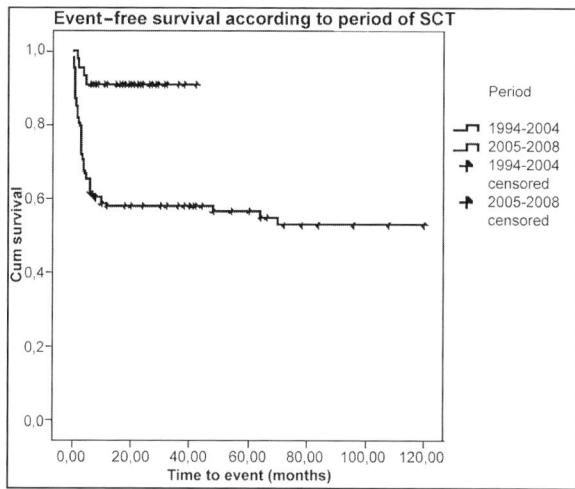

Fig. 1. Event-free survival (defined as 'alive and engrafted') of Hurler syndrome patients after stem cell transplantation.
The line showing the period 1994–2004 (n = 146) depicts the group of HS patients undergoing transplantation between 1994 and 2004, as described by Boelens et al. (2007). The upper line shows patients (n = 44) who underwent transplantation between January 2005 and January 2008 according to the new ESH-EBMT (2008) guidelines. These new guidelines include a graft hierarchy of unrelated cord blood after matched sibling donor and a conditioning including busulphan (16 to 20 mg intravenously using therapeutic drug monitoring if possible) in combination with cyclophosphamide (200 mg). Mixed chimerism was observed in 29 per cent of the patients undergoing transplantation between 1994 and 2004, whereas mixed chimerism occurred in only 2/40 (5 per cent) of the patients undergoing transplantation in the 2005 to 2008 period (90 per cent and 94 per cent donor chimerism, respectively).

2004), as well as in other forms of inborn errors of metabolism (Escolar et al., 2005; Martin et al., 2006; Prasad et al., 2008; Stein et al., 2007). Since full-donor chimerism and higher enzyme levels after SCT have been suggested to positively influence the neurocognitive outcome after SCT, cord blood might be a preferential stem cell source for HS patients (Aldenhoven et al., 2008).

Because it was still unknown which risk factors could influence the graft outcome in HS patients receiving unrelated cord blood transplants, a collaborative retrospective analysis of unrelated cord blood transplantation performed in HS patients was initiated (Boelens et al., 2009). This Eurocord–Duke University collaborative study demonstrated that a shorter interval between diagnosis and transplantation ($P = 0.007$) and a conditioning regimen containing busulphan and cyclophosphamide ($P = 0.002$) was associated with a significantly higher event-free survival ('alive and successful engraftment') rate. Importantly, almost all 'alive and engrafted' patients achieved full-donor chimerism and normal enzyme levels in circulating leukocytes. Despite small numbers, 6/6 human leukocyte antigen-matched cord blood grafts may improve the outcome as well ($P = 0.06$). The relatively high rate of chronic graft-versus-host disease observed in this study, although mainly of limited severity, might be a concern (Boelens et al., 2009).

The use of cord blood for SCT has several other important advantages compared to other stem cell sources (bone marrow, peripheral blood) (Aldenhoven et al., 2008). Cord blood is readily available (often within a month), significantly reducing the time between diagnosis and SCT (Chao et al., 2004; Escolar et al., 2005; Staba et al., 2004). This is particularly important for the rapidly progressive central nervous system involvement in HS patients. Furthermore, donors with a higher human leukocyte antigen mismatch can be used, increasing the possibility of finding a suitable donor (Kurtzberg et al., 1996; Staba et al., 2004). Other advantages of cord blood that have been reported are the lower rates of acute and chronic graft-versus-host disease and the reduced likelihood of transmitting viral infections (Boelens, 2006; Kurtzberg et al., 1996). Finally, although highly speculative, there are suggestions of transdifferentiation into cell types such as osteoblasts, chondroblasts, and neurons because of the more primitive stem cell population in cord blood (Chen et al., 2005; Kogler et al., 2005; Meier et al., 2006).

Since the introduction of the new EBMT guidelines (2005), including a standardized busulphan/cyclophosphamide conditioning regimen and the use of unrelated cord blood high in the hierarchy (after a non-carrier-matched sibling donor), the graft outcomes have been significantly improved with event-free survival rates above 90 per cent (Fig. 1).

Long-term clinical outcome: variability between Hurler syndrome patients

SCTs in HS patients have clearly been shown to be clinically effective, evidenced by an increased life expectancy and improvement of various important clinical outcome parameters. Donor engraftment after SCT in HS patients leads to a rapid reduction of obstructive airway symptoms and hepatosplenomegaly. In addition, hearing, linear growth, and psychomotor development improve in many cases. Hydrocephalus is either prevented or stabilized, and the natural history of cardiovascular pathology after SCT is altered beneficially (Aldenhoven et al., 2008). Unfortunately, there are still some limitations: successful engraftment does not prevent disease progression in all organ systems (Aldenhoven et al., 2008). Despite successful engraftment, progression of retinal degeneration, continued thickening of cardiac valves, and mainly musculoskeletal deterioration have been reported by various authors (Aldenhoven et al., 2008). Additionally, many of these manifestations appeared to be irreversible, leading to residual disease such as mild corneal clouding and variable neurocognitive dysfunction (Aldenhoven et al., 2008). It is, however, important to mention that these results should be placed in the perspective of an experimental procedure. A significant part of the patients studied so far received transplants at an older age, and were significantly affected. Additionally, outdated transplantation techniques and carrier donors were used at that time, and a large percentage of these patients achieved only mixed chimerism, associated with lower enzyme levels.

Overall, the long-term clinical outcome appears to be promising, but is nevertheless highly variable among HS patients, presumably because of factors such as genotype, age and clinical situation at SCT, donor status (carrier *versus* unaffected), donor chimerism (mixed *versus* full donor), stem cell source (cord blood *versus* bone marrow or peripheral blood), and enzyme activity (normal *versus* heterozygous), all of which have been suggested to influence the long-term outcome, although this conclusion was based primarily on small study populations (Aldenhoven et al., 2008). Unfortunately, standardized long-term follow-up studies performed in HS patients are lacking to confirm these suggestions. To evaluate the natural course and the influence of various patient, donor, and transplantation characteristics on the long-term outcome of HS patients after successful SCT, an international long-term collaborative follow-up study (EBMT, CIBMTR, Eurocord, Duke University, and the University of Minnesota) has recently been initiated. This study will focus on those outcome parameters that are of most importance to the patient. The neurocognitive/developmental outcome and the functional outcome are thus considered as the primary outcome parameters. In addition, this study offers a unique chance to describe the overall long-term outcome/natural course regarding the various organ systems (orthopaedic, cardiac, respiratory, ophthalmologic, *etc.*) of HS patients after successful SCT and to analyse the quality of life, needs, and processes of care of HS patients after successful SCT. The primary and secondary outcome parameters are outlined in Table 1.

This international observational study will include 'alive and engrafted' HS patients, with a follow-up period of at least 3 years after SCT. These approximately 200 HS patients (about 80 per cent of the patients successfully receiving transplants worldwide) have undergone transplantation between 1980 and 2005 in the larger transplantation centres within Europe as well as the United States.

The main goals of this international study are (1) to evaluate the natural course of HS after successful SCT (*e.g.*, what are the remaining problems? what is the impact on the quality of life?); (2) to optimize the selection criteria (which patients are eligible for transplantation?); (3) to optimize the transplantation techniques (*e.g.*, questions about the conditioning regimen, source of stem cells, optimal timing of SCT); and (4) to develop an international follow-up protocol for HS patients after SCT, including international multidisciplinary guidelines for patient care and follow-up procedures. Furthermore, the outcome and guideline adaptations might also have an impact on patients with other inborn errors of metabolism.

Table 1. Primary and secondary outcome parameters used in the international long-term follow-up study[a] of Hurler syndrome patients after successful stem cell transplantation

Primary outcome parameters	
Neurocognitive/developmental outcome	WISC – Wechsler Intelligence Scale for Children Mullen Scales of early learning
Functional outcome	POSNA – Musculoskeletal functional health questionnaire
Secondary outcome parameters	
Physical characteristics	Amsterdam Dysmorphology Database
Orthopaedic outcome	Complications (kyphosis, hip dysplasia, carpal tunnel syndrome, *etc.*) Required intervention
Cardiac outcome	Complications (cardiomyopathy, valve abnormalities, *etc.*) Required intervention
Respiratory outcome	Complications (obstruction, infections, overnight hypoxia, *etc.*) Required intervention
Ophthalmologic outcome	Complications (decreased visual acuity, corneal opacity, retinopathy, *etc.*) Required intervention
Audiologic outcome	Complications (hearing loss) Required intervention
Endocrinologic outcome	Complications (reduced linear growth, abnormal sexual development, *etc.*) Required intervention
Biochemical parameters	Enzyme activity, urinary GAG excretion, donor chimerism
Work-up	Cerebral and spinal MRI/CT, cardiac ultrasound, skeletal X-ray, EMG, *etc.*
Quality of life	CHQ – Child Health Questionnaire
Processes of care	MPOC – Measurement of Processes of Care
Potential new biomarkers	Measured in serum and urine

[a] International multicentre study evaluating the long-term outcome of successful stem cell transplantation in Hurler syndrome patients. (Sponsored by the University Medical Center Utrecht, Utrecht, the Netherlands)

Conclusions

Thanks to the progress in SCT techniques that has been achieved during recent years, SCT in HS has become a much safer procedure, resulting in survival rates above 90 per cent over the last three to four years. Some transplantation techniques, such as T-cell depletion and reduced-intensity conditioning, have been shown to be associated with graft failure and are therefore less frequently used, while busulphan-targeting (to a certain level of exposure) protected against graft failure. Furthermore, the use of unrelated cord blood was associated with higher rates of full-donor chimerism and normal enzyme levels and is being used more frequently. The interval between diagnosis and SCT appeared to be important for higher survival rates in HS patients receiving an unrelated cord blood graft. International studies and collaborations have resulted in international guidelines. Additional international collaborations are needed to further optimize these techniques and study new developments in the near future.

The long-term clinical outcomes after successful SCT are encouraging: they result in an increased life expectancy with a significantly improved quality of life. Nevertheless, the outcomes are inexplicably widely variable among HS patients. Various factors, patient-, donor-, and transplantation-associated, may influence these outcomes. In order to improve the prognosis of HS patients after successful SCT, focus on the long-term clinical outcome is of utmost importance. Recently, an international multicentre study has been initiated to gain insight into the natural course of HS after successful SCT and to provide predictors that will further optimize the protocols.

Acknowledgments: We would like to thank in particular Dr. M.L. Escolar (University North Carolina, Chapel Hill, NC, USA), Dr. J. Kurtzberg (Duke University, Durham, NC, USA), Dr. J. Tolar and Dr. P. Orchard (University of Minnesota Medical Center, Minneapolis, MN, USA), and Dr. J.E. Wraith and Dr. R.F. Wynn (Royal Manchester Children's Hospital, Manchester, UK) for the interesting discussions and close collaboration that improve the practices, strategies, and knowledge concerning stem cell transplantations for inborn errors of metabolism. Additionally, we would like to acknowledge all participating medical doctors, (research) nurses, statisticians, data managers, and all others involved in the various collaborative studies performed on SCT in HS during recent years.

References

Aldenhoven, M., Boelens, J.J. & de Koning, T.J. (2008): The clinical outcome of Hurler syndrome after stem cell transplantation. *Biol. Blood Marrow Transplant.* **14**, 485–498.

Aldenhoven, M., Sakkers, R., Boelens J.J., de Koning, T.J. & Wulffraat, N. (2009): Musculoskeletal manifestations of lysosomal storage disorders. *Ann. Rheum. Dis.* **68**, 1659–1665.

Boelens, J.J. (2006): Trends in haematopoietic cell transplantation for inborn errors of metabolism. *J. Inherit. Metab. Dis.* **29**, 413–420.

Boelens, J.J., Wynn, R.F., O'Meara, A., Veys, P., Bertrand, Y., Souillet, G., Wraith, J.E., Fischer, A., Cavazzana-Calvo, M., Sykora, K.W., Sedlacek, P., Rovelli, A., Uiterwaal, C.S.P.M. & Wulffraat, N. (2007): Outcomes of hematopoietic stem cell transplantation for Hurler's syndrome in Europe: a risk factor analysis for graft failure. *Bone Marrow Transplant.* **40**, 225–233.

Boelens, J.J., Rocha, V., Aldenhoven, M., Wynn, R., O'Meara, A., Michel, G., Ionescu, I., Parikh, S., Prasad, V., Szabolcs, P., Escolar, M., Gluckman, E., Cavazzana-Calvo, M. & Kurtzberg, J. (2009): Risk factor analysis of outcomes after unrelated cord blood transplantation in patients with Hurler syndrome. *Biol. Blood Marrow Transplant.* **15**, 618–625.

Chao, N.J., Emerson, S.G. & Weinberg, K.I. (2004): Stem cell transplantation (cord blood transplants). *Hematology* [American Society of Hematology Education Program], pp. 354–371.

Chen, N., Hudson, J.E., Walczak, P., Misiuta, I., Garbuzova-Davis, S., Jiang, L. Sanchez-Ramos, J., Sanberg, P.R., Zigova, T. & Willing, A.E. (2005): Human umbilical cord blood progenitors: the potential of these hematopoietic cells to become neural. *Stem Cells* **23**, 1560–1570.

Church, H., Tylee, K., Cooper, A., Thornley, M., Mercer, J., Wraith, E., Carr, T., O'Meara, A. & Wynn, R.F. (2007): Biochemical monitoring after haemopoietic stem cell transplant for Hurler syndrome (MPSIH): implications for functional outcome after transplant in metabolic disease. *Bone Marrow Transplant.* **39,** 207–210.

EBMT Registry (2007): <http://www.ebmt.org/4Registry/registry1.html>

ESH-EBMT (2008): *ESH-EMBT handbook on haematopoietic stem cell transplantation*, eds. J. Apperley, E. Carreras, E. Gluckman, A. Gratwohl & T. Masszi. Paris: ESH.

Escolar, M.L., Poe, M.D., Provenzale, J.M., Richards, K.C., Allison, J., Wood, S., Wenger, D.A., Pietryga, D., Wall, D., Champagne, M., Morse, R., Krivit, W. & Kurtzberg, J. (2005): Transplantation of umbilical-cord blood in babies with infantile Krabbe's disease. *N. Engl. J. Med.* **352,** 2069–2081.

IBMTR Registry (2007): <http://www.cibmtr.org>

Kakkis, E.D., Muenzer, J., Tiller, G.E., Waber, L., Belmont, J., Passage, M., Izykowski, B., Philips, J., Doroshow, R., Walot, I., Hoft, R. & Neufeld, E.F. (2001): Enzyme-replacement therapy in mucopolysaccharidosis I. *N. Engl. J. Med.* **344,** 182–188.

Kogler, G., Enczmann, J., Rocha, V., Gluckman, E. & Wernet, P. (2005): High-resolution HLA typing by sequencing for HLA-A, -B, -C, -DR, -DQ in 122 unrelated cord blood/patient pair transplants hardly improves long-term clinical outcome. *Bone Marrow Transplant.* **36,** 1033–1041.

Kurtzberg, J. Laughlin, M., Graham, M.L., Smith, C., Olson, J.F., Halperin, E.C., Ciocci, G., Carrier, C., Stevens, C.E. & Rubinstein, P. (1996): Placental blood as a source of hematopoietic stem cells for transplantation into unrelated recipients. *N. Engl. J. Med.* **335,** 157–166.

Martin, P.L., Carter, S.L., Kernan, N.A., Sahdev, I., Wall, D., Pietryga, D., Wagner, J.E. & Kurtzberg, J. (2006): Results of the cord blood transplantation study (COBLT): outcomes of unrelated donor umbilical cord blood transplantation in pediatric patients with lysosomal and peroxisomal storage diseases. *Biol. Blood Marrow Transplant.* **12,** 184–194.

Meier, C., Middelanis, J., Wasielewski, B., Neuhoff, S., Roth-Haerer, A., Gantert, M., Dinse, H.R., Dermietzel, R. & Jensen, A. (2006): Spastic paresis after perinatal brain damage in rats is reduced by human cord blood mononuclear cells. *Pediatr. Res.* **59,** 244–249.

Neufeld, E.F. & Muenzer, J. (2001): The mucopolysaccharidoses. In: *The metabolic and molecular basis of inherited disease*, eds. C. Scriver, A. Beaudet, W. Sly & D. Valle, pp. 3421–3452. New York: McGraw-Hill.

Prasad, V.K., Mendizabal, A., Parikh, S.H., Szabolcs, P., Driscoll, T.A., Page, K., Lakshminarayanan, S., Allison, J., Wood, S., Semmel, D., Escolar, M.L., Martin, P.L., Carter, S. & Kurtzberg, J. (2008): Unrelated donor umbilical cord blood transplantation for inherited metabolic disorders in 159 pediatric patients from a single center: influence of cellular composition of the graft on transplantation outcomes. *Blood* **112,** 2979–2989.

Staba, S.L., Escolar, M.L., Poe, M., Kim, Y., Martin, P.L., Szabolcs, P., Allison-Thacker, J., Wood, S., Wenger, D.A., Rubinstein, P., Hopwood, J.J., Krivit, W. & Kurtzberg, J. (2004): Cord-blood transplants from unrelated donors in patients with Hurler's syndrome. *N. Engl. J. Med.* **350,** 1960–1969.

Stein, J., Zion, G.B., Dror, Y., Fenig, E., Zeigler, M. & Yaniv, I. (2007): Successful treatment of Wolman disease by unrelated umbilical cord blood transplantation. *Eur. J. Pediatr.* **166,** 663–666.

Wraith, J.E. (2005): The first 5 years of clinical experience with laronidase enzyme replacement therapy for mucopolysaccharidosis I. *Expert. Opin. Pharmacother.* **6,** 489–506.

Chapter 17

Haematopoietic stem cell gene therapy for metachromatic leukodystrophy

Alessandra Biffi and Luigi Naldini

San Raffaele Telethon Institute for Gene Therapy, via Olgettina 58, 20132 Milan, Italy, and H. San Raffaele Scientific Institute, Milan, Italy
a.biffi@hsr.it

Summary

Metachromatic leukodystrophy (MLD) is a rare, fatal, inherited autosomal recessive lysosomal storage disorder (LSD), characterized by severe and progressive demyelination affecting the central and peripheral nervous system. Despite initial expectations for the efficacy of haematopoietic stem cell transplantation (HSCT), and despite ameliorative supportive therapy, MLD remains a life-threatening disease, with an extremely poor quality of life and a poor prognosis for all affected patients. Prospectively, in children affected by MLD who have no other therapeutic options and an extremely poor prognosis, the potential risks associated with the use of a novel technology, such as gene therapy, might be balanced by the potential benefit of a positive outcome. Thus, MLD might be considered an optimal candidate disease for testing innovative and potentially efficacious therapeutic approaches. Among different gene therapy approaches currently being developed for MLD, we will here discuss recent advances in hematopoietic stem cell–based gene therapy, which will enter clinical testing in the near future.

Introduction

Metachromatic leukodystrophy (MLD) is a rare, fatal inherited autosomal recessive lysosomal storage disorder (LSD), with an estimated frequency of 1:40,000.

Most LSDs are caused by loss of function of specific lysosomal acid hydrolases, which act to degrade complex substrates that have been targeted for degradation to the lysosomes after endocytosis or autophagy. Undegraded substrate accumulation within lysosomes is responsible for distention of the organelle, cellular malfunction, and subsequent apoptosis of affected cells. Despite sharing a similar pathogenic mechanism, the more-than 40 different LSDs that have been described differ in several disease-specific features. The main differences are represented by the pattern of visceral organ involvement and by the presence and severity of nervous system (NS) involvement. It has been reported that neurodegeneration in the central NS (CNS) and/or dysmyelination affecting the entire NS are the hallmarks of roughly 60 per cent of LSDs (Neufeld, 1991). The severity of NS disease varies among different types of LSDs and among different forms of the same LSD, and it ranges from mild mental retardation with minimal alteration of cognitive function to severe and rapidly progressing disability and death. MLD is an example of LSD with NS involvement.

The lysosomal enzyme arylsulphatase A (ARSA), which is involved in sulphatide metabolism through the hydrolysis of the 3–O ester bond of galactosyl and lactosyl sulphatides, is defective in MLD. Pathology is characterized by massive accumulation of nonmetabolized sulpholipids primarily in white matter cells, and subsequently in neurons and microglia, leading to extensive demyelination in the CNS and peripheral nervous system (PNS) and late-onset neuronal degeneration.

Major signs and symptoms are due to the severe and progressive involvement of both the CNS and PNS. The severity of the clinical syndrome varies from infantile regression, hypotonia, peripheral neuropathy, seizures, and cognitive deterioration, to late adult onset behavioural disturbance, followed by spastic paraparesis and dementia. Minor involvement of visceral organs occurs, but it does not significantly affect patients' prognosis. The early-onset variants are the most frequent; in these patients progression of symptoms is extremely rapid since onset and death occur within the first decade of life (Aicardi, 1998; Neufeld & Muenzer, 2001). Currently, therapy is only supportive. As in the case of several other LSDs with NS involvement, no efficacious treatment is currently available that can reverse the fatal outcome of this devastating disease (Neufeld, 1991; Aicardi, 1998). The severity of the disease and the absence of effective therapies emphasize the need for testing innovative therapeutic approaches.

Among the diverse experimental approaches that have been explored to fulfill this unmet medical need, gene therapy presently constitutes one of only a few with potential for clinical success. Gene therapy, according to the route of administration, may provide: (1) direct metabolic correction of specific cell types representing major disease targets, such as oligodendrocytes and neurons, upon vector administration into the CNS; (2) replacement of specific cell subsets in the affected tissues by genetically corrected cells or progenitors, such as *ex vivo* transduced haematopoietic or neural stem cells; these cells also give rise to a local source of functional enzyme for cross-correction of the affected nervous tissue. Because of its very promising preliminary results (Biffi *et al.*, 2004, 2006), haematopoietic stem cell (HSC) gene therapy is very close to clinical testing. Therefore, the state of the development of this gene therapy approach in the murine model and efforts towards its clinical application are reviewed in this chapter.

General description

ARSA is a 62kDA polypeptide whose coding region spans 8 exons and predicts a primary protein sequence of 507 amino acids. The first 18 amino acids constitute the leader sequence and are missing from the mature enzyme, which contains 3 *N*-glycosylation sites. The ARSA enzyme is devoted to the hydrolysis of galactose-3-sulphate from sulphatides. Thus far, more than 140 MLD-related *ARSA* mutations have been described according to the Human Gene Mutation Database (Eng *et al.*, 2003; Berna *et al.*, 2004; Marcao *et al.*, 2005; Lugawska *et al.*, 2005). The biological and clinical effects of the mutations vary. MLD mutations can be functionally divided into two broad groups: null (0) alleles associated with no enzymatic activity, and R alleles, which are associated with some residual enzyme activity (von Figura & Jaeken, 2001). Although most mutant alleles are extremely rare or private mutations, the occurrence of a genotype–phenotype correlation has been recently suggested (Rauschka *et al.*, 2006; Sevin *et al.*, 2007; Biffi *et al.*, 2008; Cesani *et al.*, 2009).

The main pathologic features of MLD are demyelination and the deposition of metachromatic granules in both the CNS and the PNS. The demyelination in the CNS is widespread, whereas the peripheral nerves show segmental demyelination. The metachromatic granules, which under the electron microscope consist of lamellae and vacuoles, are present not only in the nervous system, where they are prominent in microglial cells, oligodendrocytes, and Schwann cells, but also in the kidney, gallbladder, retina, rectal tissue, and other tissues. The mechanisms responsible for the demyelination are not clearly defined and are still a matter of debate, although many theories have been proposed. Sulphatide accumulation may induce alterations within the cells responsible for myelin maintenance, the oligodendrocyte in the CNS and the Schwann cell in the PNS. An abnormally high content of sulphatide may cause instability of myelin. The accumulation of sulphogalactosylsphingosine, which is thought to be highly cytotoxic, is present in abnormally high concentration in the tissues of MLD patients and may have a role in demyelination. More recently, data obtained in mouse models suggest a pathogenic role of microglial activation in MLD and other lysosomal storage disorders (Hess *et al.*, 1996; Ohmi *et al.*, 2003).

Clinically, MLD is classified into four main variants according to the age of onset: late infantile (LI), early and late juvenile (EJ and LJ), and adult (AD) forms, the LI and EJ forms being the most common. The prognosis and quality of life are extremely poor for all described clinical forms of this disease. The LI form manifests most commonly between the first and second year of life. Affected children develop a rapidly progressive neurologic disease leading in all cases to decerebration, blindness, deafness, and loss of speech or volitional movement and of meaningful contact with the surroundings. Death occurs invariably within 5 years from onset of symptoms. The juvenile variant manifests between 4 and 14 years of age and is further subdivided into early and late juvenile variants based on onset before or after 6 years of age. The EJ and LJ forms are characterized by a progressive evolution of the disease, leading to very severe neurologic impairment. The prognosis is poor, most patients dying before the age of 20. In the AD form, onset may occur around the age of 15, but often the disorder is not diagnosed until adulthood. Initial symptoms typically affect behaviour, manifesting as a change in personality or in poor school or work performance. Dystonic postures may develop. In the later and final stages, there may be bulbar and spastic tetraparesis or decorticate posturing. Most commonly, the duration of the illness varies between 5 and 10 years, but in some patients it extends over decades.

A 'knockout' mouse model of MLD has been developed Hess *et al.* (1996). Affected mice have the expected deficiency of ARSA activity and accumulate sulphatide in neuronal and non-neuronal tissues (Yaghootfam *et al.*, 2005). They exhibit a delay in myelination in the first 2 to 3 weeks of life, but only during the second year of life do they develop focal demyelinating lesions. Furthermore, extensive neuronal degeneration is a constant feature in the hippocampus of 1-year-old MLD mice. Neurologic examination and behavioural tests reveal impairment of motor coordination and learning abilities in affected mice after 6–8 months of age. More recently, transgenic $Arsa^{-/-}$ mice overexpressing the sulphatide-synthesizing enzyme galactose-3-*O*-sulphotransferase-1 in myelinating cells were generated. These mice display a significant increase in sulphatide storage in brain and peripheral nerves, an impaired nerve conduction velocity due to a hypomyelinating peripheral neuropathy and hypo/demyelination in the central nervous system, and they develop severe neurologic symptoms by 1 year of age. Thus, increased sulphatide storage in $Arsa^{-/-}$ mice led to a phenotype more reminiscent of human MLD (Ramakrishnan *et al.*, 2005). Moreover, transgenic $Arsa^{-/-}$ mice overexpressing the galactosyltransferase (GCT) and cerebroside sulphotransferase (CST) in neurons were generated to provoke storage in neurons. These mice, as compared to the original 'knockouts', developed a more severe neuromotor coordination defect and weakness of forelimbs and hindlimbs, thus better reproducing the human disease (Eckhardt et al., 2007). Availability of these animal models has provided insights into the histopathologic and cellular consequences of sulphatide storage. Moreover, they represent important models for testing conventional and new therapeutic interventions, including gene therapy.

Conventional therapeutic approaches for the treatment of metachromatic leukodystrophy

Lysosomal enzyme replacement

Most lysosomal enzymes, including ARSA, are sorted to the lysosomes as inactive proenzymes from the Golgi apparatus through a specific pathway controlled by the mannose-6-phosphate receptor (M6PR). A fraction of proenzyme escapes the lysosomal sorting pathway and is secreted into the extracellular space (Neufeld, 1991). The secreted proenzyme may then be endocytosed by neighbouring cells via M6PR molecules expressed on the cell membrane and sorted to the lysosomes. Because of this feature, most treatment strategies for LSD are based on providing an exogenous supply of the missing or defective lysosomal enzyme in the appropriate target tissue or in the systemic circulation. The exogenous enzyme can be up-taken by the deficient cells, leading to cross-correction of the metabolic defect. The therapeutic relevance of this phenomenon relies on the small quantities of enzyme, which are presumed to be sufficient to correct the metabolic defect. Because of its potential to compensate for the deficiency, enzyme replacement therapy (ERT)–parenteral administration of purified recombinant proenzyme–has become one of the most promising therapeutic options for some LSDs (Barranger & O'Rourke, 2001; Desnick et al., 2001; Eng et al., 2001; and Kakkis et al., 2001). ERT is considered the standard therapy for patients with non-neuropathic Gaucher or Fabry disease, and it was approved or is being evaluated for the treatment of Pompe disease, mucopolysaccharidoses type I (MPS I), MPS II, and MPS VI (Brady & Schiffman, 2004) and, more recently, of MLD. However, protein delivery poses serious challenges when the NS is the major disease target, as in the case of MLD. Indeed, the blood–brain barrier severely limits access of systemically administered therapeutic molecules to the nervous tissue, severely affecting the therapeutic impact of this strategy (Matzner, 2005). Further, recurring parenteral administration of an exogenous protein carries the risk of inducing an immune response against the therapeutic enzyme, as was indicated by some recent preclinical and clinical studies (van den Hout et al., 2004; Kakkis et al., 2004; Miebach, 2005). A large-scale manufacturing process of human recombinant ARSA has been developed, and an ERT phase I trial has been recently accomplished. Results from clinical testing will clarify whether ERT could have a role in alleviating CNS and/or PNS disease manifestations in MLD patients.

Haematopoietic stem cell transplantation

Over the past two decades, haematopoietic stem cell (HSC) transplantation (HSCT) has been used to treat LSD patients with the aim of replacing the intra- and extravascular haematopoietic compartments with cell populations expressing a functional enzyme (Krivit et al., 1995, 1999). Macrophages and microglia represent major effectors of the catabolism of the storage material, and their replacement by donor-derived cells has the potential to restore a critical scavenger function. Furthermore, gene-corrected macrophages and microglia may represent a local source of functional enzyme for cross-correction of resident neurons and oligodendrocytes. The therapeutic impact of HSCT in LSDs depends on the specific enzymatic deficiency, on the involvement of the CNS, and on the stage of the disease at the time of the transplant. Clinical evidence supporting HSCT for LSDs with CNS involvement has been recently obtained in patients affected by globoid cell leukodsytrophy (GLD), an LSD related to MLD and consequent to the deficiency of the enzyme involved in the downstream reaction after ARSA in the catabolism of myelin lipids. If performed in the neonatal period, cord blood HSCT may favorably alter the natural history of infantile forms by delaying onset and progression. On the contrary, it did not result in any substantial neurologic improvement if performed in symptomatic babies (Escolar *et al.*, 2005). In the case of MLD, however, little evidence in favor of efficacy of HSCT is available (Peters & Steward, 2003; Bredius *et al.*, 2007). Moreover, the high risk of rejection (Bredius *et al.*, 2007), and the high morbidity and mortality associated with the allogeneic transplant procedure, mainly due to the risk of graft-versus-host disease (GVHD), further reduce the indication for haematopoietic stem cell transplantation for MLD patients.

Gene therapy approaches for the treatment of metachromatic leukodystrophy

Gene therapy approaches for the treatment of MLD can consist of: (1) direct vector administration into the CNS, which may allow metabolic correction of specific cell types representing major disease targets, such as oligodendrocytes and neurons; and (2) replacement of specific cell subsets in the affected tissues by genetically corrected cells or progenitors, such as *ex vivo* transduced hematopoietic stem cells; these cells might also constitute a local source of functional enzyme for cross-correction of the affected nervous tissue.

Gene-based delivery may allow establishing a sustained source of therapeutic protein within the NS, overcoming the anatomic barriers which limit enzyme diffusion from the circulation (Kay *et al.*, 2001; Glorioso *et al.*, 2003). Currently, a number of vector delivery systems exists that can be used for direct *in vivo* gene transfer into the CNS. Among other vectors, lentiviral vectors (LVs) and adeno-associated vectors (AAVs), which are able to efficiently transduce several cell types both *in vitro* and *in vivo*, represent profitable tools for these purposes. Moreover, with the discovery and characterization of different AAV serotypes, the potential patterns of *in vivo* vector transduction have been expanded substantially, offering alternatives to the more studied AAV2 and AAV5 serotypes (Sondhi *et al.*, 2007). Direct injection of gene transfer vectors into the CNS has achieved long-term protein expression and therapeutic benefit in several disease models of LSD (Skorupa *et al.*, 1999; Stein *et al.*, 1999; Bosch *et al.*, 2000; Consiglio *et al.*, 2001; Stein *et al.*, 2001; Cressant *et al.*, 2004; Desmaris *et al.*, 2004; Ciron *et al.*, 2006; Sevin *et al.*, 2006; Sevin *et al.*, 2007b). Efficient transduction of the neurons of adult rodent brains was observed with all generations of LVs (Naldini *et al.*, 1996; Blomer *et al.*, 1997; Zufferey *et al.*, 1997; Zufferey *et al.*, 1998) and AAVs (Skorupa *et al.*, 1999; Desmaris *et al.*, 2004), and effective gene transfer was also observed in brain neurons of large animal models and nonhuman primates (Kordower *et al.*, 1999; Ciron *et al.*, 2006). The main cellular targets of both LV and AAV gene transfer in the CNS are neurons, in which long-term, stable transgene expression can be obtained with minor toxicity. Glial cells are transduced *in vivo* to a lower efficiency. Cross-correction from transduced neurons may have the advantage of achieving a widespread enzyme distribution within the CNS thanks to the long-range reach of neural processes (Luca *et al.*, 2005).

The pioneering work of Consiglio and co-workers demonstrated the possibility of achieving sustained expression of active enzyme throughout a large portion of the brain and long-term protection from the development of neuropathology and hippocampus-related learning impairments in MLD mice upon unilateral, single injection of LVs carrying the *ARSA* cDNA (Consiglio et al., 2001). These initial studies have been reproduced with other vector systems on several disease models (Haskell et al., 2003; Desmaris et al., 2004; Griffey et al., 2004), demonstrating that direct CNS gene delivery by viral vectors is an effective strategy to restore biologic functions of LSD brains. In particular, sustained long-term ARSA expression and prevention of disease manifestations were also demonstrated using AAV5 administered in presymptomatic MLD mice (Sevin et al., 2006). However, some recent observations indicate that this strategy might not only arrest disease progression, but also partially reverse the disease phenotype once it has been established. Sevin and colleagues have shown that multiple intraparenchymal injections of AAV5 encoding for the ARSA cDNA can provide partial correction of neuropathology and sulphatide storage, but are unable to arrest the progression of neuromotor impairment in symptomatic MLD mice (Sevin et al., 2007b). On the contrary, Kurai and colleagues have shown that a single injection of AAV1 encoding for ARSA and SUMF1 cDNAs allows partial correction of behavioral impairments at rotarod test in MLD mice treated when already symptomatic (Kurai et al., 2007). Despite these promising results showing enhancing effects of SUMF1 co-delivery on ARSA activity (Fraldi et al., 2007; Kurai et al., 2007), the actual requirement for SUMF1 co-expression with ARSA for achieving widespread, robust enzyme reconstitution in the affected brain upon direct viral gene transfer and for achieving disease correction and therapeutic efficacy still need to be formally proven. Overall, these data suggest that gene transfer in MLD brains might have the potential to reverse some neurologic deficit in mice with established disease if robust enzymatic reconstitution is achieved.

Clinical protocols for CNS-directed gene therapy with AAV have been approved for other LSDs (Janson et al., 2002; Crystal et al., 2004). Unfortunately, some adverse events have been observed: in the LINCL trial, one patient died after developing epileptic seizures, while another one showed a humoral response against the transgene (Worgall et al., 2008). In the Canavan disease clinical trial, three of 10 patients developed a low level of neutralizing antibodies. Besides these adverse events, direct CNS gene delivery did not provide overt clinical benefit, likely because of the modest distribution of the vector and/or enzyme throughout the brain (Janson et al., 2002).

Therefore, the likely requirement for multiple injection sites affecting the safety of the procedure, as well as the need for additional treatments to be administered to the patients in order to deliver the functional enzyme to the peripheral nervous system whose involvement is critically affecting patients' survival, limit the clinical applicability of this approach.

Hematopoietic stem cell gene therapy

HSC gene therapy has long been considered an attractive option for the treatment of LSDs, and in particular for NS manifestations. On the basis of preclinical and clinical experience with HSCT, we might expect autologous HSC gene therapy to be able to: (1) exploit the unique properties of HSCT, capable of repopulating affected tissues with donor-derived myeloid cells, which then become an effective tissue source of the functional enzyme (Priller et al., 2001); (2) further improve the therapeutic potential of HSCT, since autologous cells may be genetically-modified to constitutively express higher levels of the therapeutic enzyme and become a quantitatively more effective source of enzyme than wild-type cells, possibly also at the level of the NS (Biffi *et al.*, 2006); and (3) reduce allogeneic HSCT side effects since the autologous procedure is expected to be associated with a reduced transplant-related morbidity and mortality, and it avoids the risks of GVHD.

Therapeutic efficacy of HSC gene therapy approaches in controlling disease manifestations has been shown in preclinical experiments on LSD models (Leiming *et al.*, 2002; Zheng *et al.*, 2003). However, the proof of the therapeutic potential of this strategy for MLD and, more generally, for LSD characterized by extensive CNS and PNS involvement came more recently. Microglial cells have been implicated in the pathogenesis of several LSDs, including MLD (Hess *et al.*, 1996; Wada *et al.*, 2000; German *et al.*, 2002; Ohmi *et al.*, 2003). They are considered a primary site of lipid storage, resulting in cell activation and secretion of cytokines and pro-inflammatory molecules, which trigger the focal inflammation, demyelination, and neurodegeneration. Thus, microglia represent a primary target cell type in therapeutic strategies for MLD. Formal proof of HSC contribution to the turnover of CNS-resident microglia in adult mice came from gene-marking studies (Eglitis & Mezey, 1997; Kennedy & Abkowitz, 1997; Priller *et al.*, 2001; Biffi *et al.*, 2004), which showed progressive reconstitution of a significant fraction of well-differentiated resting microglia a few months after HSCT. Of interest, while microglia replacement by HSC-derived cells seems to occur independently from the conditioning regimen applied prior to HSCT (Yeager *et al.*, 1991; Yeager *et al.*, 1993), the disease setting, and in particular neuroinflammation and microglial activation, promotes recruitment of bone marrow–derived cells to the CNS (Biffi *et al.*, 2004; Sano *et al.*, 2005; Visigalli *et al.*, 2009). Similar findings can be also observed monitoring the progeny of human $CD34^+$ HSC in hemato-chimeric mice (Asheuer *et al.*, 2004; Hofling *et al.*, 2004). Remarkably, reconstitution by gene-modified cells was also demonstrated in the PNS of transplanted mice, in which donor-derived cells progressively replaced endoneurial macrophages (Biffi *et al.*, 2004). The frequency of transgene-expressing monocyte lineage cells found in the PNS approached that observed in the BM and peripheral blood, indicating a faster turnover of endoneurial macrophages as compared to CNS microglia, and possibly reflecting the more permeable blood–nerve barrier. This significant recruitment provides a new avenue for gene therapy to 'vehicle' the therapeutic product to the widespread and hardly accessible PNS.

Despite some initial difficulties, evidence of the efficacy of this approach in preventing and/or correcting NS manifestations of MLD is progressively increasing. Matzner and colleagues showed that gene therapy with bone marrow cells expressing the human ARSA cDNA from a retroviral vector (RV) resulted in the expression of high levels of enzyme and prevention of sulphatide storage in liver and kidney. Only a partial correction of the lipid metabolism was detectable in the brain (Matzner *et al.*, 2000, 2001), and modest amelioration of the neuropathology and of the performance of treated animals on behavioral tests was observed. The limited success of this approach suggests that unexpectedly high levels of ARSA are required for the correction of the metabolic defect in the CNS. This requirement could be met only upon high-frequency HSC transduction and robust therapeutic gene expression in their progeny. LVs enable efficient gene marking of mouse and human HSCs (the latter ones being assayed in mouse xenografts) with minimal *in vitro* manipulation and cell perturbation, allowing for full maintenance of stem cell properties and multiclonal repopulation of chimeric hosts (Miyoshi *et al.*, 1999; Guenechea *et al.*, 2000, 2001; Ailles *et al.*, 2002). Further, upon LV transduction of HSCs, robust, long-term transgene expression in the HSC differentiated progeny has been demonstrated *in vivo* (Biffi *et al.*, 2004). Thus, LVs may provide the opportunity of achieving high enzyme expression levels in affected tissues. Indeed, by transplanting HSC transduced with LV carrying the ARSA cDNA, enzyme activity was reconstituted in the hematopoietic system of MLD mice at supra-normal levels, and the development of CNS and PNS disease manifestations was prevented. Remarkably, gene therapy had a significantly better therapeutic impact than wild-type HSC transplantation (Biffi *et al.*, 2004). More recently, we demonstrated correction of already established neurologic deficit upon genetically corrected HSC transplantation into symptomatic mice (Biffi *et al.*, 2006). Overall, this preclinical experience demonstrated that HSC gene therapy based on LV has the potential to halt MLD disease progression. The degree of efficacy of gene therapy is dependent on the levels of enzyme activity in HSCs and in their differentiated progeny. This evidence strengthens the concept that the primary advantage of gene therapy is likely due to the expression of the functional enzyme in HSCs and in their progeny largely above normal donors' levels.

HSC gene therapy for metachromatic leukodystrophy toward clinical development

In the case of HSC gene therapy, the therapeutic efficacy observed in the animal model relies on: (1) efficient repopulation of CNS microglia and PNS macrophages by the gene-corrected HSC progeny; and (2) robust expression of functional ARSA in HSC and in their progeny. These requirements pose some relevant issues for clinical application. Regarding enzyme expression, our recent work has demonstrated that the degree of efficacy of HSC gene therapy is dependent on the levels of enzyme activity in HSCs and their differentiated progeny. Few data regarding the potential toxicity induced by the overexpression of lysosomal enzymes in different cells and tissues are currently available. In this regard, different aspects should be considered. Enzyme overexpression might *per se* perturb intracellular homeostasis, thus affecting cell viability and function. In particular, the maintenance of the unique and long-term function of human HSCs upon LV-mediated enzyme overexpression should be demonstrated in adequate models. Further, the metabolic consequences of ARSA overexpression deserve in-depth evaluation. Sulphatases are a large family of enzymes involved in the degradation of sulphated substrates (Sardiello *et al.*, 2005). As mentioned, SUMF1 has been recently identified as a common activator of sulphatases and an essential factor for their activity (Cosma *et al.*, 2003; Dierks *et al.*, 2003). Since it has been suggested that SUMF1 might be a rate-limiting factor in the biological activation of these enzymes, the overexpression of one type of sulphatase may lead to reduced activity of other sulphatases by a competitive interaction with their common activator. Finally, although the superior proficiency of LV at integrating into HSCs provides a critical advantage over RV for gene therapy applications, it may also imply an increased risk of insertional mutagenesis (Fischer *et al.*, 2004). With the final goal of clinical translation of HSC gene therapy for the treatment of MLD patients, our group recently demonstrated the safety of ARSA overexpression with respect to the abovementioned issues (De Palma *et al.*, 2005; Montini *et al.*, 2006; Capotondo *et al.*, 2007; Montini *et al.*, 2009).

While clear indications about the turnover rate of microglial cells have been provided in rodents, few data are available in humans. Infiltration of donor-derived cells with the antigenic features of microglia have been detected in the brain of a patient with Hunter disease after transplantation of CD34[+] cells from normal cord blood (Araya *et al.*, 2009). However, lower rates of cell replacement in the CNS by hematopoietic elements have been reported to date in patients who underwent allo-HSCT for hematologic malignances (Unger *et al.*, 1993), suggesting that active CNS disease may enhance microglia turnover in humans as it does in rodents. Another important issue is whether the conditioning regimen could play any role in microglia reconstitution in humans. A conditioning-dependent toxic effect might account for both an enhancement of microglia reconstitution by donor-derived cells as well as for a direct negative effect on the disease course. Finally, it remains to be elucidated whether the turnover rate could be adequate to provide protection from disease progression. Indeed, this parameter could change considerably according to the disease and its stage. GLD, as other LSDs, is characterized by a massive inflammation in the CNS, which may favor microglia turnover *versus* disease progression and allow better therapeutic outcomes of HSC transplantation. Also, in the case of MLD, microglia activation might *per se* enhance migration of gene-corrected cells in the affected brain. However, the slow turnover of microglia might be a limiting factor in infantile forms of MLD, which are characterized by an extremely rapid disease progression. Clinical experience will allow understanding the real clinical impact of microglia and macrophage turnover with gene-corrected cells in the different disease forms.

In addition to the stringent demonstration of the feasibility and safety of the gene transfer protocols in the most appropriate models, essential steps for entering clinical testing include the development of clinical-grade large-scale vector manufacturing and quality assays, mobilization of the financial resources required to support such an endeavor, and securing the consensus and/or approval of the scientific and biomedical communities, national and international regulatory bodies, and patients' associations. Further, for clinical protocol set-up, a comprehensive knowledge of disease manifestations and evolution is crucial to allow proper assessment of the risk–benefit ratio and identification of the most appropriate candidates.

Very few studies on the natural history of MLD were available until recently, and no registries exist. In order to increase the knowledge on the natural history of the different variants of the disease, in the past several years we have carried out a detailed follow-up of a cohort of 27 MLD patients who have been molecularly characterized and evaluated with clinical and instrumental tools every 6 to 12 months for a period up to 6 years (Biffi *et al.*, 2008). We demonstrated a quite precise genotype–phenotype correlation, confirming that: (1) patients carrying at least one severe mutation of the disease-causing ARSA gene have an early disease onset (LI and EJ) and a rapid clinical progression; and (2) patients with two mild mutations have later onset (LJ and AD) disease which is relatively stable, even if these patients are more heterogeneous compared to patients with early-onset disease. Moreover, this study allowed us to validate clinical (gross motor function measure, GMFM) and instrumental (brain magnetic resonance, MR; ElectroNeuroGraphic recordings, ENG) tests to monitor disease progression.

According to the information obtained from this study and to ethical considerations applied to a disease such as MLD where a proxy has to provide the consent, and where the procedure is irreversible and associated with potential risks, we identified a patient population that could be considered as candidates for clinical testing of HSC gene therapy. Moreover, in light of the ethical considerations, we could define end-points for clinical efficacy based on validated tools.

Therefore, in view of the promising results and on the clinical considerations discussed, HSC gene therapy will enter clinical testing in the near future with a Phase I/II clinical trial based on LVs and autologous HSCs.

Conclusions

Treatment decisions for MLD patients are not as straightforward as for other LSDs. The identification of candidates for HSCT remains extremely difficult because of the overall very poor or null outcome of MLD patients receiving transplants and to the huge clinical variability of the disease. ERT is not available as a standard treatment at the moment, but a Phase I dose-escalation trial has been recently completed. Despite ameliorative supportive therapy, MLD remains an invariably fatal disease, with an extremely poor quality of life and a poor prognosis for all affected patients, the LI and EJ forms being the ones with the shortest lifespan. Prospectively, in children affected by MLD who have no other therapeutic option and an extremely poor prognosis, the potential risks associated with the use of a novel technology, such as gene therapy, might be well balanced by the potential benefit of a positive outcome. Thus, MLD might be considered an optimal candidate disease for testing the innovative and potentially efficacious therapeutic approach represented by HSC gene therapy.

Acknowledgments: We are grateful to Dr. Maria Sessa, Dr. Attilio Rovelli, and Prof. Maria Grazia Roncarolo for fruitful discussion.

References

Aicardi, J. (1998): *Disease of the nervous system in childhood*. Cambridge, UK: Cambridge University Press.

Ailles, L., Schmidt, M., Santoni de Sio, F.R., Glimm, H., Cavalieri, S., Bruno, S., Piacibello, W., von Kalle, C. & Naldini, L. (2002): Molecular evidence of lentiviral vector-mediated gene transfer into human self-renewing, multipotent, long-term NOD/SCID repopulating hematopoietic cell. *Mol. Ther.* **6,** 615–626.

Araya, K., Sakai, N., Mohri, I., Kagitani-Shimono, K., Okinaga, T., Hashii, Y., Ohta, H., Nakamichi, I., Aozasa, K., Taniike, M. & Ozono, K. (2009): Localized donor cells in brain of a Hunter disease patient after cord blood stem cell transplantation. *Mol. Genet. Metab.* [Epub ahead of print] PMID: 19556155.

Asheuer, M., Pflumio, F., Benhamida, S., Dubart-Kupperschmitt, A., Fouquet, F., Imai, Y., Aubourg, P. & Cartier, N. (2004): Human CD34+ cells differentiate into microglia and express recombinant therapeutic protein. *Proc. Natl. Acad. Sci. USA* **101,** 3557–3562.

Barranger, J.A. & O'Rourke, E. (2001): Lessons learned from the development of enzyme therapy for Gaucher disease. *J. Inherit. Metab. Dis.* **24,** 89–96.

Berna, L., Gieselmann, V., Poupetova, H., Hrebicek, M., Elleder, M. & Ledvinova, J. (2004): Novel mutations associated with metachromatic leukodystrophy: phenotype and expression studies in nine Czech and Slovak patients. *Am. J. Med. Genet.* **129A,** 277–281.

Biffi, A., de Palma, M., Quattrini, A., Del Carro, U., Amadio, S., Visigalli, I., Sessa, M., Fasano, S., Brambilla, R., Marchesini, S., Bordignon, C. & Naldini, L. (2004): Correction of metachromatic leukodystrophy in the mouse model by transplantation of genetically modified hematopoietic stem cells. *J. Clin. Invest.* **113,** 1118–1129.

Biffi, A., Capotondo, A., Fasano, S., Del Carro, U., Marchesini, S., Azuma, H., Malaguti, M.C., Amadio, S., Brambilla, R., Grompe, M., Bordignon, C., Quattrini, A. & Naldini, L. (2006): Gene therapy of metachromatic leukodystrophy reverses neurological damage and deficits in mice. *J. Clin. Invest.* **116,** 3070–3082.

Biffi, A., Cesani, M., Fumagalli, F., Del Carro, U., Baldoli, C., Canale, S., GerevinI, S., Amadio, S., Falautano, M., Rovelli, A., Comi, G., Roncarolo, M.G. & Sessa, M. (2008): Metachromatic leukodystrophy: mutation analysys provides further evidence of genotype-phenotype correlation. *Clin. Genet.* **74,** 349–357.

Blomer, U., Naldini, L., Kafri, T., Trono, D., Verma, I.M. & Gage, F.H. (1997): Highly efficient and sustained gene transfer in adult neurons with a lentivirus vector. *J. Virol.* **71,** 6641–6649.

Bosch, A., Perret, E., Desmaris, N., Trono, D. & Heard, J.M. (2000): Reversal of pathology in the entire brain of mucopolysaccharidosis type VII mice after lentivirus-mediated gene transfer. *Hum. Gene Ther.* **11,** 1139–1150.

Brady, R.O. & Schiffmann, R. (2004): Enzyme-replacement therapy for metabolic storage disorders. *Lancet Neurol.* **3,** 752–756.

Bredius, R.G., Laan, L.A., Lankester, A.C., Poorthuis, B.J., van Tol, M.J., Egeler, R.M. & Arts, W.F. (2007): Early marrow transplantation in a pre-symptomatic neonate with late infantile metachromatic leukodystrophy does not halt disease progression. *Bone Marrow Transplant.* **39,** 309–310.

Capotondo, A., Cesani, M., Pepe, S., Fasano, S., Gregori, S., Tononi, L., Venneri, M.A., Brambilla, R., Quattrini, A., Ballabio, A., Cosma, M.P., Naldini, L. & Biffi, A. (2007): Safety of arylsulphatase A overexpression for gene therapy of metachromatic leukodystrophy. *Hum. Gene Ther.* **18,** 821–836.

Cesani, M., Capotondo, A., Plati, T., Sergi, L.S., Fumagalli, F., Roncarolo, M.G., Naldini, L., Comi, G., Sessa, M. & Biffi, A. (2009): Characterization of new arylsulphatase A gene mutations reinforces genotype-phenotype correlation in metachromatic leukodystrophy. *Hum. Mutat.* [Epub ahead of print] PMID: 19606494.

Ciron, C., Desmaris, N., Colle, M.A., Raoul, S., Joussemet, B., Verot, L., Ausseil, J., Froissart, R., Roux, F., Cherel, Y., Ferry, N., Lajat, Y., Schwartz, B., Vanier, M.T., Maire, I., Tardieu, M., Moullier, P. & Heard, J.M. (2006). Gene therapy of the brain in the dog model of Hurler's syndrome. *Ann. Neurol.* **60,** 204–213.

Consiglio, A., Quattrini, A., Martino, S., Bensadoun, J.C., Dolcetta, D., Trojani, A., Benaglia, G.L., Marchesini, S., Cestari, V., Oliverio, A., Bordignon, C. & Naldini, L. (2001): In vivo gene therapy of metachromatic leukodystrophy by lentiviral vectors: correction of neuropathology and protection against learning impairment in affected mice. *Nat. Med.* **7,** 310–316.

Cosma, M.P., Pepe, S., Annunziata, I., Newbold, R.F., Grompe, M., Parenti, G. & Ballabio, A. (2003): The multiple sulphatase deficiency gene encodes an essential and limiting factor for the activity of sulphatases. *Cell* **113,** 445–456.

Cressant, A., Desmaris, N., Verot, L., Brejot, T., Froissart, R., Vanier, M.T., Maire, I. & Heard, J.M. (2004): Improved behavior and neuropathology in the mouse model of Sanfilippo type IIIB disease after adeno-associated virus-mediated gene transfer in the striatum. *J. Neurosci.* **24,** 10229–10239.

Crystal, R.G., Sondhi, D., Hackett, N.R., Kaminsky, S.M., Worgall, S., Stieg, P., Souweidane, M., Hosain, S., Heier, L., Ballon, D., Dinner, M., Wisniewski, K., Kaplitt, M., Greenwald, B.M., Howell, J.D., Strybing, K., Dyke, J. & Voss, H. (2004): Clinical protocol: administration of a replication-deficient adeno-associated virus gene transfer vector expressing the human CLN2 cDNA to the brain of children with late infantile neuronal ceroid lipofuscinosis. *Hum. Gene Ther.* **15,** 1131–1154.

de Palma, M., Montini, E., Santoni de Sio, F.R., Benedicenti, F., Gentile, A., Medico, E. & Naldini, L. (2005): Promoter trapping reveals significant differences in integration site selection between MLV and HIV vectors in primary hematopoietic cells. *Blood* **105,** 2307–2315.

Desmaris, N., Verot, L., Puech, J.P., Caillaud, C., Vanier, M.T. & Heardt, J.M. (2004): Prevention of neuropathology in the mouse model of Hurler syndrome. *Ann. Neurol.* **56,** 68–76.

Desnick, R.J., Ioannou, Y.A. & Eng, C.M. (2001): In *Metabolic and molecular bases of inherited diseases*, eds. C.R. Scriver *et al.*, pp. 3733–3774. New York: McGraw-Hill.

Dierks, T., Schmidt, B., Borissenko, L.V., Peng, J., Preusser, A., Mariappan, M. & von Figura, K. (2003): Multiple sulphatase deficiency is caused by mutations in the gene encoding the human C(alpha)-formylglycine generating enzyme. *Cell* **113,** 435–444.

Eckhardt, M., Hedayati, K.K., Pitsch, J., Lüllmann-Rauch, R., Beck, H., Fewou, S.N. & Gieselmann, V. (2007): Sulfatide storage in neurons causes hyperexcitability and axonal degeneration in a mouse model of metachromatic leukodystrophy. *J. Neurosci.* **27,** 9009–9021.

Eglitis, M.A. & Mezey, E. (1997): Hematopoietic cells differentiate into both microglia and macroglia in the brains of adult mice. *Proc. Natl. Acad. Sci. USA* **94,** 4080–4085.

Eng, C.M., Guffon, N., Wilcox, W.R., Germain, D.P., Lee, P., Waldek, S., Caplan, L., Linthorst, G.E. & Desnick, R.J. (2001): Safety and efficacy of recombinant human alpha-galactosidase A replacement therapy in Fabry's disease. *N. Engl. J. Med.* **345,** 9–16.

Eng, B., Nakamura, L.N., O'Reilly, N., Schokman, N., Nowaczyk, M.M., Krivit, W. & Waye, J.S. (2003): Identification of nine novel arylsulphatase a (ARSA) gene mutations in patients with metachromatic leukodystrophy (MLD). *Hum. Mutat.* **22,** 418–419.

Escolar, M.L., Poe, M.D., Provenzale, J.M., Richards, K.C., Allison, J., Wood, S., Wenger, D.A., Pietryga, D., Wall, D., Champagne, M., Morse, R., Krivit, W. & Kurtzberg, J. (2005): Transplantation of umbilical-cord blood in babies with infantile Krabbe's disease. *N. Engl. J. Med.* **352,** 2069–2081.

Fischer, A., Abina, S.H., Thrasher, A., Von Kalle, C. & Cavazzana-Calvo, M. (2004): LMO2 and gene therapy for severe combined immunodeficiency. *N. Engl. J. Med.* **350,** 2526–2527.

Fraldi, A., Biffi, A., Lombardi, A., Visigalli, I., Pepe, S., Settembre, C., Nusco, E., Auricchio, A., Naldini, L., Ballabio, A. & Cosma, M.P. (2007): SUMF1 enhances sulphatase activities in vivo in five sulphatase deficiencies. *Biochem J.* [Epub ahead of print] PMID: 17206939.

German, D.C., Liang, C.L., Song, T., Yazdani, U., Xie, C. & Dietschy, J.M. (2002): Neurodegeneration in the Niemann-Pick C mouse: glial involvement. *Neuroscience* **109,** 437–450.

Glorioso, J.C., Mata, M. & Fink, D.J. (2003): Therapeutic gene transfer to the nervous system using viral vectors. *Neurovirology* **9,** 165–172.

Griffey, M., Bible, E., Vogler, C., Levy, B., Gupta, P., Cooper, J. & Sands, M.S. (2004): Adeno-associated virus 2-mediated gene therapy decreases autofluorescent storage material and increases brain mass in a murine model of infantile neuronal ceroid lipofuscinosis. *Neurobiol. Dis.* **16,** 360–369.

Guenechea, G., Gan, O.I., Inamitsu, T., Dorrell, C., Pereira, D.S., Kelly, M., Naldini, L. & Dick, J.E. (2000): Transduction of human CD34+ CD38– bone marrow and cord blood-derived SCID-repopulating cells with third-generation lentiviral vectors. *Mol. Ther.* **1,** 566–573.

Guenechea, G., Gan, O.I., Dorrell, C. & Dick, J.E. (2001). Distinct classes of human stem cells that differ in proliferative and self-renewal potential. *Nat. Immunol.* **2**, 75–82.

Haskell, R.E., Hughes, S.M., Chiorini, J.A., Alisky, J.M. & Davidson, B.L. (2003): Viral-mediated delivery of the late-infantile neuronal ceroid lipofuscinosis gene, TPP-I to the mouse central nervous system. *Gene Ther.* **10**, 34–42.

Hess, B., Saftig, P., Hartmann, D., Coenen, R., Lullmann-Rauch, R., Goebel, H.H., Evers, M., Von Figura, K., D'hooge, R., Nagels, G., De Deyn, P., Peters, C. & Gieselmann, V. (1996): Phenotype of arylsulphatase A-deficient mice: relationship to human metachromatic leukodystrophy. *Proc. Natl. Acad. Sci. USA* **93**, 14821–14826.

Hofling, A.A., Devine, S., Vogler, C. & Sands, M.S. (2004): Human CD34+ hematopoietic progenitor cell-directed lentiviral-mediated gene therapy in a xenotransplantation model of lysosomal storage disease. *Mol. Ther.* **9**, 856–865.

Janson, C., Mcphee, S., Bilaniuk, L., Haselgrove, J., Testaiuti, M., Freese, A., Wang, D.J., Shera, D., Hurh, P., Rupin, J., Saslow, E., Goldfarb, O., Goldberg, M., Larijani, G., Sharrar, W., Liouterman, L., Camp, A., Kolodny, E., Samulski, J. & Leone, P. (2002): Clinical protocol. Gene therapy of Canavan disease: AAV-2 vector for neurosurgical delivery of aspartoacylase gene (ASPA) to the human brain. *Hum. Gene Ther.* **13**, 1391–1412.

Kakkis, E.D., Muenzer, J., Tiller, G.E., Waber, L., Belmont, J., Passge, M., Izykowski, B., Phillips, J., Doroshow, R., Walot, I., *et al.* (2001): Enzyme-replacement therapy in mucopolysaccharidosis I. *N. Engl. J. Med.* **344**, 182–188.

Kakkis, E., Lester, T., Yang, R., Tanaka, C., Anand, V., Lemontt, J., Peinovich, M. & Passage, M. (2004): Successful induction of immune tolerance to enzyme replacement therapy in canine mucopolysaccharidosis I. *Proc. Natl. Acad. Sci. USA* **101**, 829–834.

Kay, M.A., Glorioso, J.C. & Naldini, L. (2001): Viral vectors for gene therapy: the art of turning infectious agents into vehicles of therapeutics. *Nat. Med.* **7**, 33–40.

Kennedy, D.W. & Abkowitz, J.L. (1997): Kinetics of central nervous system microglial and macrophage engraftment: analysis using a transgenic bone marrow transplantation model. *Blood* **90**, 986–993.

Kordower, J.H., Bloch, J., Ma, S.Y., Chu, Y., Palfi, S., Roitberg, B.Z., Emborg, M., Hantraye, P., Deglon, N. & Aebischer, P. (1999): Lentiviral gene transfer to the nonhuman primate brain. *Exp. Neurol.* **160**, 1–16.

Krivit, W., Sung, J.H., Shapiro, E.G. & Lockman, L.A. (1995): Microglia: the effector cell for reconstitution of the central nervous system following bone marrow transplantation for lysosomal and peroxisomal storage diseases. *Cell Transplant.* **4**, 385–392.

Krivit, W., Peters, C. & Shapiro, E.G. (1999): Bone marrow transplantation as effective treatment of central nervous system disease in globoid cell leukodystrophy, metachromatic leukodystrophy, adrenoleukodystrophy, mannosidosis, fucosidosis, aspartylglucosaminuria, Hurler, Maroteaux-Lamy, and Sly syndromes, and Gaucher disease type III. *Curr. Opin. Neurol.* **12**, 167–176.

Kurai, T., Hisayasu, S., Kitagawa, R., Migita, M., Suzuki, H., Hirai, Y. & Shimada, T. (2007): AAV1 mediated co-expression of formylglycine-generating enzyme and arylsulphatase A efficiently corrects sulphatide storage in a mouse model of metachromatic leukodystrophy. *Mol. Ther.* **15**, 38–43.

Leiming, T., Mann, L., Del Pilar Martin, M., Bonten, E., Persons, D., Knowles, J., Allay, J.A., Cunningham, J., Nienhuis, A.W., Smeyne, R. & D'Azzo, A. (2002): Functional amelioration of murine galactosialidosis by genetically modified bone marrow hematopoietic progenitor cells. *Blood* **99**, 3169–3178.

Luca, T., Givogri, M.I., Perani, L., Galbiati, F., Follenzi, A., Naldini, L. & Bongarzone, E.R. (2005): Axons mediate the distribution of arylsulphatase a within the mouse hippocampus upon gene delivery. *Mol. Ther.* **12**, 669–679.

Lugowska, A., Amaral, O., Berger, J., Berna, L., Bosshard, N.U., Chabas, A., Fensom, A., Gieselmann, V., Gorovenko, N.G., Lissens, W., Mansson, J.E., Marcao, A., Michelakakis, H., Bernheimer, H., Ol'khovych, N.V., Regis, S., Sinke, R., Tylki-Szymanska, A. & Czartoryska, B. (2005): Mutations c.459+1G>A and p.P426L in the ARSA gene: prevalence in metachromatic leukodystrophy patients from European countries. *Mol. Genet. Metab.* **86**, 353–359.

Marcao, A.M., Wiest, R., Schindler, K., Wiesmann, U., Weis, J., Schroth, G., Miranda, M.C., Sturzenegger, M. & Gieselmann, V. (2005): Adult onset metachromatic leukodystrophy without electroclinical peripheral nervous system involvement: a new mutation in the ARSA gene. *Arch. Neurol.* **62**, 309–313.

Matzner, U., Harzer, K., Learish, R.D., Barranger, J.A. & Gieselmann, V. (2000): Long-term expression and transfer of arylsulphatase A into brain of arylsulphatase A-deficient mice transplanted with bone marrow expressing the arylsulphatase A cDNA from a retroviral vector. *Gene Ther.* **7**, 1250–1257.

Matzner, U., Schestag, F., Hartmann, D., Lullmann-Rauch, R., D'hooge, R., De Deyn, P.P. & Gieselmann, V. (2001): Bone marrow stem cell gene therapy of arylsulphatase A-deficient mice, using an arylsulphatase A mutant that is hypersecreted from retrovirally transduced donor-type cells. *Hum. Gene Ther.* **12**, 1021–1033.

Matzner, U., Herbst, E., Hedayati, K.K., Lüllmann-Rauch, R., Wessig, C., Schröder, S., Eistrup, C., Möller, C., Fogh, J. & Gieselmann, V. (2005): Enzyme replacement improves nervous system pathology and function in a mouse model for metachromatic leukodystrophy. *Hum. Mol. Genet.* **14**, 1139–1152. [E-pub 2005 Mar 16].

Miebach, E. (2005): Enzyme replacement therapy in mucopolysaccharidosis type I. *Acta Paediatr. Suppl.* **94**, 58–60.

Miyoshi, H., Smith, K.A., Mosier, D.E., Verma, I.M. & Torbett, B.E. (1999): Transduction of human CD34+ cells that mediate long-term engraftment of NOD/SCID mice by HIV vectors. *Science* **283**, 682–686.

Montini, E., Cesana, D., Schmidt, M., Sanvito, F., Ponzoni, M., Bartholomae, C., Sergi Sergi, L., Benedicenti, F., Ambrosi, A., Di Serio, C., Doglioni, C., Von Kalle, C. & Naldini, L. (2006): Hematopoietic stem cell gene transfer in a tumor-prone mouse model uncovers low genotoxicity of lentiviral vector integration. *Nat. Biotechnol.* **24**, 687–696.

Montini, E., Cesana, D., Schmidt, M., Sanvito, F., Bartholomae, C.C., Ranzani, M., Benedicenti, F., Sergi, L.S., Ambrosi, A., Ponzoni, M., Doglioni, C., Di Serio, C., Von Kalle, C. & Naldini, L. (2009): The genotoxic potential of retroviral vectors is strongly modulated by vector design and integration site selection in a mouse model of HSC gene therapy. *J. Clin. Invest.* **119**, 964–975.

Naldini, L., Blomer, U., Gallay, P., Ory, D., Mulligan, R., Gage, F.H., Verma, I.M. & Trono, D. (1996): In vivo gene delivery and stable transduction of nondividing cells by a lentiviral vector. *Science* **272**, 263–267.

Neufeld, E.F. (1991): Lysosomal disease. *Annu. Rev. Biochem.* **60**, 257–280.

Neufeld, E.F. & Muenzer, J. (2001): *The metabolic and molecular bases of inherited disease,* eds. C.R. Scriver *et al.* New York: McGraw-Hill.

Ohmi, K., Greenberg, D.S., Rajavel, K.S., Ryazantsev, S., Li, H.H. & Neufeld, E.F. (2003): Activated microglia in cortex of mouse models of mucopolysaccharidoses I and IIIB. *Proc. Natl. Acad. Sci. USA* **100**, 1902–1907.

Peters, C. & Steward, C.G. (2003). Hematopoietic cell transplantation for inherited metabolic diseases: an overview of outcomes and practice guidelines. *Bone Marrow Transplant.* **31**, 229–239.

Priller, J., Flugel, A., Wehner, T., Boentert, M., Haas, C.A., Prinz, M., Fernandez-Klett, F., Prass, K., Bechmann, I., De Boer, B.A., Frotscher, M., Kreutzberg, G.W., Persons, D.A. & Dirnagl, U. (2001): Targeting gene-modified hematopoietic cells to central nervous system; use of green fluorescent proteine uncovers microglial engraftment. *Nat. Med.* **7**, 1356–1361.

Ramakrishnan, H., Hedayati, K.K., Lüllmann-Rauch, R., Wessig, C., Fewou, S.N., Maier, H., Goebel, H.H., Gieselmann, V. & Eckhardt, M. (2007): Increasing sulphatide synthesis in myelin-forming cells of arylsulphatase A-deficient mice causes demyelination and neurological symptoms reminiscent of human metachromatic leukodystrophy. *J. Neurosci.* **27**, 9482–9490.

Rauschka, H., Colsch, B., Baumann, N., Wevers, R., Schmidbauer, M., Krammer, M., Turpin, J.C., Lefevre, M., Olivier, C., Tardieu, S., Krivit, W., Moser, H., Moser, A., Gieselmann, V., Zalc, B., Cox, T., Reuner, U., Tylki-Szymanska, A., Aboul-Enein, F., Leguern, E., Bernheimer, H. & Berger, J. (2006): Late-onset metachromatic leukodystrophy: genotype strongly influences phenotype. *Neurology* **67**, 859–863.

Sano, R., Tessitore, A., Ingrassia, A. & D'Azzo, A. (2005): Chemokine-induced recruitment of genetically modified bone marrow cells into the CNS of GM1-gangliosidosis mice corrects neuronal pathology. *Blood* **106**, 2259–2268.

Sardiello, M., Annunziata, I., Roma, G. & Ballabio, A. (2005): Sulfatases and sulphatase modifying factors: an exclusive and promiscuous relationship. *Hum. Mol. Genet.* **14**, 3203–3217.

Sevin, C., Benraiss, A., Van Dam, D., Bonnin, D., Nagels, G., Verot, L., Laurendeau, I., Vidaud, M., Gieselmann, V., Vanier, M., De Deyn, P.P., Aubourg, P. & Cartier, N. (2006): Intracerebral adeno-associated virus-mediated gene transfer in rapidly progressive forms of metachromatic leukodystrophy. *Hum. Mol. Genet.* **15**, 53–64.

Sevin, C., Aubourg, P. & Cartier, N. (2007a): Enzyme, cell and gene-based therapies for metachromatic leukodystrophy. *J. Inherit. Metab. Dis.* **30**, 175–183.

Sevin, C., Verot, L., Benraiss, A., Van Dam, D., Bonnin, D., Nagels, G., Fouquet, F., Gieselmann, V., Vanier, M.T., De Deyn, P.P., Aubourg, P. & Cartier, N. (2007b): Partial cure of established disease in an animal model of metachromatic leukodystrophy after intracerebral adeno-associated virus-mediated gene transfer. *Gene Ther.* **14**, 405–414.

Skorupa, A.F., Fisher, J.K., Wilson, J.M., Parente, M.K. & Wolfe, J.H. (1999). Sustained production of beta-glucuronidase from localized sites after AAV vector gene transfer results in widespread distribution of enzyme and reversal of lysosomal storage lesions in a large volume of brain in mucopolysaccharidosis VII mice. *Exp. Neurol.* **160**, 17–27.

Sondhi, D., Hackett, N.R., Peterson, D.A., Stratton, J., Baad, M., Travis, K.M., Wilson, J.M. & Crystal, R.G. (2007): Enhanced survival of the LINCL mouse following CLN2 gene transfer using the rh.10 rhesus macaque-derived adeno-associated virus vector. *Mol. Ther.* **15**, 481–491.

Stein, C.S., Ghodsi, A., Derksen, T. & Davidson, B.L. (1999): Systemic and central nervous system correction of lysosomal storage in mucopolysaccharidosis type VII mice. *J. Virol.* **73**, 3424–3429.

Stein, C.S., Kang, Y., Sauter, S.L., Townsend, K., Staber, P., Derksen, T.A., Martins, I., Qian, J., Davidson, B.L. & McCray, P.B.J. (2001): In vivo treatment of hemophilia A and mucopolysaccharidosis type VII using nonprimate lentiviral vectors. *Mol. Ther.* **3**, 850–856.

Unger, E.R., Sung, J.H., Manivel, J.C., Chenggis, M.L., Blazar, B.R. & Krivit, W. (1993): Male donor-derived cells in the brains of female sex-mismatched bone marrow transplant recipients: a Y-chromosome specific in situ hybridization study. *J. Neuropathol. Exp. Neurol.* **52**, 460–470.

Van Den Hout, J.M., Kamphoven, J.H., Winkel, L.P., Arts, W.F., de Klerk, J.B., Loonen, M.C., Vulto, A.G., Cromme-Dijkhuis, A., Weisglas-Kuperus, N., Hop, W., van Hirtum, H., Van Diggelen, O.P., Boer, M., Kroos, M.A., Van Doorn, P.A., Van Der Voort, E., Sibbles, B., Van Corven, E.J., Brakenhoff, J.P., van Hove, J., Smeitink, J.A., De Jong, G., Reuser, A.J. & van Der Ploeg, A.T. (2004): Long-term intravenous treatment of Pompe disease with recombinant human alpha-glucosidase from milk. *Pediatrics* **113**, 448–457.

Visigalli, I., Moresco, R.M., Belloli, S., Politi, L.S., Gritti, A., Ungaro, D., Matarrese, M., Turolla, E., Falini, A., Scotti, G., Naldini, L., Fazio, F. & Biffi, A. (2009): Monitoring disease evolution and treatment response in lysosomal disorders by the peripheral benzodiazepine receptor ligand PK11195. *Neurobiol Dis.* **34**, 51–62.

Von Figura, K. & Jaeken, J. (2001): Metachromatic leukodystrophy. In: *The metabolic and molecular bases of inherited diseases*, eds. C.R. Scriver *et al.*, pp. 3695–3724. New York: McGraw-Hill.

Wada, R., Tifft, C.J. & Proia, R.L. (2000): Microglial activation precedes acute neurodegeneration in Sandhoff disease and is suppressed by bone marrow transplantation. *Proc. Natl. Acad. Sci. USA* **97**, 10954–10959.

Worgall, S., Sondhi, D., Hackett, N.R., Kosofsky, B., Kekatpure, M.V., Neyzi, N., Dyke, J.P., Ballon, D., Heier, L., Greenwald, B.M., Christos, P., Mazumdar, M., Souweidane, M.M., Kaplitt, M.G. & Crystal, R.G. (2008): Treatment of late infantile neuronal ceroid lipofuscinosis by CNS administration of a serotype 2 adeno-associated virus expressing CLN2 cDNA. *Hum. Gene Ther.* **19**, 463–474.

Yaghootfam, A., Gieselmann, V. & Eckhardt, M. (2005): Delay of myelin formation in arylsulphatase A-deficient mice. *Eur. J. Neurosci.* **21**, 711–720.

Yeager, A.M., Shinohara, M. & Shinn, C. (1991): Hematopoietic cell transplantation after administration of high-dose busulphan in murine globoid cell leukodystrophy (the twitcher mouse). *Pediatr. Res.* **29**, 302–305.

Yeager, A.M., Shinn, C., Shinohara, M. & Pardoll, D.M. (1993): Hematopoietic cell transplantation in the twitcher mouse: the effects of pretransplant conditioning with graded doses of busulphan. *Transplantation* **56**, 185–190.

Zheng, Y., Rozengurt, N., Ryazantsev, S., Kohn, D.B., Satyake, N. & Neufeld, E.F. (2003): Treatment of the mouse model of mucopolysaccharidosis I with retrovirally tyransduced bone marrow. *Mol. Genet. Metab.* **79**, 233–244.

Zufferey, R., Nagy, D., Mandel, R.J., Naldini, L. & Trono, D. (1997): Multiply attenuated lentiviral vector achieves efficient gene delivery in vivo. *Nat. Biotechnol.* **15**, 871–875.

Zufferey, R., Dull, T., Mandel, R.J., Bukovsky, A., Quiroz, D., Naldini, L. & Trono, D. (1998): Self-inactivating lentivirus vector for safe and efficient in vivo gene delivery. *J. Virol.* **72**, 9873–9880.

Mariani Foundation
Paediatric Neurology Series

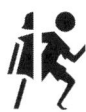

1: Occipital Seizures and Epilepsies in Children
Edited by: *F. Andermann, A. Beaumanoir, L. Mira, J. Roger and C.A. Tassinari*

2: Motor Development in Children
Edited by: *E. Fedrizzi, G. Avanzini and P. Crenna*

3: Continuous Spikes and Waves during Slow Sleep – Electrical Status Epilepticus during Slow Sleep
Edited by: *A. Beaumanoir, M. Bureau, T. Deonna, L. Mira and C.A. Tassinari*

4: Metabolic Encephalopathies: Therapy and Prognosis
Edited by: *S. Di Donato, R. Parini and G. Uziel*

5: Neuromuscular Diseases during Development
Edited by: *F. Cornelio, G. Lanzi and E. Fedrizzi*

6: Falls in Epileptic and Non-Epileptic Seizures during Childhood
Edited by: *A. Beaumanoir, F. Andermann, G. Avanzini and L. Mira*

7: Abnormal Cortical Development and Epilepsy – From Basic to Clinical Science
Edited by: *R. Spreafico, G. Avanzini and F. Andermann*

8: Limbic Seizures in Children
Edited by: *G. Avanzini, A. Beaumanoir and L. Mira*

9: Localization of Brain Lesions and Developmental Functions
Edited by: *D. Riva and A. Benton*

10: Immune-Mediated Disorders of the Central Nervous System in Children
Edited by: *L. Angelini, M. Bardare and A. Martini*

11: Frontal Lobe Seizures and Epilepsies in Children
Edited by: *A. Beaumanoir, F. Andermann, P. Chauvel, L. Mira and B. Zifkin*

12: Hereditary Leukoencephalopathies and Demyelinating Neuropathies in Children
Edited by: *G. Uziel, F. Taroni*

13: Neurodevelopmental Disorders: Cognitive/Behavioural Phenotypes
Edited by: *D. Riva, U. Bellugi and M.B. Denckla*

14: Autistic Spectrum Disorders
Edited by: *D. Riva and I. Rapin*

15: Neurocutaneous Syndromes in Children
Edited by: *P. Curatolo and D. Riva*

16: Language: Normal and Pathological Development
Edited by: *D. Riva, I. Rapin and G. Zardini*

17: Movement Disorders in Children: a Clinical Update, with video recordings
Edited by: *N. Nardocci and E. Fernandez-Alvarez*

18: Mental Retardation
Edited by: *D. Riva, S. Bulgheroni and C. Pantaleoni*

19: Perinatal Brain Damage: From Pathogenesis to Neuroprotection
Edited by: *L.A. Ramenghi, P. Evrard and E. Mercuri*

20: Genetics of Epilepsy and Genetic Epilepsies
Edited by: *G. Avanzini and J. Noebels*

21: Neurology of the Infant
Edited by: *F. Guzzetta*

22: Brain Lesion Localization and Developmental Functions
Edited by: *D. Riva and C. Njiokiktjien*